Reducing the Burden of

Injury

ADVANCING PREVENTION AND TREATMENT

Richard J. Bonnie, Carolyn E. Fulco, and
Catharyn T. Liverman, Editors

Committee on Injury Prevention and Control
Division of Health Promotion and Disease Prevention

INSTITUTE OF MEDICINE

NATIONAL ACADEMY PRESS
Washington, D.C. 1999

NATIONAL ACADEMY PRESS • 2101 Constitution Avenue, N.W. • Washington, DC 20418

NOTICE: The project that is the subject of this report was approved by the Governing Board of the National Research Council, whose members are drawn from the councils of the National Academy of Sciences, the National Academy of Engineering, and the Institute of Medicine. The members of the committee responsible for the report were chosen for their special competences and with regard for appropriate balance.

The Institute of Medicine was chartered in 1970 by the National Academy of Sciences to enlist distinguished members of the appropriate professions in the examination of policy matters pertaining to the health of the public. In this, the Institute acts under both the Academy's 1863 congressional charter responsibility to be an advisor to the federal government and its own initiative in identifying issues of medical care, research, and education. Dr. Kenneth I. Shine is president of the Institute of Medicine.

Support for this project was provided by the W.K. Kellogg Foundation, the John D. and Catherine T. MacArthur Foundation, and the Robert Wood Johnson Foundation. The views presented are those of the Institute of Medicine Committee on Injury Prevention and Control and are not necessarily those of the funding organization.

Library of Congress Cataloging-in-Publication Data

Reducing the burden of injury : advancing prevention and treatment
/ Richard J. Bonnie, Carolyn E. Fulco, Catharyn T. Liverman,
editors ; Committee on Injury Prevention and Control, Division of
Health Promotion and Disease Prevention, Institute of Medicine.
    p. cm.
Includes bibliographical references and index.
ISBN 0-309-06566-6 (pbk.)
    1. Accidents--United States--Prevention. 2. Wounds and
injuries--United States--Prevention. I. Bonnie, Richard J. II.
Fulco, Carolyn. III. Liverman, Catharyn T. IV. Institute of
Medicine (U.S.). Committee on Injury Prevention and Control.
    HV676.A2 R44 1999
    363.11'5--dc21
                            98-40288

The serpent has been a symbol of long life, healing, and knowledge among almost all cultures and religions since the beginning of recorded history. The image adopted as a logotype by the Institute of Medicine is based on a relief carving from ancient Greece, now held by the Staatliche Museen in Berlin.

Staff

CAROLYN E. FULCO, Study Director
CATHARYN T. LIVERMAN, Study Director
SANDRA AU, Project Assistant/Research Assistant
KATHLEEN STRATTON, Director, Division of Health Promotion and
    Disease Prevention

Acknowledgments

The committee's efforts were supported by the work and dedication of the project staff and consultants and numerous individuals named in Appendix A who shared their thoughts and expertise with the committee. The committee benefited from the project staff's direction and commitment to the study; Carolyn Fulco and Cathy Liverman contributed constructively to the committee's deliberations and provided necessary guidance in informing the committee of our responsibilities in developing the report. Sandra Au provided the committee with excellent attention to detail, exceptional concern for the study process, and dedication to the production of the report. Institute of Medicine summer intern, Ann St. Claire, in consultation with many individuals, produced an informative timeline of the development of the injury field and provided assistance with numerous other activities; we appreciate her efforts on our behalf. We also thank Kysa Christie for her diligent work on producing the camera-ready copy of the report.

We are indebted to Kathleen Stratton for her insight, assistance, and guidance as we negotiated our way through various difficult issues, and especially to Elena Nightingale for her thoughtful comments that kept us true to our task. They both contributed constructively to the committee's deliberations and provided guidance to make the report responsive to the charge.

Miriam Davis, consultant to the committee, provided exceptional background information and research for our deliberations and extensive written material for the committee's consideration. Lois Fingerhut, National Center for Health Statistics, provided considerable technical assistance and information on injury statistics and injury surveillance systems and we are very grateful for her help. Finally, we appreciate the careful editing by Florence Poillon who has enhanced the readability of the report, and to all the reviewers whose thoughtful comments have improved the quality of our work.

This report has been reviewed in draft form by individuals chosen for their diverse perspectives and technical expertise, in accordance with procedures approved by the National Research Council's Report Review Committee. The purpose of this independent review is to provide candid and critical comments that will assist the institution in making the published report as sound as possible and to ensure that the report meets institutional standards for objectivity, evidence, and responsiveness to the study charge. The review comments and draft manuscript remain confidential to protect the integrity of the deliberative process. We wish to thank the following individuals for their participation in the review of this report:

Susan Baker, Johns Hopkins University School of Hygiene and Public Health;
Barbara Barlow, Columbia University, Harlem Hospital Injury Prevention Program;
Enriqueta Bond, Burroughs Wellcome Foundation;
James Ebert, Marine Biological Laboratory, Johns Hopkins University;
Lois Fingerhut, National Center for Health Statistics;
John Graham, Harvard University School of Public Health;
Robert Haggerty, University of Rochester School of Medicine;
David Hoyt, University of California, San Diego, Medical Center;
Alexander Kelter, California Department of Health Services;
Mark Moore, Harvard University;
Barry Myers, Duke University;
Fred Rivara, University of Washington; and
Gerald Strauch, American College of Surgeons.

While the individuals listed above have provided constructive comments and suggestions, it must be emphasized that responsibility for the final content of this report rests entirely with the authoring committee and the institution.

The committee expresses its appreciation to the sponsors of this study: the W.K. Kellogg Foundation, the John D. and Catherine T. MacArthur Foundation, and the Robert Wood Johnson Foundation.

Preface

The Committee on Injury Prevention and Control was appointed by the Institute of Medicine in March 1997, with funding from the Robert Wood Johnson, W.K. Kellogg, and John D. and Catherine T. MacArthur foundations, and was directed to "make recommendations intended to further develop the field of injury prevention and control and to reduce the burden of injury in America." In carrying out this charge, the 17-member committee was standing on the shoulders of two predecessor committees of the Institute of Medicine (IOM) and the National Research Council (NRC), whose efforts laid the foundation for the field of injury prevention and treatment, as distinct spheres of specialization within public health and clinical medicine, more than a decade ago. Accordingly, the reports of these earlier committees—*Injury in America* (NRC, 1985) and *Injury Control* (NRC, 1988)—have been taken as the starting point for this work. William H. Foege, who chaired both of these committees, correctly observed that future historians would regard this formative period as a "turning point" for the field, "when science began defining injury, measuring determinants [and] devising interventions" and public and private efforts were galvanized to address injury problems. Although much has been accomplished since the publication of *Injury in America*, the aspirations of the previous IOM-NRC committees have not yet been fully realized.

Injury prevention and treatment encompass a vast terrain and touch on the interests of numerous disciplines and constituencies. To open the process to as many voices as possible, the committee convened a public hearing in Washington, D.C., conducted three scientific workshops, invited written comments and suggestions from hundreds of organizations and individuals, and conducted surveys of researchers and practitioners about the needs of the field. The level and intensity of the response provide compelling evidence of the growth and

Institutes of Health (NIH) budget, and funding outside NIH (e.g., Centers for Disease Control and Prevention, Agency for Health Care Policy and Research) for extramural research in all aspects of injury prevention and treatment should be increased. The committee also concluded that there is a yawning gap between what we already know about preventing or ameliorating injuries and what is being done in our communities, workplaces, and clinics. Thousands of lives could be saved every year if interventions already known to be successful were more widely implemented. Funding for prevention program support, emergency medical services and trauma systems, and public health infrastructure should be significantly increased. Although the committee has not attempted to develop cost estimates for its recommendations, carrying them out will clearly require the investment of new funds. The committee has provided adequate support for the programmatic goals and objectives of its recommendations; additional funds and resources must be forthcoming from the Congress for the relevant federal agencies and the states. Echoing Dr. Foege's prefatory claim in *Injury in America*, adequate investment in injury research and program implementation "could yield an unprecedented public health return." It is time for the country to make the necessary investment.

Richard J. Bonnie, LL.B.
Chair
Committee on Injury Prevention and Control

REFERENCES

IOM (Institute of Medicine). 1988. *The Future of Public Health*. Washington, DC: National Academy Press.

IOM (Institute of Medicine). 1996. *Healthy Communities: New Partnerships for the Future of Public Health*. Washington, DC: National Academy Press.

Lasker RD, Committee on Medicine and Public Health. 1997. *Medicine and Public Health: The Power of Collaboration*. New York: New York Academy of Medicine.

Mechanic D. 1998. Topics for our times: Managed care and public health opportunities. *American Journal of Public Health* 88(6):874–875.

NRC (National Research Council). 1985. *Injury in America: A Continuing Public Health Problem*. Washington, DC: National Academy Press.

NRC (National Research Council). 1988. *Injury Control: A Review of the Status and Progress of the Injury Control Program at the Centers for Disease Control*. Washington, DC: National Academy Press.

Thompson B. 1998. The science of violence: Guns, politics, and the public health. *Washington Post Magazine*. March 20.

Contents

EXECUTIVE SUMMARY 1

1   THE INJURY FIELD 18
    Study Background, 18
    Origins of the Injury Field, 20
    Injury as a Public Health Problem, 23
    The Mission and Boundaries of the Injury Field, 23
    Vocabulary of the Injury Field, 28
    Development of the Injury Field, 30
    Organization of the Report, 36

2   MAGNITUDE AND COSTS 39
    Overall Burden of Injury: Mortality Rates, 44
    Overall Burden of Injury: Morbidity, 48
    Patterns of Injury in the Population, 49
    The Cost of Injury, 53

3   SURVEILLANCE AND DATA 60
    Coding Issues, 62
    Existing Data Sources 64
    Data Linkages, 78
    Summary, 78

4   PREVENTION RESEARCH 82
    Research Accomplishments, 83

Research Opportunities, 95
Summary, 106

5   **CASE STUDIES ON PREVENTION**... 115
Motor Vehicle Injuries, 115
Firearm Injuries, 124
Summary, 134

6   **TRAUMA CARE** 138
Overview of Trauma Care Systems, 139
Role of Trauma Systems in Primary Prevention, Surveillance,
    and Research, 146
Growth in Trauma Care Systems, 148
Outcomes of Trauma Care Systems, 150
Research on Treatment Outcomes and Clinical Effectiveness, 152
Costs of Trauma Care Systems, 156
Financing of Trauma Systems, 159
Advent of Managed Care, 164
Summary, 167

7   **STATE AND COMMUNITY RESPONSE**... 178
Strengthening the Public Health Infrastructure, 186
Training and Technical Assistance, 194
Integrating Research and Practice, 197
Public Awareness and Advocacy, 198
Summary, 201

8   **FEDERAL RESPONSE**.. 204
National Highway Traffic Safety Administration, 205
Consumer Product Safety Commission, 212
Occupational Safety and Health Administration, 217
National Institute for Occupational Safety and Health, 223
National Institutes of Health, 227
Maternal and Child Health Bureau, 230
Office of Justice Programs, 234
National Center for Injury Prevention and Control, 239
Coordination and Leadership, 251

9   **CHALLENGES AND OPPORTUNITIES**... 258
Coordination and Collaboration, 260
Strengthening Capacity for Research and Practice, 262
Integrating the Field, 264
Nurturing Public Support, 265
Promoting Informed Policy Making, 266

APPENDIXES

A   Acknowledgments, 273
B   Timeline, 284
C   Public Meeting Agenda, 296
D   Acronyms, 300

INDEX 305

TABLES, FIGURES, AND BOXES

Tables

1.1 Mission and Vocabulary of the Injury Field, 30
2.1 Leading Causes of Injury Death, Trends, 1985–1995, 46
2.2 Leading Causes of Years of Potential Life Lost, 54
3.1 U.S. Federal Data Systems for Injury Surveillance, Research, and Prevention Activities, 66
4.1 Examples of Effective Unintentional Injury Prevention Interventions, 87
6.1 Chronology of Trauma System Legislation, 144
6.2 Essential Criteria to Identify Regional Trauma Systems, 150
7.1 State and Local Government Agencies and Organizations, 184
8.1 Federal Agencies Involved in Injury Prevention and Treatment, 206
9.1 Leading Causes of Death and Disability in the United States, 263

Figures

1.1 Years of potential life lost, 19
1.2 Haddon matrix, 22
2.1 Ten leading causes of death, 1995, 42
2.2 Burden of injury: United States, 1995, 44
2.3 Leading causes of injury death by manner of death, United States, 1995, 45
2.4 Age-adjusted death rates for leading causes of injury: United States, 1985–1995, 47
2.5 Hospital discharge rates for injury by age and sex: United States, 1993–1994, 51
5.1 Motor vehicle traffic injury deaths in the United States, 1950–1996, 116
6.1 Reimbursement profile for all service areas, 163

Boxes

1 The Federal Response, 11
2 Summary of Recommendations, 15
4.1 Harlem Hospital Injury Prevention Program, 85

4.1 Harlem Hospital Injury Prevention Program, 85
5.1 Brief Overview of Federal Firearm Laws and Regulations, 127
6.1 The Continuum of Care, 140
6.2 Levels of Trauma Centers, 141
7.1 Child Passenger Safety Seats: An Example of the Lessons Learned, 179
7.2 Examples of Nonprofit Organizations, 181
7.3 Examples of Professional Organizations, 183

Reducing the Burden of
Injury

Executive Summary

THE INJURY FIELD

Injury morbidity and mortality have been persistent problems in the United States. Recent findings report that in 1995 alone, injuries were responsible for 147,891 deaths, 2.6 million hospitalizations, and over 36 million emergency room visits (Fingerhut and Warner, 1997). Societal costs of injury-related morbidity and mortality were estimated at $260 billion in FY 1995.[1] Unintentional injuries and violence account for about 30 percent of all lost years of productive life before age 65, exceeding losses from heart disease, cancer, and stroke combined (CDC, 1991; Waller, 1994). Given the staggering costs of injury morbidity and mortality, the Robert Wood Johnson, W.K. Kellogg, and John D. and Catherine T. MacArthur foundations, requested that the Institute of Medicine (IOM) establish a committee to make recommendations for advancing the injury field and reducing the burden of injury in America. In this report, the IOM Committee on Injury Prevention and Control characterizes the injury problem in the United States, assesses the current response by the public and private sectors, and presents recommendations for reducing the burden of injury in America.[2]

---

[1]The 1985 cost-of-injury estimates were updated to 1995 separately by type of cost. Direct costs were inflated using the appropriate component of the Consumer Price Index (hospital and related services, physicians' services, prescription drugs, professional medical services, and medical care services). Indirect costs were inflated using the index of hourly compensation in the business sector.

[2]The recommendations are presented in order of appearance in the text and are not placed in priority order.

1

The Mission and the Boundaries of the Injury Field

The mission of the injury field is prevention, amelioration, and treatment of injury and the reduction of injury-related disability and death. The field is defined by its focus on the injury, whatever the mechanism by which it was immediately caused and regardless of the contributing role of human intent. This understanding, which emerges clearly from *Injury in America* (NRC, 1985), has profoundly important implications for the boundaries of the field because, by drawing no distinction between unintentional and intentional injuries (i.e., homicide, assaultive injuries), it broadens the reach of prevention research and practice beyond the traditional domain of "accident prevention."

Despite its emphasis on the need for greater attention to assaultive and self-inflicted injuries, *Injury in America* focused mainly on unintentional injuries, primarily those caused by motor vehicle crashes. Three years later [with the publication of *Injury Control*; (NRC, 1988)], the IOM reviewed the status and progress of the injury control programs at the Centers for Disease Control and Prevention (CDC); that report reiterated the need to intensify the study of intentional injury.

The committee decided, unanimously, to reaffirm the views expressed in *Injury in America* and *Injury Control* regarding the scope and mission of the injury field. Despite important differences associated with intentionality, the committee strongly endorses the continued integration of all injury prevention activities within a common framework of research and program development. The injury field has much to contribute to scientific understanding of firearm injuries and to the prevention of violence, complementing the contributions made by criminal justice, mental health, and other approaches. The public health investment in these areas should be strengthened, not abandoned or diminished.

The committee notes that there have been major accomplishments in the injury field over the past 25 years. Future advancements are dependent on the continued development and support of the infrastructure of the field. Investment in priority areas (discussed below) will ensure further advances in injury science and practice.

• *Improving coordination and collaboration:* Coordinating the diverse efforts currently devoted to injury prevention and treatment, promoting collaboration among interested agencies and constituencies, and clarifying the roles of the main federal agencies.

• *Strengthening capacity for research and practice:* Strengthening the infrastructure of the injury field for developing knowledge and for translating knowledge into practice.

• *Integrating the field:* Infusing the injury field with a common sense of purpose and a shared understanding of its methods and perspectives, and promoting new channels of communication.

• *Nurturing public understanding and support*: Broadening public understanding of the feasibility and value of efforts to prevent and ameliorate injuries and promoting investment in injury prevention by managed care organizations.

• *Promoting informed policy making:* Improving the information systems used for identifying and evaluating injury risks and setting priorities for research and intervention.

SURVEILLANCE AND DATA NEEDS

Surveillance data are needed at the national, state, and local (community) levels. National data are critical for drawing attention to the magnitude of an injury problem, for monitoring the impact of federal legislation, and for examining variations in injury rates by region of the country and by rural versus urban or suburban environments. They are also useful in aggregating sufficient numbers of rare cases of a particular type of injury to identify patterns and mechanisms of injury. State and local data better reflect injury problems in specific communities and are therefore more useful in setting program priorities and evaluating the impact of local policies and expenditures.

As the availability, accessibility, and quality of the data have improved, they have played an increasingly important role in the development and evaluation of interventions at national, state, and local levels. However, significant impediments to effective injury surveillance remain, notably the high costs of development and maintenance of surveillance systems. Therefore, priority attention should be given to the improvement or expansion of existing data systems and to the development of efficient strategies for linking data across systems to gather additional and more complex information. Additionally, surveillance systems are dependent upon the quality of coded data.

The committee recommends that a high priority be directed at ensuring uniform and reliable coding of both the external cause and the nature of the injury using the International Classification of Diseases (ICD) on all health systems data, particularly on hospital and emergency department discharge records. Special efforts should be directed at training to ensure optimal use of the tenth revision of the ICD.

An important source of information on product-related injuries is the National Electronic Injury Surveillance System (NEISS) maintained for 25 years by the Consumer Product Safety Commission (CPSC). NEISS obtains statistical information through surveillance of 101 hospital emergency departments and through follow-up studies. The committee believes that an expansion of NEISS data collection to include all injuries treated in emergency departments will increase knowledge of the causes and severity of nonfatal injuries. Furthermore,

The committee strongly recommends the utilization of rigorous analytical methods in injury research. Collaborations between research centers are critical for assembling populations and cohort groups necessary for conducting large-scale randomized control trials, cohort studies, and case-control studies.

The committee also recommends intensified research in three promising areas for the injury field, specifically:

• **the continued development of physical, mathematical, cellular, and biofidelic models of injury, particularly for high-risk populations (such as children and small women) while continuing to use animals and cadavers to validate biomechanical models of injury;**
• **the pathophysiology and reparative processes necessary to further the understanding of nonfatal injury causes and consequences, in particular, those that result in long-term disability; and**
• **differences in risk perception, risk taking, and behavioral responses to safety improvements among different segments of the population, particularly among those groups at highest risk of injury.**

The lack of research training is a major barrier to the development of the field of injury prevention research. Training attracts young people to a field and equips them for a lifelong commitment to research and education. A cadre of talented young researchers ensures the growth, innovation, and continuity of a field, yet funding has not been forthcoming to train injury researchers.

In addition to funds for training, the maintenance of a vital extramural research community will require adequate funding for investigator-initiated, peer-reviewed research grants. It is necessary to ensure viable careers for the country's best young researchers and to sustain experienced investigators. Investigator-initiated research should be encouraged to ensure the emergence of innovative approaches to injury research. To ensure the scientific rigor of this research, proposed projects should be peer reviewed by scientists outside the sponsoring federal agencies.

The committee recommends the expansion of research training opportunities by the relevant federal agencies (e.g., NCIPC, the National Institute for Occupational Safety and Health [NIOSH], and NHTSA). This includes an increase in the number of individual and institutional training grants for injury prevention; research grant proposals should have independent peer review. Adequate federal funding must be forthcoming to sustain careers in the injury field.

A national, long-term commitment to the expansion of training and interdisciplinary research in injury prevention is essential to public health. Without this commitment, injury research will not achieve the sophistication necessary for effective intervention development; talented new researchers will not be attracted to the field; and existing injury researchers may be forced to leave the field. In short, without a national commitment, the field of injury science will stagnate and the unnecessary toll of injury will persist.

CASE STUDIES ON PREVENTION

The two leading mechanisms causing fatal injury in the United States are motor vehicles and firearms; in 1995, 42,452 people died from motor vehicle traffic injuries and 35,957 people died as a result of firearm injuries (Fingerhut and Warner, 1997). Over the past three decades, dramatic progress has been made in reducing motor vehicle injuries by understanding the factors that increase the risk of injury; designing interventions to reduce these risks; implementing and evaluating a wide array of interventions; assessing their benefits and costs; and providing a scientific foundation for individual and business choices and public policy judgments. However, a similar comprehensive multidisciplinary approach has not been taken in relation to firearm injuries.

Over the long term, an effective national policy directed at reducing the risk and severity of firearm-related injury requires a strong federal presence. The multipronged approach used to develop federal motor vehicle safety policy—surveillance, regulatory action, multidisciplinary research, support for state and local prevention initiatives, and public support—provides a useful model.

The committee recommends the implementation of a comprehensive approach for preventing and reducing firearm injuries that includes firearm surveillance, firearm safety regulation, multidisciplinary research, enforcement of existing restrictions on access by minors and other unlawful purchasers, prevention programs at the state and local levels, and mobilization of public support.

A workable political consensus has not yet developed on the balance that should be struck between the prerogatives of firearm ownership and the reduction of firearm-related injuries, especially in a social context in which about 192 million firearms, including 65 million handguns, are in circulation (Cook and Ludwig, 1996). In the committee's view, a workable consensus is most likely to emerge if the discussion is focused less on ownership issues and more on the steps that can be taken to reduce the adverse health consequences of firearms use and to strengthen the scientific basis of policy making. In short, the points of departure for national firearms policy should be harm reduction and better science.

Within the overall framework, initial priority should be given to measures that reduce the risk of harm to the most vulnerable segments of the population, particularly children and adolescents and that curtail the risk of firearm injury caused by children and adolescents. Even in the absence of a broad consensus about the aims of national policy, few people are likely to contest the ethical legitimacy of aggressive measures designed to reduce gun-related injuries to and by youths.

A youth-centered injury prevention strategy is needed that would have several components: reducing the number of locations in which youth have access to guns; restricting their ability to gain access to the guns and ammunition in these settings; building features into guns that will reduce the risk of accidental or unauthorized use if the gun does get into the hands of youth; and building community coalitions to make youth environments safer.

The committee recommends the development of a national policy on the prevention of firearm injuries directed toward the reduction of morbidity and mortality associated with unintended or unlawful uses of firearms. An immediate priority should be a strategic focus on reduction of firearm injuries caused by children and adolescents.

To ensure the success of a youth-centered prevention initiative, Congress and relevant federal agencies (e.g., the Departments of Health and Human Services [DHHS] and Justice) should set national goals for reducing assaultive injuries, suicide, and unintentional injuries by young people using firearms. As a long-term commitment to this goal, consideration should be given to appointing a high-level task force for implementing and evaluating such an initiative.

TRAUMA CARE

Great strides have been made over the past decades in developing trauma systems covering a continuum of prehospital, acute care, and rehabilitation services. Public health organizations and providers have embraced the need for a broader, more inclusive philosophy that shifts the focus from the trauma center to a system of trauma care that attends to the needs of all trauma patients over the full course of treatment.

A focal point at the federal level has to be reinstated to support research and to cultivate the growth of state and regional trauma systems. A federal program had been in place until 1995, when budget pressures led to the program's demise. Consequently, there is no longer a focal point at the federal level to cultivate trauma systems development.

The committee supports a greater national commitment to, and support of, trauma care systems at the federal, state, and local lev-

els, and recommends the reauthorization of trauma care systems planning, development, and outcomes research at the Health Resources and Services Administration (HRSA).

To ensure the success of this recommendation, resources should be provided to stimulate the development and evaluation of trauma systems in states and regions with the greatest need for systems development.

Trauma care is lifesaving, yet expensive. The costs of trauma systems development should be shared by federal, state, and local governments. About half of the states report having some kind of trauma system, although their nature and extent are not well documented. Some of the most successful statewide trauma systems have flourished with dedicated sources of funding through motor vehicle fees and other creative approaches. Research has begun to demonstrate that the investment in systems of care can be cost-effective in terms of long-term health care costs and productivity.

The committee recommends intensified trauma outcomes research, including research on the delivery and financing of acute care services and rehabilitation. The committee envisions that HRSA and other appropriate federal agencies (e.g., NCIPC, and the Agency for Health Care Policy and Research [AHCPR]) will collaborate on this research.

Specific areas of research that have to be addressed include the following:

• the cost-effectiveness of specific clinical and service interventions to establish best practices in trauma care;
• the most efficient and effective strategies for organizing and financing the delivery of both acute care services and rehabilitation, including the impact of managed care arrangements on access to services, quality of care, and outcomes; and
• the development of improved methods for measuring the severity of injury, particularly for those at high risk of adverse outcomes.

STATE AND COMMUNITY RESPONSE

Further progress in reducing the burden of injuries not only depends on concerted research and treatment efforts but also requires a strengthened focus on prevention implementation. Great strides have been made in developing injury prevention strategies that have been shown to be successful in promoting safety and reducing injury morbidity and mortality. In most cases, injury prevention is best achieved through a multifaceted approach that utilizes the range of available prevention strategies. However, the state and community response is often hampered by federal and state funding constraints and a lack of awareness of injury prevention measures. The committee has identified five areas that, if successfully addressed, could optimize proven strategies for prevention: (1) strengthening the public health infrastructure; (2) building and encouraging collaboration and coalitions of state and local safety agencies and organizations; (3) improving training and technical assistance; (4) better translating of research findings into practice; and (5) increasing public awareness and advocacy.

Although it is difficult to quantify the total extent of government, community, and private-sector endeavors in the injury field, there is a wide range of ongoing efforts, many of which have begun or expanded within the past 20 years. Although the current response is impressive, it is also fragmented. A core injury prevention program is needed in each state that can implement (and assist other agencies and organizations in implementing) injury prevention interventions. State injury prevention programs require a sustained federal commitment to funding and to providing technical assistance to the states.

The committee recommends strengthening the state infrastructure in injury prevention by development of core injury prevention programs in each state's department of health. To accomplish this goal, funding, resources, and technical assistance should be provided to the states. Support for such programs should be provided by the NCIPC in collaboration with state and local governments.

Additionally, training opportunities for state and local injury prevention practitioners should be expanded. Consideration should be given by multiple federal agencies to the expansion of training opportunities for state and local injury prevention professionals.

The committee recommends the expansion of training opportunities for injury prevention practitioners by the relevant state and federal agencies (e.g., NCIPC, NHTSA, the Maternal and Child Health Bureau [MCHB], and NIOSH) in partnership with key stakeholders such as the State and Territorial Injury Prevention Directors' Association (STIPDA). Training should emphasize program development, implementation, and evaluation as well as participation in program research.

As new prevention interventions are developed and evaluated, ongoing information exchange between researchers and practitioners is needed that will facilitate the implementation of new interventions and the refinement of these interventions to meet real-world demands. A final component of strengthening the state and local response is raising public awareness and increasing advocacy efforts. Both the general public and policy makers need information on the effectiveness of injury prevention measures in order to make informed decisions and choices.

FEDERAL RESPONSE

It is important to clarify the roles of federal agencies and to facilitate coordination among them. Injury prevention and treatment cover a vast terrain. Numerous federal agencies play important roles in supporting injury science or carrying out the national agenda in injury prevention and treatment. This potpourri of federal responsibilities emerged piecemeal over several decades rather than as components of a coordinated national plan. This is not to say that the federal response has been weak or wasteful. To the contrary, the key federal agencies have accomplished a great deal over the past three decades in building a new scientific field and reducing the burden of injury. The problem is one of missed opportunities due to lack of focus, cohesion, and coordination. The committee believes that the federal response could be strengthened significantly by several important refinements of the present organizational architecture of injury prevention and treatment, in the following key agencies, NHTSA, CPSC, NIOSH, NIH, NIJ, and the NCIPC. The refinements are listed as recommendations in Box 1.

BOX 1
The Federal Response

NHTSA

The committee recommends that NHTSA expand its investigator-initiated research program, conduct periodic and independent peer review of its research and surveillance programs, and provide training and research support to sustain careers in the highway traffic safety field.

CPSC

The committee recommends that CPSC's capacity to conduct product safety research be significantly strengthened.

NIOSH

The committee recommends that NIOSH, working in collaboration with other federal partners, implement the National Occupational Research Agenda research priorities for traumatic and other injury-related occupational injuries, and give higher priority to injury research.

NIH

The committee supports a greater focus on trauma research and training at the National Institutes of Health (NIH) and recommends that the National Institute of General Medical Sciences (NIGMS) elevate its existing trauma and burn program to the level of a division.

NIJ

The committee recommends that NIJ continue to give explicit priority to the prevention of violence, especially lethal violence, within its overall activity in crime prevention research and program evaluation, and that NIJ establish new institutional training grants for violence prevention research at academic institutions.

Continued

BOX 1 *Continued*

NCIPC

The committee recommends that NCIPC establish an ongoing and open process for refining its research priorities in the areas of biomechanics, residential and recreational injuries, and suicide and violence prevention, in close coordination with its stakeholders and federal partners.

The committee reasserts the need for training of injury professionals and strongly recommends that NCIPC expand training opportunities for injury prevention practitioners and researchers.

The committee recommends that the NCIPC support the development of core injury prevention programs in each state's department of health and provide greater technical assistance to the states.

The committee recommends that the NCIPC continue to nurture the growth and development of the public health effort in injury prevention and treatment through information exchange, collaboration with injury practitioners and researchers, and leveraging available resources to promote the effectiveness of programs and research.

COORDINATION AND LEADERSHIP

In 1985, *Injury in America* recommended that an injury center at the CDC be established to serve as a "lead agency among federal agencies and private organizations" (NRC, 1985). By using this formulation, the 1985 report appears to have envisioned that the CDC would provide leadership in two ways: (1) by nurturing the public health community's commitment to and interest in the injury field and (2) by coordinating the efforts of the multiple federal agencies involved in injury prevention and treatment. The committee believes that the NCIPC should continue to be a focal point for the public health commitment to the injury field (see recommendation in Box 1). However, when Congress enacted the Injury Control Act in 1990, it properly recognized that no single agency could "lead" such a diverse federal effort, and instead authorized the CDC to create a program to "work in cooperation with other Federal agencies, and with public and nonprofit private entities, to promote injury control" (P.L. 101-558). Congress envisioned a cooperative effort because, as a practical matter, an agency in one cabinet department has no authority to direct other agencies in the same department, much less in other departments.

It became apparent to the committee during numerous discussions and meetings with individuals representing diverse perspectives[3] that characterization of the NCIPC as "the lead Federal agency" should be redefined by the NCIPC in collaboration with other relevant federal agencies, as it has led to unrealistic expectations about what NCIPC can accomplish with its resources. It also has impeded collaboration by spawning institutional rivalries and resentments, especially from federal agencies whose funding is similar to, or greater than, that of NCIPC. Although there are certainly stellar examples of coordination—for example, between NHTSA and HRSA on the Emergency Medical Services for Children Program, and between CPSC and NCIPC on the expansion of emergency department injury surveillance—these examples are more the exception than the rule.

An effective federal response to injury requires many agencies to play a leadership role in their areas of strength and jurisdiction. Playing a leadership role means taking the initiative to persuade and induce others to join in collective action toward a common goal. Yet playing a lead role is not an exclusive role; it involves collaboration with other agencies to reduce injuries, promote synergies, and harness limited resources. Leadership, or playing a lead role, requires each agency to forge partnerships with other federal agencies in a collaborative manner to meet the overall objective of preventing injuries and improving safety. The committee recommends that federal agencies with injury-related programs create mechanisms to promote coordination and interagency collaboration.

The crosscutting nature of the injury problem, as well as of injury research and interventions, has been highlighted throughout this report. Through collaboration and coordination, federal agencies can work jointly to combat related and sometimes overlapping problems and to overcome fragmentation. They can link activities and pool resources, which take the form of expertise, funds, databases, access to patient populations, and technology. They also can avoid unnecessary duplication of effort, although duplication does not currently appear to be a major problem across federal injury programs (U.S. DHHS, 1992; GAO, 1994). Although the committee is not naive about the difficulties facing federal agencies when attempting collaboration and coordination, there are effective mechanisms that may ensure success, such as memoranda of understanding, interagency task forces and committees, and funding for joint projects

CONCLUSIONS

Since 1985, significant strides have been taken to implement the vision outlined in *Injury in America* (NRC, 1985). The national investment in injury re-

---

[3]The committee met with numerous federal, state, and local government representatives, researchers, practitioners, and public and private organizations during the course of the study.

search has increased, albeit not as markedly as the report recommended. The field of injury science has developed and matured, attracting the interest of investigators from a wide range of disciplines. Important advances have been made in delivering emergency services and treatment to injured patients, saving lives, and reducing disability. Recent research is beginning to provide information about how cells respond to injury and how their normal functioning can be preserved. Important advances have also been made in demonstrating the efficacy and cost-effectiveness of preventive interventions in the field so that they can be successfully implemented on a wide scale.

One of the most impressive achievements over the past two decades has been a "political" one—through communication, advocacy, and constituency building, a national "community of interest" in promoting safety and preventing injury has emerged. Although injury prevention has achieved higher visibility in government at all levels, most of the energy for social action has come from the private sector and through the recruitment of individuals, businesses, foundations, community groups, and other organizations interested in preventing injuries and implementing safety programs. Future advances in the injury field depend on the continued development of the infrastructure of the field through public and private partnerships. The main challenge for the nation, in the view of the committee, is to consolidate the gains that have been made over the past 25 years, and particularly over the past decade, and to secure the foundation for further advances in injury science and practice.

This report emphasizes, as did *Injury in America* and *Injury Control*, that the nation's current investment in injury research is not commensurate with the magnitude of the problem. Throughout the report, the committee has recommended additional funding for surveillance, research, training, and program evaluation supported by a variety of federal agencies. Abundant opportunities for scientific advances in all aspects of the field fully justify a substantially higher level of funding for injury research. Trauma research (basic and applied) should receive a higher share (compared with current allocations) of increases in the NIH budget, and funding outside NIH (e.g., CDC, AHCPR) for extramural research in all aspects of injury prevention and treatment should be increased. The committee also concluded that there is a yawning gap between what we already know about preventing or ameliorating injuries and what is being done in our communities, workplaces, and clinics. Funding for prevention program support, emergency medical services and trauma systems, and public health infrastructure should be significantly increased. Thousands of lives could be saved every year if interventions already known to be successful were more widely implemented. Although the committee has not attempted to develop cost estimates for its recommendations, carrying them out will clearly require the investment of new funds. The committee has provided adequate support for the programmatic goals and objectives of its recommendations; additional funds and resources must be forthcoming from the Congress for the relevant federal agencies and the states. For a summary of all recommendations, see Box 2.

The challenge confronting us today is to enhance the impact and effectiveness of the field. Doing so requires a broad matrix of collaboration with other agencies and constituencies, and careful priority setting within the field in order to focus efforts and resources on areas of research and action that optimize the specialized contribution of public health.

BOX 2
Summary of Recommendations

Surveillance Systems (see Chapter 3)
- Ensure uniform and reliable coding of both the external cause and nature of the injury using the ICD on all health systems data and ensure training on optimal use of ICD-10.
- Expand the NEISS system by CPSC to gather nationally representative data on all injuries treated in emergency departments.
- Develop a fatal intentional injury surveillance system, modeled after FARS, for all homicides and suicides; explore the feasibility of establishing such a system (by NCIPC, NCEH, and NCHS) as an extension of the medical examiner and coroner systems.

Training and Research (see Chapter 4)
- Expand research training opportunities by the relevant federal agencies (e.g., NCIPC, NIOSH, NHTSA).
- Utilize rigorous analytical methods in injury research.
- Conduct research in injury biomechanics, especially for high-risk populations, while continuing to use animals and cadavers to validate biomechanical models; in the pathophysiology and reparative processes necessary to further the understanding of injury causes and consequences; and on differences in risk perception, risk taking, and behavioral responses to safety improvements among different segments of the population.

Firearm Injury Prevention (see Chapter 5)
- Implement a comprehensive approach for preventing and reducing firearm injuries.
- Develop a national policy on the prevention of firearm injuries directed toward the reduction of morbidity and mortality associated with unintended or unlawful uses of firearms. A strategic focus on reduction of firearm injuries to and by children and adolescents should be an immediate priority.

Trauma Care Systems (see Chapter 6)
- Reauthorize trauma care systems planning, development, and outcomes research at HRSA.
- Intensify trauma outcomes research, including research on the delivery and financing of acute care services and rehabilitation, through collaboration of HRSA and other appropriate federal agencies (e.g., NCIPC, AHCPR).

Continued

BOX 2 *Continued*

Training and State Infrastructure (see Chapter 7)
- Strengthen the state infrastructure in injury prevention by development of core injury prevention programs in each state's department of health.
- Expand training opportunities for injury prevention practitioners by the relevant state and federal agencies (e.g., NCIPC, NHTSA, MCHB, NIOSH) in partnership with key stakeholders (e.g., STIPDA).

Federal Recommendations (see Box 1 and Chapter 8)
- Expand **NHTSA's** investigator-initiated research program, conduct periodic and independent peer review of its research and surveillance programs, and provide training and research support to sustain careers in the highway traffic safety field.
- Strengthen **CPSC's** capacity to conduct product safety research.
- Implement the NORA research priorities for traumatic and other injury-related occupational injuries by **NIOSH** working in collaboration with other federal partners; give higher priority to injury research.
- Support a greater focus on trauma research and training at NIH and elevate **NIGMS's** existing trauma and burn program to the level of a division.
- Support by **NIJ** for the prevention of violence, especially lethal violence, and establish new institutional training grants for violence prevention research at academic institutions.
- Establish an ongoing and open process for refining **NCIPC's** research priorities in the areas of biomechanics, residential and recreational injuries, and suicide and violence prevention, in close coordination with its stakeholders and federal partners.
- Expand training opportunities for injury prevention practitioners and researchers with **NCIPC** support.
- Support the development of core injury prevention programs in each state's department of health by **NCIPC**, and provide greater technical assistance to the states.
- Nurture the growth and development of the public health effort in injury prevention and treatment by **NCIPC** through information exchange, collaboration with injury practitioners and researchers, and leveraging available resources to promote the effectiveness of programs and research.

REFERENCES

Baker SP, O'Neill B, Ginsburg MJ, Li G. 1992. *The Injury Fact Book*. New York: Oxford University Press.

CDC (Centers for Disease Control and Prevention). 1991. Update: Years of potential life lost before age 65—United States, 1988 and 1989. *Morbidity and Mortality Weekly Report* 40:60–62.

Cook PJ, Ludwig J. 1996. *Guns in America: Results of a Comprehensive National Survey on Firearms Ownership and Use*. Washington, DC: Police Foundation.

Fingerhut LA, Warner M. 1997. *Injury Chartbook. Health, United States, 1996–97*. Hyattsville, MD: National Center for Health Statistics.

GAO (General Accounting Office). 1994. *Agencies Use Different Approaches to Protect the Public Against Disease and Injury*. Washington, DC: GAO. GAO/HEHS-9-85BR.

NRC (National Research Council). 1985. *Injury in America: A Continuing Public Health Problem*. Washington, DC: National Academy Press.

NRC (National Research Council). 1988. *Injury Control: A Review of the Status and Progress of the Injury Control Program at the Centers for Disease Control*. Washington, DC: National Academy Press.

U.S. DHHS (U.S. Department of Health and Human Services). 1992. *Injury Control*. Washington, DC: U.S. DHHS Office of the Inspector General. OEI-02-92-00310.

Waller JA. 1994. Reflections on a half century of injury control. *American Journal of Public Health* 84(4):664–670.

1

The Injury Field

Injury morbidity and mortality have been persistent problems in the United States. Recent findings report that in 1995 alone, injuries were responsible for 147,891 deaths, 2.6 million hospitalizations, and more than 36 million emergency room visits (Fingerhut and Warner, 1997). It has been estimated that injury accounts for 12 percent of all medical spending (Miller et al., 1994). In 1995, approximately $260 billion was spent on injury and its consequences (E. MacKenzie, Johns Hopkins University, personal communication, 1998).[1] Unintentional injury and violence account for about 30 percent of all lost years of productive life before age 65, exceeding losses from heart disease, cancer, and stroke combined (CDC, 1991; Waller, 1994). Yet, the federal investment for injury research has not been sommensurate with the problem (Figure 1.1).

STUDY BACKGROUND

In 1966, the National Academy of Sciences' Division of Medical Sciences and the National Research Council (NRC) issued *Accidental Death and Disability: The Neglected Disease of Modern Society*, recommending that the nation's public and private resources be mobilized to reduce accidental death and injury in an effort equivalent to the recent assaults on polio and cancer (NRC, 1966). The recommendations in the report focused mainly on improving emergency

---

[1]The 1985 estimates of the costs of injury in the United States were updated to 1995 separately by type of cost. Direct costs were inflated using the appropriate component of the Consumer Price Index (hospital and related services, physicians' services, prescription drugs, professional medical services, and medical care services). Indirect costs were inflated using the index of hourly compensation in the business sector.

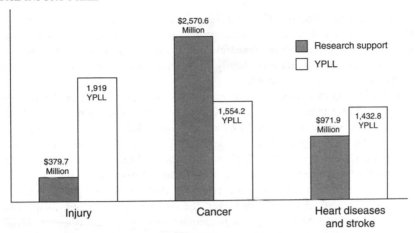

FIGURE 1.1 Years of potential life lost versus the federal research investment. NOTE: Age-adjusted years of potential life lost (YPLL) before age 75 in 1996 was calculated per 100,000 population. Injury includes unintentional injury, homicide, and suicide. The research support for injury is for FY 1995; research support for cancer, heart diseases, and stroke is NIH support for FY 1996. SOURCES: NCIPC (1997); IOM (1998); NCHS (1998).

medical care, but the committee also addressed trauma research and injury prevention, recommending creation of a National Institute on Trauma at the National Institutes of Health (to sponsor and conduct a program of injury treatment research) and a National Council on Accident Prevention in the executive branch (to coordinate and advise federal regulatory agencies and to provide support for research and program development).

Nearly 20 years later, the Committee on Trauma Research established by the NRC and the Institute of Medicine (IOM) conducted a new study at Congress's direction and issued what has become a landmark report, *Injury in America* (NRC, 1985). That committee recommended a major national program of research to address "serious, but remediable, inadequacies in the understanding of and approach to injury as a health problem." The significance of *Injury in America* lies both in its intellectual contribution and in its influence on national policy. Intellectually, the committee set forth the rationale for conceptualizing "injury prevention and control" as a distinct field of interdisciplinary research, drawing together what had been separate strands of scientific study within the framework of public health. In terms of public policy, the committee recommended a major investment in injury research, commensurate with the magnitude of the problem, and proposed creation of a center for injury research within the Centers for Disease Control, now the Centers for Disease Control and Prevention (CDC). The committee envisioned that the new center would (1) conduct and support research in biomechanics, injury epidemiology and prevention, and treatment and rehabilitation; (2) establish injury surveillance systems and support prevention activities; (3) promote professional education and training; (4) establish interdisciplinary injury research centers; and (5) serve as clearinghouse, coordinator, and lead agency on injury prevention and control among federal agencies and private organizations.

Soon after *Injury in America* was released, Congress appropriated funds for a pilot program for injury control at CDC, and two years later, a new IOM-NRC committee reviewed its progress. In *Injury Control* (NRC, 1988), the committee concluded that the program had been sufficiently successful to warrant permanent support. It commended the CDC program for establishing five interdisciplinary research centers; sponsoring a new program of extramural research; and building staff expertise for intramural research, database development, coordination, and technical assistance. However, the committee expressed disappointment that the program had been given inadequate resources to carry out its broad mission and noted that the program had underemphasized acute care and biomechanics during its start-up phase. During the intervening years, there have been several efforts to determine priorities for injury prevention and treatment (e.g., National Committee [1989]; NCIPC [1993]; NIH [1994]; IOM [1997]).

In 1997, the current Committee on Injury Prevention and Control was established by the IOM with funding from the Robert Wood Johnson, W.K. Kellogg, and John D. and Catherine T. MacArthur foundations, to review the present status and direction of the field in light of earlier IOM-NRC reports and to make appropriate recommendations for advancing the field and for reducing the burden of injury in America. The committee's charge, however, is broader than those of the earlier IOM-NRC committees, encompassing "opportunities and barriers" for practice as well as research (*Injury in America* focused exclusively on research) and "the response by public and private agencies," not only the activities of the CDC program. Recognizing the breadth of its charge, the committee decided not to replicate the work of its predecessors, choosing instead to focus on areas that had not received attention in prior reports and on current issues or challenges confronting the injury field as a whole.

This report characterizes the injury problem in the United States, assesses the current response by the public and private sectors, and presents recommendations for reducing the burden of injury in America. To introduce the issues addressed by the committee, this chapter outlines the history of the injury field, discusses the public health approach to injury prevention and treatment, and assesses progress in the development of the injury field.

ORIGINS OF THE INJURY FIELD

For centuries, human injuries have been regarded either as random and unavoidable occurrences ("accidents" or "acts of God") or as untoward consequences of human malevolence or carelessness. From this perspective, the main strategies for prevention are prayer and human improvement. With the advent of industrialization in the nineteenth century, the environmental risk factors for injury became more discernible, and the challenges of "accident prevention" and industrial safety began to receive sustained attention. Railroad, textile, and mining industries began recording work-related injuries in the early 1800s (Loimer et al., 1996). Political movements for worker protection developed in Europe in the mid-nineteenth century and later in the United States. Early developments include the creation of the National Safety Council in the United States in 1913 and the Royal Society for the Prevention of Accidents in England in 1916.

Although interest in worker safety, child safety, and driver safety grew over the course of the twentieth century, systematic scientific inquiry was rare, and the ameliorative efforts undertaken by interested private constituencies were episodic and unconnected. This situation changed dramatically during the 1960s and 1970s when two developments converged to establish the intellectual and programmatic foundation for a new field of research and social action: (1) a substantial social investment in injury prevention, spurred by a burst of federal regulatory action and (2) the emergence of injury science as a distinct interdisciplinary field of research within the domain of public health (Baker, 1989; also, see the following discussion).

The Highway Safety Act of 1966 signaled a national commitment to reducing injuries and deaths on the nation's highways In this path-breaking legislation, Congress empowered a federal agency, the National Highway Safety Bureau (now the National Highway Traffic Safety Administration [NHTSA]), to set motor vehicle safety standards and to make grants for research and programs promoting highway safety. Four years later, the federal Occupational Safety and Health Act established a regulatory agency (Occupational Safety and Health Administration) to set and enforce workplace safety standards, and a separate research agency (National Institute for Occupational Safety and Health). This period of federal regulatory innovation was consummated with the enactment of the Consumer Product Safety Act and companion legislation in 1972 that established the Consumer Product Safety Commission. Throughout this formative period, diverse initiatives were undertaken by a variety of other federal agencies, state governments, foundations, and citizen activists to promote safety and ameliorate the burden of injury. Examples include Kellogg Foundation grants for home accident prevention in the 1950s and 1960s, the founding of the American Trauma Society in 1968, the establishment of 600 poison control centers in the 1960s and 1970s, the creation of a federal program on emergency medical services in the 1970s, the funding of state injury prevention programs by the Division of Child and Maternal Health of the Department of Health, Education, and Welfare in 1979, and the founding of Remove Intoxicated Drivers in 1978 and Mothers Against Drunk Driving in 1980. Although these activities were not coordinated, they reflected a common aspiration and a shared recognition of the potential benefits of concerted social action to reduce injury. Taken together, they substantially increased the number of individuals and organizations engaged in injury prevention research and practice, and thereby began to build the infrastructure for a new field. For additional historical information, see the time line in Appendix B.

Modern injury science began to take shape as a distinct field in the mid-1960s. Perhaps the key conceptual development was the recognition that patterns of injury distribution and causation can be analyzed using the epidemiological tools of public health and that the etiology of injury includes environmental factors and interactions between human and environmental factors. The formulation of the prevailing scientific paradigm for studying the causes and prevention of injury is generally attributed to William Haddon, a public health physician. Building on the work of John Gordon (1949) and James Gibson (1961), Haddon (1968) observed that all injury events are attributable to the uncontrolled release of one of five forms of physical energy (kinetic, chemical, thermal, electrical, and radiation). From a preventive or ameliorative standpoint, interventions can be made during three temporal phases in relation to the injury event: (1) a pre-event phase, during which the energy becomes uncontrolled; (2) a brief event phase in which the uncontrolled energy is transferred to the individual, resulting in injury if the energy transfer exceeds the tolerance of the body to absorb it; and (3) a post-event phase, during which attempts can be made to restore homeostasis and repair the damage. This three-phase conceptualization of injury causation can be combined with the traditional public health categorization of risk factors and intervention opportunities— host (the potential injured person), agent (the energy and the vehicle through which it is transferred), and environment (both physical and social)—to create a 12-cell matrix that can be modified to apply to any circumstance of injury (Figure 1.2). Using this model to identify risk factors and potential interventions during all three temporal phases, Haddon summarized the range of interventions as follows: (1) preventing or limiting energy buildup; (2) controlling the circumstances of energy use to prevent uncontrolled release; (3) modifying the energy transfer phase to limit damage; and (4) improving emergency response, treatment, and rehabilitative care to limit disability and promote recovery.

	Factors			
	Individual Behavior	Agent	Physical environment	Socio-economic environment
Phases Pre-event				
Event				
Post-event				

FIGURE 1.2 Haddon matrix. SOURCE: Adapted from Haddon (1980).

INJURY AS A PUBLIC HEALTH PROBLEM

The subtitle of *Injury in America* was "A Continuing Public Health Problem" (NRC, 1985). What exactly does it mean to say that injury is a public health problem? Injuries constitute a major public health problem because, in the aggregate, they produce such an enormous toll of disability and premature death, draining health care dollars and weakening the nation's productive capacity. Fortunately, these consequences can be reduced or ameliorated by using the analytic tools and preventive perspectives of public health. Indeed, because the public health paradigm can embrace all etiologic factors bearing on prevention, it has been widely accepted by analysts in all disciplines, even though many of the interventions lie outside the expertise and capacity of public health agencies.

This is not to say that the public health approach is the only useful perspective for thinking about injuries. Some perspectives are remedial rather than preventive and normative rather than empirical. Conceptually, issues concerning the remediation of injuries (compensation of injured persons, corrective justice or the punishment of persons or entities responsible for "causing" or failing to prevent injuries) are extrinsic to issues of prevention. Operationally, however, they may converge (e.g., punishment of wrongdoers or imposition of liability can achieve preventive effects through deterrence) or diverge (e.g., the risk of tort liability faced by companies often reduces hazards, but sometimes creates disincentives to disclose safety information and may thereby retard safety innovation).

To say that injury is a public health problem should not be understood to mean that the social response should be mounted primarily or exclusively by public health agencies; nor does it imply that a public health response is superior to other forms of response. Public health agencies lack expertise and command over most of the interventions suggested by the Haddon matrix. Injuries represent a complex set of social problems. Prevention and remediation of these problems are and should be the responsibility of a wide variety of social institutions, including medicine, alcohol control, fire safety, mental health, criminal justice, the tort system, and many others. As discussed in Chapters 7 and 8, public health agencies should be playing a much more substantial role in injury prevention than they are now, but their role should be understood as a contributory one, in collaboration with other agencies.

THE MISSION AND BOUNDARIES OF THE INJURY FIELD

The mission of the injury field is prevention, amelioration, and treatment of injury and the reduction of injury-related disability and death. The field is defined by its focus on the injury, whatever the mechanism by which it was immediately caused and regardless of the contributing role of human intent. This understanding, which emerges clearly from *Injury in America*, has profoundly important implications for the boundaries of the field because, by drawing no distinction between unintentional and intentional injuries (i.e., homicide, assaultive injuries), it broadens the reach of prevention research and practice beyond the traditional domain of "accident prevention."

From "Accident Prevention" to "Injury Prevention"

Injury in America (NRC, 1985) explicitly recognized that the public health paradigm could be usefully applied to the prevention of intentional injuries as well as unintentional ones. The report identified knowledge about assaultive injuries as a major gap in current research: "Nonfatal assaultive injuries and homicides have been subjected to little prevention-oriented research. Typically, they have been regarded as a 'crime problem,' rather than as a health problem, and blame and punishment of the perpetrators have been emphasized, rather than measures to reduce the frequency and severity of such injuries." After identifying several potentially useful interventions for the prevention of firearm-related injuries, the report noted that "assaultive injuries involving other weapons or personal force are virtually unresearched." Similarly, although *Injury in America* recognized that much research had focused on the diagnosis and treatment of depressed or suicidal people, the report observed that little attention had been paid to public health approaches, such as modifying products or environments to reduce the lethality of means of suicide. It encouraged research into the "validity of the widespread assumption that nonfatal suicide attempts represent a lack of desire to kill oneself, and therefore involve the choice of less lethal means" and on "reducing the lethality of common means of committing suicide."

Despite its emphasis on the need for greater attention to assaultive and self-inflicted injuries, *Injury in America* focused mainly on unintentional injuries, primarily those caused by motor vehicle crashes. Three years later (with the publication of *Injury Control*), the IOM-NRC committee reviewed the status and progress of the injury control programs at CDC; that report reiterated the need to intensify the study of intentional injury: "The study of intentional injury can be characterized as a neglected but potentially productive research field. . . . The nation now has hundreds of programs aimed at reducing the incidences of suicide, homicide, and other intentional injuries, but there is no commensurate effort to evaluate the effectiveness of the programs" (NRC, 1988).

A Broader Field

Ten years have elapsed since the publication of *Injury Control*. Over this period, research and program development within the injury field have been expanded to give greater attention to the study of intentional injuries, reflecting a broader movement within medicine and public health embracing the cause of violence[2] prevention (see, e.g., *Surgeon General's Workshop on Violence and Public Health* [U.S. DHHS, 1986]; *Violence in America: A Public Health Approach* [Rosenberg and Fenley, 1991]; *Understanding and Preventing Violence* [NRC, 1993]; *Violence in Families: Assessing Prevention and Treatment Programs* [NRC, 1998]). The salience of intentional injuries in the collective consciousness of public health has also drawn the attention of injury scientists to the mechanisms of these injuries, principally firearms (see, e.g., Karlson and Hargarten [1997]). However, these developments have exposed some critical tensions within the injury field about its identity, mission, and future direction. Some believe this trend to be a deviation from the core scientific mission of the field and worry about the diversion of limited resources from the chronically neglected problems of unintentional injuries to areas in which the potential contributions of the field are limited. They also believe that it is a strategic mistake for the injury field to take on the daunting, complex, and highly politicized subject of violence. Others believe that the scientific and programmatic advantages of integrating the field, and its potential contributions to the cause of violence prevention, require steadfast continuation of the present course.

From the internal perspective of the injury field, the issue can be posed either as one of boundaries or as one of priorities: Does the prevention of intentional injuries lie within the domain of the field? If so, how should the priorities for research and action be set within such a diverse array of important social problems? From a societal perspective, the argument raises questions about the added value of public health to the prevention of suicide and violence, problems traditionally understood to lie within the respective domains of mental health and criminal justice.

This controversy signifies an important stage in the development of the injury field. Arguments for disaggregating the prevention of violence and suicide from the prevention of unintentional injuries have some force, especially in light of the greater importance of motivational factors and individual vulnerabilities in understanding and responding to violence and suicide and of the traditional roles played by criminal justice and mental health disciplines in these areas. However, despite the important differences associated with intentionality, the committee strongly endorses and reaffirms continued integration of all injury prevention activities within a common framework of research and program development for several reasons. First, the surveillance systems that undergird injury prevention collect data on all injuries regardless of intent and

---

[2]In this report the committee uses the term violence to denote interpersonal violence. A major 1993 report defined violence as "behavior by persons against persons that intentionally threatens, attempts, or actually inflicts physical harm. . . . [The definition] excludes consideration of human behavior that inflicts physical harm unintentionally. Also excluded are certain behaviors that inflict physical harm intentionally: violence against oneself, as in suicides and attempted suicides . . . " (NRC, 1993, pp. 35–36).

focus on the mechanism of injury because the information regarding intent may be subjective and unavailable. Second, even though differences in intentionality are often associated with different risk factors and different targets of intervention, responsibilities for carrying out preventive interventions in the field often converge on the same programs and agencies, particularly in public safety, emergency medical and other health care, and public health. Finally, epidemiologic evidence highlights the powerful etiological role of several factors that cut across all injury categories, whatever the mechanism and regardless of intention. Prominent examples are alcohol use and adolescent impulsivity. Reflecting this, some interventions tend to reduce the incidence and severity of both unintentional and intentional injuries. Examples of interventions shown to have a broad impact include reducing alcohol availability (Chiu et al., 1997; Landen et al., 1997), home visitation for first-time new mothers (Kitzman et al., 1997; Olds et al., 1997), and eliminating the carbon monoxide content of domestically used coal gas (Hassall and Trethowan, 1972).

Viewed in this way, injury prevention is necessarily a collaborative undertaking. The main contributions of injury science lie in its population-based perspective; its capacity to identify and frame interventions for a broad array of risk factors, particularly environmental ones; and its tools for measuring outcomes. However, injury scientists and prevention practitioners need partners in order to mount any successful preventive intervention. Interventions targeted at product design and the physical environment require collaboration with product manufacturers, safety engineers, and so forth. Interventions targeted on human behavior or the social environment require collaboration with schools, family service agencies, mental health agencies, and alcohol control agencies, among others. Interventions aiming to reduce self-inflicted injuries, assaults, and various types of unintentional injuries require different collaborators, but the basic approach is the same: The injury field provides the wide-angle lens, while the specific focus is provided by specialists from pertinent disciplines in adjacent fields.

In summary, by proclaiming that "violence is a public health problem," leaders in medicine and the public health establishment have summoned a growing body of researchers and practitioners to the cause of violence prevention. Perhaps an analogous effort will be undertaken for suicide prevention. However, it is important to clarify the implications of this declaration for the future of the injury field. Conceptually and scientifically, the prevention and treatment of injury (whether intentional or unintentional) may be productively studied and understood from a public health perspective. However, organizing a successful social response to injury is not a conceptual and scientific challenge; it is a political one. To say that violence is a public health problem is not necessarily to say that the public health community should be at the center of the social response to violence. Nor is it to say that the public health infrastructure has any comparative advantage in organizing the social response to violence. What is required is a coordinated effort to harness social energies for a more effective program of studying and preventing violence. The tools and resources of public health should be allocated prudently to this effort.

Boundaries

The recent emphasis on violence prevention has raised some additional questions about the conceptual boundaries of the injury field. At issue are the subtle but important differences between its defining mission—preventing and ameliorating traumatic physical injury—and the more sweeping aims of violence prevention. Physical injuries are among the most serious consequences of violence. However, definitions of violence (and "abuse") focus on the behavior (typically, force or threats of force) rather than the outcome. Moreover, the ultimate harm associated with violent relationships—including psychological distress and developmental harm—is more diffuse than physical harm, affecting both the immediate victim and those who witness the violence (Osofsky, 1995).

This difference in focus has two implications for the mission and boundaries of the injury field. First, violence prevention is a broader mission than prevention of the injury inflicted. The focus of the injury field should remain on preventing injuries, and in identifying and modifying risk factors for injuries. The committee recognizes that targeting abusive relationships and styles of violent interaction can often be effective means of reducing injuries (in the short term and across generations), but the challenge for the injury field is to promote collaboration with violence researchers and intervention agencies without losing sight of its own primary mission. In the final analysis, the value of the injury field's investment will be determined by the impact on injury morbidity and mortality. Second, the focus of the injury field should be on physical injury rather than emotional or developmental harms. One could say that all harmful outcomes from traumatic exposures, including emotional and developmental harm, are "injuries" within the domain of the injury field. However, in the committee's view, the tasks of measuring, understanding, and preventing these psychological harms are best viewed as being within the domain of mental health. This is not to say that psychological trauma is irrelevant to the injury field—emotional sequelae to physical injuries have a direct bearing on treatment, for example, and on the measurement of outcomes; but these concerns call for collaboration between injury and mental health, not for an extension of the boundaries of the injury field. In sum, although the perspectives and tools of the injury field have much to contribute to the study and prevention of violent injuries, the prevention of violence and the amelioration of its consequences comprise a much larger domain. Keeping this distinction in mind helps to shape the priorities of the injury field.

VOCABULARY OF THE INJURY FIELD

In reports of this kind, choices of terminology often signify positions on disputed issues of perspective or policy. Although the vocabulary of the injury field is less contentious than in many fields, a few terms are laden with policy significance and require clarification.

Injury and Accident

Architects of the injury field in the United States have made a concerted effort to displace the term "accident," which implies random events and bad luck, with the term "injury," implying predictability in the epidemiological sense and therefore amenability to prevention. Injury, moreover, refers to the health outcome being addressed. By focusing the attention on result or outcome, the term "injury" is neutral with respect to causation, intentionality, and fault. The terminology has thereby facilitated scientific communication and helped disentangle issues of description from assumptions about etiology and fault.

Erasing the term "accident" from the vocabulary of the field has not erased it from everyday speech, however, and the general public and policy makers seem to understand the phrase "accident prevention" much better than they understand "injury prevention." Moreover, as noted by Bijur (1995), abandoning the term accident has left the field without a generic term for the events that may or may not result in bodily injury. Instead, many such terms are used to describe specific events (e.g., crash, collision, fire, poisoning, fall, shooting, fight). Interestingly, the phrase "accident prevention" continues to be used in the United Kingdom without the implications of fatalism feared by the field in this country, and Avery (1995) has proposed that this term be revived throughout the field to refer to interventions aiming to reduce events that present a significant risk of injury. However, the committee agrees with Bijur (1995) that this approach is inadvisable, not only because of its inescapable etiological connotations but also because it leaves no room for injury events that are intentionally caused (and are in no sense accidents).

Intentionality

Although the injury field focuses on preventing and treating a condition (the "injury") and ameliorating its consequences, intentionality (e.g., the actor's purpose and awareness of the risk of injury) is an important variable in studying the causes and prevention of injuries. According to the standard practice, injuries are divided into two categories: The term "unintentional" is used to refer to injuries that were unplanned ("accidents" in the earlier terminology), whereas the term "intentional" is used to refer to injuries resulting from purposeful human action (whether directed at oneself or others). This nomenclature is embodied in the

International Classification of Diseases, which requires a determination on intentionality before any other coding decisions.

Some injury scientists, however, are increasingly dissatisfied with this terminology. Among other concerns, they point out that the focus on intentionality can divert attention to issues relating to individual moral and legal responsibility and away from the broad array of risk factors and interventions represented in the Haddon matrix, many of which can prevent both intentional and unintentional injuries. Intentionality is more sensibly understood as a continuum, ranging from inadvertence to conscious risk taking to purposeful harming, rather than as two categories; and assigning cases to one of the two categories for coding purposes often requires complex judgments based on inadequate information. The committee agrees that these characterizations cannot bear too much weight, and that coding decisions will be imperfect in many cases. Notwithstanding these shortcomings, however, the committee believes that whether an injury is "intentional" or not is reasonably ascertainable in many cases, and that these terms are useable—if oversimplifying—categories for aggregating and interpreting injury data. In the absence of any alternative conceptualization, this terminology will be retained. Among intentional injuries, greater refinement can be achieved by using the terms "assaultive injuries" (including intentional homicide if death occurs) and "self-inflicted injuries" (including suicides if death occurs). Although the category of unintentional injuries encompasses a wide variety of risk-creating behavior (ranging from inattention to gross recklessness), greater refinement cannot reasonably be achieved outside a courtroom.

Prevention and Treatment

In this report, the committee has decided to simplify its vocabulary by using two terms—prevention and treatment—to refer to the array of activities variously described as prevention, control, acute care, and rehabilitation. The term "prevention" is used to refer to efforts to reduce the risk or severity of injury. This can be accomplished by preventing injury-causing events ("pre-event" interventions) or altering the circumstances or impact of the injury-causing event ("event" interventions). The term "treatment" is used to refer to post-event efforts to ameliorate the effects of the injury through acute care and rehabilitation (Table 1.1).

Control

The committee can see no use for the term "control," borrowed from the vocabulary of infectious disease, which has been deployed in the injury field to refer mainly to the idea of ameliorating the consequences of injury-causing events. Prevention and treatment, as defined above, appear to express these ideas adequately, and adding the term "control" can only sow confusion because it implies a preference for coercive interventions. The phrase "injury field" (rather than "injury control") is used to refer to the entire domain of injury prevention and treatment.

DEVELOPMENT OF THE INJURY FIELD

The committee was assigned the task of reviewing the progress of the injury field since publication of *Injury in America* and *Injury Control* and making recommendations to further develop the field and reduce the burden of injury. The entire report is meant to be responsive to this charge. However, in light of the role of previous IOM-NRC committees in nurturing the development of the field over the past 30 years, the committee wanted to comment on measures of growth and maturity. Based on its public and scientific workshops and on discussions with researchers and practitioners, the committee has concluded that the field has grown in size, has achieved a significant degree of cohesion, and has matured in perspective. However, further development of the field has been hampered by inadequate opportunities for training and scientific communication (see Chapters 4, 7, and 8).

Growth and Cohesion

The authors of *Injury in America* (NRC, 1985) envisioned an interdisciplinary field of science and practice with five components: (1) epidemiology, (2) prevention, (3) biomechanics, (4) acute care, and (5) rehabilitation. In the follow-up report, *Injury Control* (NRC, 1988), the IOM-NRC committee referred to these components as the "five core disciplines" of injury control. The current committee has found it helpful to distinguish between the applications of knowledge (prevention and treatment) and the scientific disciplines that provide the methods and analytic tools for acquiring such knowledge. From this perspective, the range of contributing disciplines is far broader than one might infer from *Injury in America*. In addition to epidemiology, biomechanics, acute care, and rehabilitation, for example, contributing disciplines include psychology, criminology, economics, health outcomes research, and other social and behavioral sciences.

TABLE 1.1 Mission and Vocabulary of the Injury Field

Injury Prevention		Injury Treatment	
Pre-Event	Event	Acute Care	Rehabilitation
Preventing injury-causing event	Preventing injury or minimizing severity of injury	Minimizing severity of outcome	Restoring optimum functioning

Increasing numbers of individuals, from a wide variety of disciplines and occupational settings, identify themselves as participants in the field of injury prevention and treatment rooted in the intellectual perspectives and methods of public health. When the CDC and the Johns Hopkins University convened the First National Conference on Injury Control in 1981, it was attended by approximately 25 individuals, representing about half of all of those working in the field at the time. In comparison, more than 900 people participated in the November 1997 Safe America Conference. The National Directory of Injury Prevention Professionals lists 1,234 individuals in its 1992 edition (Children's Safety Network, 1992).

It also appears that the injury field has achieved a significant degree of cohesion, notwithstanding the diversity of disciplines and the variety of specialized spheres of interest. The field has drawn together specialists interested in various domains of prevention (e.g., highway safety, fire safety, product safety, occupational safety, child injury, and violence and suicide prevention) as well as basic scientists and clinicians interested in various types of trauma (e.g., burns, orthopedic injuries, and head injuries). As has occurred in the cancer field, these specialists have come to see scientific, programmatic, and political advantages to characterizing injury as a single "disease." The growing cohesion of the field (within public health) is evidenced by the growth of the Injury Control and Emergency Health Services section within the American Public Health Association, and the development of the field is reflected in, and symbolized by, the 10 multidisciplinary injury control research centers (ICRCs) established over the past decade by the CDC (see Chapter 8).

Links between researchers and practitioners are also developing. National conferences in the field draw together science and practice in both prevention and treatment. The ICRCs have played an important role in this effort, holding conferences for practitioners and facilitating the implementation and evaluation of interventions. In addition, several journals are now devoted exclusively to the field, including the *Journal of Safety Research, Injury Prevention, Accident Analysis and Prevention,* and the *Journal of Trauma,* and an increasing amount of space is devoted to injury-related articles in journals with general professional readerships, including the *American Journal of Public Health, Pediatrics,* the *Journal of the American Medical Association,* and the *New England Journal of Medicine.*

Another intriguing aspect of the emergence and composition of the injury field has been the close collaboration of prevention and treatment. An analogous development has occurred in the fields of cancer and heart disease. One might say that these partnerships can be explained entirely as expressions of political self-interest. Voices raised in support of injury prevention (including fire prevention, violence and suicide prevention, etc.) and in support of trauma care and rehabilitation are most likely to be heard if they are raised in unison. But the committee believes that much more than political strength would be lost if the prevention and treatment communities were to lose their sense of common identity. Injury epidemiology straddles prevention and treatment, serving as a bridge and source of information and insight in both directions. Designing strategies for protecting people from the effects of injury-causing events requires ongoing scientific communication between scientists in biomechanics, molecular biology, and clinical pathology. Implementation of public education and other prevention programs requires participation of surgeons and rehabilitation specialists to convey information about consequences. Although the task of drawing together specialists in injury prevention and treatment is unfinished, remarkable progress has been made.

A recent example is the Crash Injury Research and Engineering Network (CIREN) established by NHTSA in 1996. CIREN links trauma center clinicians and crash investigators in a nationwide computerized network. This enables engineers to better understand injury-producing mechanisms and to develop better criteria for vehicle safety design, while informing clinicians about emerging injury patterns, and thereby facilitating triage, diagnosis, and treatment of crash injuries.

Of course, not all people interested in preventing or treating injuries (e.g., violence and suicide prevention, highway engineering, fire safety, emergency medical services) identify themselves with the injury field. All of these groups have an interest in safety, which is more a common cause than a recognizable field of scientific study or professional practice. However, many people within these specialized spheres have increasingly recognized their common interests with specialists in the injury field and have embraced its conceptual paradigms, intellectual perspectives, and methods. One of the challenges facing the field in the coming years is to develop and implement strategies for injecting injury science into the training curricula of the many disciplines that participate in and contribute to the injury field.

The injury field (including the many specialized spheres of interest within it) overlaps with other fields whose knowledge and practice affect injury prevention and treatment. These adjacent fields include substance abuse, disability prevention, criminal justice, child development, and mental health. Another important challenge facing leaders of the injury field in the coming years is to facilitate collaboration with scientists and practitioners from these many overlapping and adjacent fields.

Maturity

A vibrant interdisciplinary field, encompassing biomedical, engineering, and social and behavioral sciences cannot thrive in the face of intellectual orthodoxy. In the injury field, the challenge has been to open a discourse between environmental and behavioral perspectives. Until the 1960s, the predecessor field of accident prevention was dominated by a behavioral perspective, and proposed interventions relied heavily on changing individual behavior, primarily through education and persuasion. Partly in reaction to the perceived failure of health education, Haddon (1968) and others highlighted the importance of mechanical and environmental factors. What Haddon had in mind was an extension of injury prevention from one cell of the matrix in Figure 1.2 (pre-event, individual behavior) to all the cells. However, during the late 1960s and early 1970s, the pendulum swung in the other direction, and the developing injury field was characterized by a strong emphasis on environmental intervention (and passive protection) and a deep skepticism about the efficacy of behavioral intervention. This perspective has long been regarded as axiomatic in the literature, and behavioral perspectives (e.g., of economists or health educators) have often been discounted or strongly criticized. In recent years, however, this intellectual tension has receded and behavioral perspectives are now increasingly viewed as complementary rather than antagonistic to environmental perspectives. Since 1985, knowledge about human judgment and decision making has made significant advances, integrating the perspectives of cognitive psychologists and economists. People have also recognized that behavioral interventions may sometimes be cheaper and more cost-effective than environmental ones even if they are more circumscribed in scope. Moreover, educational efforts have increasingly focused on changing the behaviors of those with opportunities to influence policy, such as legislators and the media, rather than on merely educating for the purpose of changing individual behavior.

Like other fields in public health, such as infectious disease control and substance abuse prevention, the injury field is defined by a preventive mission. Injury specialists are not "neutral" about whether injuries occur or whether their impact is ameliorated. However, this mission must be pursued in a social and cultural context where the message (that injuries are preventable) competes for attention with other concerns and where people have widely divergent attitudes about what risks are acceptable or what interventions are appropriate. One sign of the maturation of the injury field is the growing appreciation of the ethical and cultural context of injury prevention and treatment.

Injury prevention is not free. All preventive interventions have costs, including possible trade-offs with other important social values. In the early years of the field, injury specialists were almost reflexively inclined toward regulation, particularly of consumer products and environmental risks. This orientation was understandable in light of the weaknesses of legal regulation at the time. In recent years, however, the field has begun to incorporate the perspectives of economists, particularly the need to consider all of the behavioral effects of an intervention, to measure costs, and to seek a reasonable balance between benefits and costs. A complementary phenomenon has also occurred within the allied disciplines, as some economists and public policy experts have embraced the perspectives and vocabulary of public health (Cook, 1991; Zimring and Hawkins, 1997).

A related development is recognition of the need to embrace different perspectives on the weighing of risks. A developing literature on risk analysis has described the factors that affect people's judgments about what risks are acceptable (e.g., whether they are voluntarily assumed) and how different types of risks are compared with one another, and has helped to highlight the ways in which the benefits and burdens of risk-taking behavior are differentially distributed (Fischhoff et al., 1981). Those contributions have enriched our understanding of the ethical dimensions of preventive interventions and have located the injury field in the larger landscape of risk regulation.

Controversies in the Field

Because the injury field is mission driven and action oriented, some controversies concerning the ethics and politics of prevention tend to recur. A continuing challenge for participants in the public debate, and particularly for leaders of the field, is to develop rhetorical strategies for promoting public consensus on controversial issues.

Regulation and Freedom

Injury prevention interventions often aim at protecting people from the consequences of their own risk taking. In some instances, critics may characterize these interventions as "paternalistic" because they curtail people's freedom "for their own good," rather than to protect other people. The most clear-cut examples are mandatory motorcycle helmet laws and other regulations requiring that people use safety precautions to protect themselves. More ambiguous examples include prohibiting manufacturers from selling products thought to be too risky (e.g., three-wheel all-terrain vehicles [ATVs]) or requiring manufacturers to protect adult consumers from their own negligence (e.g., machine guards) when doing so increases the product's cost or reduces its utility.

The argument that an intervention is impermissibly paternalistic can be contested on a variety of grounds. First, it might be argued that the intervention is designed to offset irremediable deficits in information that prevent people from appreciating the risks they face or otherwise making informed risk-benefit judgments. Everyone would agree that such information deficits, if proven, provide an ethically appropriate basis for regulation. The disagreement arises when the government restricts peoples' choices (by banning three-wheel ATVs for use by adults or requiring adult car occupants to wear safety belts) on the ground that people sometimes do not make "rational" choices based on the information at hand. Libertarian critics would find this argument unpersuasive because it substitutes the government's values and preferences for the individual's. Proponents might also defend supposedly paternalistic regulation by arguing that the person injured as a result of his or her own risk taking rarely "internalizes" the cost of the injury and that everyone therefore has a stake in reducing the social costs of injury. Finally, some might argue that even if the intervention is paternalistic, it still may be justified as long as some other criterion is met (e.g., that the aggregate social benefits of the intervention outweigh its costs). Recent studies have shown, for example, that mandatory helmet laws and mandatory safety-belt use laws substantially reduce injury costs (Graham et al., 1997; Max et al., 1998). In the final analysis, opposition to mandatory safety-belt laws virtually evaporated in the face of unequivocal evidence that the safety gains (lives saved and disability avoided) far outweigh the costs of enforcement and the slight reduction in freedom.

Regardless of one's views on the issue of paternalism, injury prevention interventions always require attention to costs and benefits, and a restriction of individual freedom must sometimes be "weighed" as one of the "costs" of the intervention. One example is the argument that reducing the blood alcohol level (BAL) that constitutes conclusive evidence of drunk driving (from 0.10 g/dL to 0.08 g/dL) will curtail the opportunity for social drinking in bars and restaurants by many people who would not have posed a higher crash risk. How does one quantify the "costs" of this reduced freedom to drink and weigh them against the safety gains effected by the 0.08 BAL laws? Another contentious example is the argument that reducing access to handguns in the home poses a trade-off between the value of the lives that would be saved by reduced access and the value of a reduced sense of security for homeowners. One of the important challenges facing the field is to promote rational discourse about the empirical issues and value judgments raised by these recurrent conflicts between safety regulation and personal freedom (see Chapter 5).

Federalism and Priority Setting

As in many areas of public health, an ongoing dispute concerns the role of the federal government in priority setting. Some argue that the most useful role of the federal government in the sphere of injury prevention is to support states and communities in their efforts to set and implement local priorities. The counterargument is that limited federal dollars should be used to generate new knowledge and to spur states and communities to implement policies and programs that have been identified as federal priorities. This dispute is evident in debates between those who want federal money to be used for capacity building in state health departments and those who prefer that the money be used to support the implementation and evaluation of programs identified as federal priorities.

Another dimension of this controversy is the degree of pressure that should be brought to bear on states to implement federal priorities. Sometimes Congress uses the "carrot," making grants available for the specific purpose of implementing a new program. In other contexts, however, Congress uses a "stick," withholding funding for ongoing federally supported state activities, such as highway construction. For example, a provision of the National Highway System Act of 1995 directed the Department of Transportation to withhold federal highway construction monies from states that failed to enact "zero tolerance" laws for drivers under 21 by 1998. The dispute over the use of "conditional" federal funding was evident in the 1998 congressional debate over the .08 BAL laws, when the battle lines were drawn between those who wanted to withhold federal highway monies from noncomplying states and those who wanted to offer an incentive for adoption rather than use a penalty.

Science and Advocacy

In any value-laden field where research is highly susceptible to political bias, special efforts are required to preserve the integrity of the scientific process through peer review of proposals and publications and through the corrective effects of replication and reinterpretation of scientific findings. (The distortion of tobacco research is described by Bero and colleagues [1994].) Research can never be value free, of course. Inevitably, a researcher's values influence the topics he or she chooses to investigate and the discussion of the possible implications of study findings. Yet every reasonable effort should be made to minimize the influence—and the appearance—of bias on the study methods and the analysis of results.

It is also important for investigators to avoid becoming so invested in a particular policy position that they compromise public confidence in the objectivity and integrity of the scientific process. Some investigators try to do this by eschewing advocacy altogether, and the committee believes that the injury field would benefit from a stronger cadre of "pure scientists" who try to maintain an objective stance on their work. However, it would go too far to insist that all injury scientists abstain from advocacy. As noted in Chapter 7, advocacy on behalf of injury prevention is a key component of public health practice, and injury scientists may properly want to assume the burdens—and risks—of advocacy. How to balance the demands of science and advocacy is one of the ongoing challenges for the field.

ORGANIZATION OF THE REPORT

It is customary to summarize the knowledge, activities, and challenges of the injury field by categorizing injuries according to mechanism (motor vehicle, firearm, fall, fire, etc.), intentionality (unintentional, assaultive, and self-inflicted), or context (transportation, residential, recreational, and occupational). The committee decided not to use any of these customary devices to organize this report. For one thing, other reports and reviews have recently synthesized knowledge and opportunities in the component parts of the field (see, e.g., National Committee [1989]; IOM [1997]; Rivara et al. [1997a,b]). More importantly, the committee's charge was to assess the injury field as a whole and to make recommendations for advancing the field as a whole. Rather than compiling particular recommendations for each of the component areas, the committee wanted to highlight the potential contributions of injury science and practice to a diverse, collaborative effort to achieve a safer society.

Chapter 2 describes the magnitude and costs of injury in the United States. Chapter 3 reviews existing injury data systems and makes recommendations for improving injury surveillance as a necessary foundation for further advances in risk analysis, prevention research, and program evaluation. Chapter 4 highlights opportunities for strengthening injury prevention research. Chapter 5 presents two case studies of injury prevention—motor vehicles and firearms—in an effort to identify the successful components from motor vehicle injury prevention that may be applied to reducing firearm injuries. Chapter 6 reviews progress in trauma systems development.

Chapters 7 and 8 present recommendations for strengthening society's capacity to prevent and treat injuries. Chapter 7 focuses on state and community action, with a particular emphasis on the implementation of injury prevention programs. Chapter 8 addresses the federal response, with a series of recommendations for strengthening federal support for research and program development and for coordinating the federal effort. Chapter 9 provides the main conclusions of this report and discusses future opportunities for reducing the burden of injury in America. Finally, there are four appendices in the report: Appendix A provides a list of those individuals who shared their insights and knowledge with committee members, attended meetings, and the public or scientific workshop. Appendix B provides a timeline of selected historical events in the injury field. Appendix C details the agenda for the committee's public workshop. Appendix D contains a list of acronyms used in the report.

REFERENCES

Avery JG. 1995. Accident prevention—injury control—injury prevention—or whatever? *Injury Prevention* 1(1):10–11.

Baker SP. 1989. Injury science comes of age. *Journal of the American Medical Association* 262(2):2284–2285.

Bero LA, Glantz SA, Rennie D. 1994. Publication bias and public health policy on environmental tobacco smoke. *Journal of the American Medical Association* 272(2): 133–136.

Bijur PE. 1995. What's in a name? Comments on the use of the terms "accident" and "injury." *Injury Prevention* 1(1):9–11.

CDC (Centers for Disease Control and Prevention). 1991. Update: Years of potential life lost before age 65—United States, 1988 and 1989. *Morbidity and Mortality Weekly Report* 40:60–62.

Children's Safety Network. 1992. *Injury Prevention Professionals: A National Directory*, 3rd edition. Washington, DC: National Center for Education in Maternal and Child Health.

Chiu AY, Perez PE, Parker RN. 1997. Impact of banning alcohol on outpatient visits in Barrow, Alaska. *Journal of the American Medical Association* 278(21):1775–1777.

Cook PJ. 1991. The technology of personal violence. In: Tonry M, ed. *Crime and Justice: A Review of Research.* Chicago, IL: University of Chicago Press. Pp. 1–71.

Fingerhut LA, Warner M. 1997. *Injury Chartbook. Health, United States, 1996–97.* Hyattsville, MD: National Center for Health Statistics.

Fischhoff B, Lichtenstein S, Slovic P, Derby SL, Keeney RL. 1981. *Acceptable Risk.* New York: Cambridge University Press.

Gibson JJ. 1961. The contribution of experimental psychology to the formulation of the problem of safety: A brief for basic research. In: *Behavioral Approaches to Accident Research.* New York: Association for the Aid of Crippled Children. Pp. 77–89.

Gordon JE. 1949. The epidemiology of accidents. *American Journal of Public Health* 39:504–515.

Graham JD, Thompson KM, Goldie SJ, Segui-Gomez M, Weinstein MC. 1997. The cost-effectiveness of air bags by seating position. *Journal of the American Medical Association* 278(17):1418–1425

Haddon W Jr. 1968. The changing approach to the epidemiology, prevention, and amelioration of trauma: The transition to approaches etiologically rather than descriptively based. *American Journal of Public Health* 58(8):1431–1438.

Haddon W Jr. 1980. Options for the prevention of motor vehicle crash injury. *Israel Journal of Medicine* 16:45–68.

Hassall C, Trethowan WH. 1972. Suicide in Birmingham. *British Medical Journal* 1(5802):717–718.

IOM (Institute of Medicine). 1997. *Enabling America: Assessing the Role of Rehabilitation Science and Engineering.* Washington, DC: National Academy Press.

IOM (Institute of Medicine). 1998. *Scientific Opportunities and Public Needs: Improving Priority Setting and Public Input at the National Institutes of Health.* Washington, DC: National Academy Press.

Karlson TA, Hargarten SW. 1997. *Reducing Firearm Injury and Death: A Public Health Sourcebook on Guns.* New Brunswick, NJ: Rutgers University Press.

Kitzman H, Olds DL, Henderson CR Jr, Hanks C, Cole R, Tatelbaum R, McConnochie KM, Sidora K, Luckey DW, Shaver D, Engelhardt K, James D, Barnard K. 1997. Effect of prenatal and infancy home visitation by nurses on pregnancy outcomes, childhood injuries and repeated childbearing: A randomized control trial. *Journal of the American Medical Association* 278(8):644–652.

Landen MG, Beller M, Funk E, Propst M, Middaugh J, Moolenaar RL. 1997. Alcohol-related injury death and alcohol availability in remote Alaska. *Journal of the American Medical Association* 278(21):1755–1758.

Loimer H, Driur M, Guarnieri M. 1996. Accidents and acts of God: A history of the terms. *American Journal of Public Health* 86(1):101–107.

Max W, Stark B, Root S. 1998. Putting a lid on injury costs: The economic impact of the California motorcycle helmet law. *Journal of Trauma* 45(3):550–556.

Miller TR, Lestina DC, Galbraith MS, Viano DC. 1994. Medical-care spending—United States. *Morbidity and Mortality Weekly Report* 43(32):581–586.

National Committee (National Committee for Injury Prevention and Control). 1989. *Injury Prevention: Meeting the Challenge.* New York: Oxford University Press. Published as a supplement to the *American Journal of Preventive Medicine* 5(3).

NCHS (National Center for Health Statistics). 1998. *Health, United States, 1998 with Socioeconomic Status and Health Chartbook.* Hyattsville, MD: NCHS. DHHS Publication No. (PHS) 98-1232.

NCIPC (National Center for Injury Prevention and Control). 1993. *Injury Control in the 1990s: A National Plan for Action. A Report to the Second World Conference on Injury Control.* Atlanta, GA: Centers for Disease Control and Prevention.

NCIPC (National Center for Injury Prevention and Control). 1997. *Inventory of Federally Funded Research in Injury Prevention and Control, FY 1995.* Atlanta, GA: NCIPC.

NIH (National Institutes of Health). 1994. *A Report of the Task Force on Trauma Research.* Bethesda, MD: NIH.

NRC (National Research Council). 1966. *Accidental Death and Disability: The Neglected Disease of Modern Society.* Washington, DC: National Academy Press.

NRC (National Research Council). 1985. *Injury in America: A Continuing Public Health Problem.* Washington, DC: National Academy Press.

NRC (National Research Council). 1988. *Injury Control: A Review of the Status and Progress of the Injury Control Program at the Centers for Disease Control.* Washington, DC: National Academy Press.

NRC (National Research Council). 1993. *Understanding and Preventing Violence.* Washington, DC: National Academy Press.

NRC (National Research Council). 1998. *Violence in Families: Assessing Prevention and Treatment Programs.* Washington, DC: National Academy Press.

Olds DL, Eckenrode J, Henderson CR Jr, Kitzman H, Powers J, Cole R, Sidora K, Morris P, Pettitt LM, Luckey D. 1997. Long-term effects of home visitation on maternal life course and child abuse and neglect. *Journal of the American Medical Association* 278(8):637–643.

Osofsky JD. 1995. The effects of exposure to violence on young children. *American Psychologist* 50(9):782–788.

Rivara FP, Grossman DC, Cummings P. 1997a. Injury prevention. First of two parts. *New England Journal of Medicine* 337(8):543–548.

Rivara FP, Grossman DC, Cummings P. 1997b. Injury prevention. Second of two parts. *New England Journal of Medicine* 337(9):613–618.

Rosenberg ML, Fenley MA, eds. 1991. *Violence in America. A Public Health Approach.* New York: Oxford University Press.

U.S. DHHS (Department of Health and Human Services), Department of Justice. 1986. *Surgeon General's Workshop on Violence and Public Health. October 27–29, 1985.* Rockville, MD: DHHS, Public Health Service. DHHS Publication No. HRS-D-MC-86-1.

Waller JA. 1994. Reflections on a half century of injury control. *American Journal of Public Health* 84(4):664–670.
Zimring FE, Hawkins G. 1997. *Crime Is Not the Problem: Lethal Violence in America.* New York: Oxford University Press.

2

Magnitude and Costs

Injury is a major public health problem in America (see Figure 2.1). Consider the following: In 1995 in the United States,

- 59 million episodes of injuries were reported;
- 2.6 million hospital discharges and 37 million emergency department (ED) visits were for the treatment of injuries;
- 147,891 individuals died as a result of an injury;
- 77 percent of all deaths and 10 percent of the hospitalizations among 15 to 24-year-olds were caused by injuries; and
- 52 percent of all deaths and 17 percent of the hospitalizations among 5- to 14-year-olds were caused by injuries. Additionally,
- injury and its consequences accounted for 12 percent of all medical spending and
- the cost of injury was estimated at $260 billion[1] (Miller et al., 1994, 1995; Fingerhut and Warner, 1997; E. MacKenzie, Johns Hopkins University, personal communication, 1998; see Figure 2.2).

---

[1]The 1985 cost-of-injury estimates were updated to 1995 separately by type of cost. Direct costs were inflated using the appropriate component of the Consumer Price Index (hospital and related services, physicians' services, prescription drugs, professional medical services, and medical care services). Indirect costs were inflated using the index of hourly compensation in the business sector.

41

	Age Groups				
Rank	<1	1-4	5-9	10-14	15-24
1	Congenital Anomalies 6,554	Unintentional Injuries 2,280	Unintentional Injuries 1,612	Unintentional Injuries 1,932	Unintentional Injuries 13,842
2	Short Gestation 3,933	Congenital Anomalies 695	Malignant Neoplasms 523	Malignant Neoplasms 503	Homicide 7,284
3	SIDS 3,397	Malignant Neoplasms 488	Congenital Anomalies 242	Homicide 405	Suicide 4,784
4	Respiratory Distress Synd. 1,454	Homicide 452	Homicide 157	Suicide 330	Malignant Neoplasms 1,642
5	Maternal Complications 1,309	Heart Disease 251	Heart Disease 130	Congenital Anomalies 207	Heart Disease 1,039
6	Placenta Cord Membranes 962	HIV 210	HIV 123	Heart Disease 164	HIV 629
7	Perinatal Infections 788	Pneumonia & Influenza 156	Pneumonia & Influenza 73	Bronchitis Emphysema Asthma 105	Congenital Anomalies 452
8	Unintentional Injuries 787	Perinatal Period 87	Benign Neoplasms 50	HIV 66	Bronchitis Emphysema Asthma 246
9	Pneumonia & Influenza 492	Septicemia 80	Bronchitis Emphysema Asthma 38	Benign Neoplasms 55	Pneumonia & Influenza 207
10	Intrauterine Hypoxia 475	Cerebro-vascular 57	Anemias 31	Pneumonia & Influenza 55	Cerebro-vascular 172

FIGURE 2.1 Ten leading causes of death by age group, 1995. SOURCE: NCIPC, 1998.

Age Groups					
25-34	35-44	45-54	55-64	65+	Total
Unintentional Injuries 13,435	HIV 18,860	Malignant Neoplasms 44,186	Malignant Neoplasms 87,898	Heart Disease 615,426	Heart Disease 737,563
HIV 11,894	Malignant Neoplasms 17,110	Heart Disease 34,498	Heart Disease 68,240	Malignant Neoplasms 381,142	Malignant Neoplasms 538,455
Suicide 6,292	Unintentional Injuries 14,225	Unintentional Injuries 9,261	Bronchitis Emphysema Asthma 9,988	Cerebro-vascular 138,762	Cerebro-vascular 157,991
Homicide 6,162	Heart Disease 13,603	HIV 8,179	Cerebro-vascular 9,735	Bronchitis Emphysema Asthma 88,478	Bronchitis Emphysema Asthma 102,899
Malignant Neoplasms 4,875	Suicide 6,467	Cerebro-vascular 5,473	Diabetes 8,188	Pneumonia & Influenza 74,297	Unintentional Injuries 93,320
Heart Disease 3,461	Homicide 4,118	Liver Disease 5,247	Unintentional Injuries 6,743	Diabetes 44,452	Pneumonia & Influenza 82,923
Cerebro-vascular 720	Liver Disease 3,705	Suicide 4,532	Liver Disease 5,356	Unintentional Injuries 29,099	Diabetes 59,254
Pneumonia & Influenza 622	Cerebro-vascular 2,772	Diabetes 3,996	Pneumonia & Influenza 3,458	Alzheimer's Disease 20,230	HIV 43,115
Diabetes 614	Diabetes 1,844	Bronchitis Emphysema Asthma 2,756	Suicide 2,804	Nephritis 20,182	Suicide 31,284
Liver Disease 604	Pneumonia & Influenza 1,480	Pneumonia & Influenza 2,079	HIV 2,320	Septicemia 16,899	Liver Disease 25,222

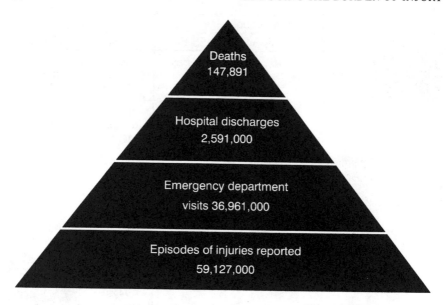

FIGURE 2.2 Burden of injury: United States, 1995. SOURCE: Fingerhut and Warner, 1997.

Measuring the overall magnitude of injury as a major public health problem is crucial in the development of a rational basis for resource allocation, for defining strategies for prevention interventions, and for determining their outcomes. As surveillance efforts have continued to improve, we have gained increasing knowledge about the magnitude of the injury problem and the costs to society; however, knowledge is sparse regarding nonfatal injuries, the settings in which they occur, and the total costs associated with injury morbidity.

This chapter focuses on the impact of injury in terms of mortality, morbidity, and societal costs. Patterns of injury over time and within and across specific demographic subgroups are briefly described. The statistics and discussion presented in this chapter are based primarily on the work of Fingerhut and Warner (1997), unless otherwise noted.

OVERALL BURDEN OF INJURY: MORTALITY RATES

In 1995, 90,402 people died from unintentional injuries[2] (61 percent of all injury fatalities, at a rate of 34.4 deaths per 100,000 persons); there were 22,552

---

[2]Excludes 2,918 deaths due to adverse events.

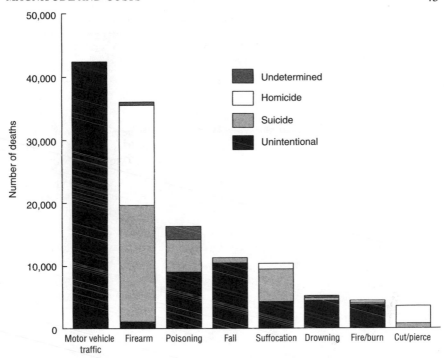

FIGURE 2.3 Leading causes of injury death by manner of death, United States, 1995. SOURCE: Fingerhut and Warner, 1997.

homicides (15 percent of all injury deaths, at a rate of 8.6 per 100,000) and 31,284 suicides (21 percent of injury fatalities, at a rate of 11.9 per 100,000).

For at least the past 30 years, motor vehicle and firearm injuries have been the two leading causes of injury death (see Chapter 5). In 1995, motor vehicle traffic-related injuries accounted for 29 percent of all injury deaths, or 42,452 deaths. Firearm injuries accounted for 24 percent of all injury deaths and claimed a total of 35,957 lives. Motor vehicle deaths are generally classified as unintentional, whereas firearm injuries have been classified primarily as intentional. Of deaths due to firearms, 51 percent were suicides, 43 percent homicides, 3 percent unintentional, and approximately 3 percent other.

Poisonings were the third leading cause of injury death (11 percent), followed by falls and suffocation (8 and 7 percent, respectively); drownings, fires and burns, and cutting and piercing injuries accounted for another 9 percent of all injury deaths (see Figure 2.3) (Fingerhut and Warner, 1997).

TABLE 2.1 Leading Causes of Injury Death, Trends, 1985–1995

Cause of Death	Number of Deaths (all age groups), 1995	Trends, 1985–1995
Motor vehicle traffic	42,452	Decrease 15% from 1985 to 1993, increase 2% from 1993 to 1995
Firearm	35,957	Increase 22% from 1985 to 1993, decrease 11% from 1993 to 1995
Poisoning	16,307	Stable from 1985 to 1991 at about 5/100,000, increase 18% from 1991 to 1995
Falls	11,275	Decrease 11% from 1985 to 1995
Suffocation	10,376	Stable from 1985 to 1995 at about 3/100,000

SOURCE: Fingerhut and Warner (1997).

Trends in Injury Mortality Rates: 1985 to 1996

Although the leading causes of injury death have not changed over the past decade, some trends are important to note; these are described in detail by Fingerhut and Warner (1997) and illustrated in Figure 2.4 and Table 2.1. The age-adjusted unintentional injury death rate declined 12 percent between 1985 and 1995, whereas the suicide rate remained relatively constant, and the overall homicide rate increased 12 percent. The increase in the homicide rate has not been steady; there was a 32 percent increase between 1985 and 1991, followed by a decrease of 15 percent from 1991 to 1995.

Age-adjusted motor vehicle traffic-related death rates declined 15 percent from 1985 to 1993, but increased 2 percent from 1993 to 1995.[3] In 1995, 18,428 persons 15 to 34 years of age died of a motor vehicle traffic injury, comprising 43 percent of all motor vehicle traffic injury deaths. The death rate in this age group declined about 18 percent from 1985 to 1993, to about 24 per 100,000 individuals (Fingerhut and Warner, 1997). From 1985 to 1995, the alcohol-related fatality rate for those 15–34 declined 32 percent, and the nonalcohol

---

[3]In 1995, Congress repealed the national maximum speed limit (effective December 8, 1995). Subsequently, 32 states also repealed their 55 mile per hour speed limits. Estimates suggest that these two actions have resulted in hundreds of additional deaths, but the full effect of the repeals has not yet been quantified (NHTSA, 1998).

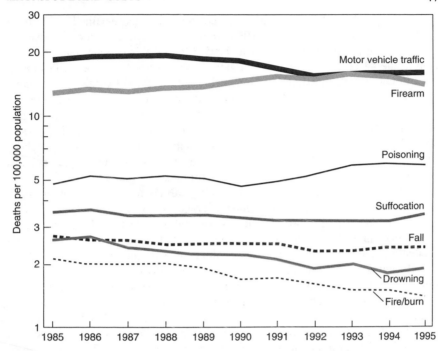

FIGURE 2.4 Age-adjusted death rates for leading causes of injury: United States, 1995. SOURCE: Fingerhut and Warner, 1997.

fatality rate increased 13 percent. The National Highway Traffic Safety Administration (NHTSA) estimates that minimum-age drinking laws have reduced traffic fatalities of 18- to 20-year-olds by 13 percent since 1975 and have saved about 15,700 lives (Fingerhut and Warner, 1997). In 1995, 50 percent of all motor vehicle traffic fatalities among 15- to 34-year-olds were alcohol related.

The age-adjusted firearm death rate increased by 22 percent from 12.8 per 100,000 in 1985 to 15.6 per 100,000 in 1993, followed by an 11 percent decline from 1993 to 1995 to 13.9 per 100,000. The increase in firearm death rates can be attributed almost exclusively to an increase in firearm homicides among adolescents and young adults ages 15 to 34. From 1985 to 1993, there was an increase of 83 percent in the firearm homicide rate of 15- to 34-year-olds, followed by a decline of 14 percent from 1993 to 1995 to 13.7 per 100,000 (Fingerhut and Warner, 1997).

The firearm suicide rate for 15- to 34-year-olds increased by 10 percent from 1984 to 1994 and then declined by about 6 percent in 1995. The increase is attributed to an increase in firearm suicides among males by 13 percent from 1985 to 1994 (followed by a decline of 5 percent in 1995). During 1985–1995, the suicide rate of women declined 13 percent (Fingerhut and Warner, 1997).

The age-adjusted injury death rate due to poisonings remained stable from 1985 to 1991 around 5 deaths per 100,000, followed by an 18 percent increase in the poisoning death rate from 1991 to 1995. Most of this increase can be attributed to the 44 percent increase in the rate among males 25–44 years. Poisoning rates in children declined during both periods. Rates for suffocation were stable from 1985 to 1995. During this same interval, drowning death rates declined 27 percent, and fire and burn death rates declined by 33 percent (Fingerhut and Warner, 1997). Mortality from falls declined by 11 percent during this period, although among the elderly, where rates are highest, the rate increased slightly. In 1995, falls accounted for 23 percent of the deaths due to injury among persons over age 65 and 34 percent of injury deaths for those 85 and older.

Occupational injuries resulted in 77,675 fatalities for civilian workers from 1980 to 1992. This represents an annual average of 5.5 per 100,000 workers. In 1994 and 1995 the rates fell to 5 deaths per 100,000 workers. It has been estimated that, in 1995, occupational injuries cost $119 billion in lost wages and productivity, administrative expenses, health care, and other costs (NSC, 1997).

Recent data indicate that, in 1996, 147,126 individuals died as a result of injury, which was a 2.5 percent decline in the injury death rate to 50.2 per 100,000 population. The motor vehicle traffic injury death rate remained unchanged at 15.8 per 100,000 and the firearm death rate declined 7 percent to 12.9 per 100,000 population. Most of the decline is attributed to the 11 percent decline in the firearm homicide rate (with a more modest decline of 3 percent in the firearm suicide rate). The death rate for poisoning, the third leading cause of injury death, increased slightly, just under 2 percent, in 1996. By manner of injury death, the age-adjusted death rates for all unintentional injury and for all suicide remained unchanged and the homicide rate declined about 11 percent (Peters et al., 1998). Preliminary data for 1997 indicate a 6 percent decline in overall injury mortality. Preliminary data, however, are subject to change once the final figures are all accounted for. Known biases in preliminary data are attributed, in part, to medical examiner and coroner cases for which amended certificates are filed later (Ventura et al., 1998).

OVERALL BURDEN OF INJURY: MORBIDITY

Whereas current surveillance and other data collection efforts provide information about the numbers and types of fatal injuries, much less is known about the incidence and patterns of nonfatal injuries (see Chapter 3). Almost one in four people in the United States sustains an injury during a single year. In 1995, injuries accounted for an estimated 8 percent of all short-stay hospital discharges and 37 percent of all emergency department visits. Injury as a first-listed diagnosis was identified in 2.6 million hospital discharges. In addition, there were 3.4 million more discharges with injury listed as a secondary diagnosis (Gillum et al., 1998). Falls are the leading cause of nonfatal injury visits to emergency departments, accounting for approximately 8 million visits to the emergency department yearly. Motor vehicles remain an important cause of injury accounting for approximately 3.8 million visits to the emergency department per year (Fingerhut and Warner, 1997).

Although most nonfatal injuries are of minor severity and do not result in more than one or two days of restricted activity, a large number result in fractures, brain injuries, major burns, or other significant disability. In 1992–1994, the average hospital discharge rates for fractures—which account for nearly 2 out of 5 injury-related discharges—was 39.3 per 10,000 persons. During this same period, the other leading injury-related discharge diagnoses were poisonings, open wounds and lacerations, intracranial injuries, and sprains and strains. These accounted for 25 percent of first-listed injury hospital discharges. Fractures typically required six to seven days of hospitalization, whereas the other diagnoses, on average, required three to four days of hospitalization (Fingerhut and Warner, 1997).

PATTERNS OF INJURY IN THE POPULATION

Social and demographic characteristics may influence the risk of injury. Surveillance systems, through ongoing and systematic collection of data, can provide information that allows the identification of patterns of injury in specific localities or nationally. Data from surveillance systems may be used to implement prevention strategies in areas designated at high risk for specific types of injuries or hazards. Analyzing cause-specific injury data by age, gender, ethnicity, or occupation helps to focus prevention planning.

Patterns of Injury by Age, Gender, Race, and Ethnicity

Mortality

The percentage of all deaths that were caused by an injury was greater for males (9 percent) than for females (4 percent). Among males ages 15–19 years and 20–24 years, 83 and 80 percent, respectively, of all deaths were caused by injuries compared with 69 and 56 percent among females. With increasing age, the percentages decrease for both males and females. For persons 65 years and over, about 2 percent of all deaths were caused by injuries.

Although injury is a leading cause of childhood death, injury death rates are lowest for children under 15 years of age. The injury death rate for infants in 1995 (29 per 100,000 population) was about 2–3 times the rate for children 1–4 years, 5–9 years, and 10–14 years of age. For persons 15–74 years of age, injury death rates ranged from 49 per 100,000 at 55–64 years to 80 per 100,000 at 20–24 years. Although injury is not a leading cause of death in the elderly, rates were higher for persons 75–84 years and 85 years of age and over, at 116 and 281 per 100,000 persons.

Injury death rates were higher for males than for females in each age group except for infancy when the rates were similar. In 1995 for children 1–9 years of age, injury death rates for males were about 1.5 times the rates for females, and the difference increases with age. The mortality sex ratio (the ratio of death rate for males to that for females) jumped from 2.1:1 at ages 10–14 years to 4.6:1 at 20–24 years. The mortality sex ratio for persons 65 years and over was about 2:1.

Injury death rates vary with race and ethnicity. The average annual injury death rate for 1993–1995 among teenagers and young adults 15–34 years of age was higher for the black population and for American Indian/Alaskan Natives (referred to as American Indians) (119 per 100,000) than for Hispanics (78 per 100,000), non-Hispanic white population (58.0 per 100,000), and Asian or Pacific Islanders (referred to as Asians) (36 per 100,000). Unintentional injury death rates and suicide rates were higher for American Indians than for other racial and ethnic groups. Homicide rates were higher for the black population than for other groups. Motor vehicle traffic injuries were the leading cause of unintentional injury in each race and ethnic group.

Hospitalization

In 1993–1994, 9 percent of all discharges had a first-listed injury diagnosis. For persons 25 years and over, 7–9 percent of discharges were for an injury. Differences by sex were greater for persons ages 15–24 years (31 percent among males compared with 4 percent among females) and for persons 25–44 years of age (17 percent for males compared with 5 percent for females) than for other ages (Figure 2.5). For both white and black males 15–44 years, 20 percent of all hospital discharges were for an injury compared with about 5 percent among females.

The age and gender patterns for injury-related hospitalization are different than those for mortality. In general, discharge rates for persons with a first-listed diagnosis of injury increase with age. In 1993–1994 the average annual rates for children under 5 years of age and 5–14 years of age were 57 percent and 42 percent of the rate for young persons ages 15–24 years (90 discharges per 10,000 persons), and that rate is about one-half the rate for persons 65–74 years of age, and about a fifth of the rate for persons 75 years of age and over (412 per 10,000 persons).

Although injury discharge rates for males and females were similar (108 and 99 per 10,000 persons) for all ages combined, gender discharge rates vary considerably by age. At ages 15–24 years the discharge rates for males were twice those for females (119 compared with 60 per 10,000), whereas for the elderly 75 years of age and over, the rate for males was about 70 percent of the rate for females (322 compared with 463 per 10,000 persons).

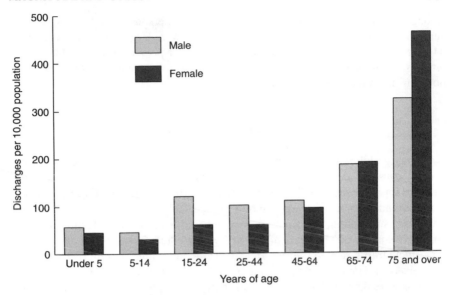

FIGURE 2.5 Hospital discharge rates for injury by age and sex: United States, 1993–1994. SOURCE: Fingerhut and Warner, 1997.

Hospitalization rates for black males under 15 years, 15–44 years, and 45–64 years of age were about twice the rates for white males. At ages 65 years and over, the rates for white and black males were similar. Among females, discharge rates for black children were about twice the rates for white children and differences narrowed with increasing age. For persons 65 years of age and over, injury discharge rates for white females were 1.4 times the rates for black females.

Emergency Department Visits

About 4 of 10 ED visits were for injuries. In 1993–1994, injury visit rates were similarly high for children under 5 years of age and for persons 15–24 years of age and were similarly lower for people aged 45–64 years and 65–74 years compared with other age groups. At ages 5–14 years, 15–24 years, and 25–44 years, injury visit rates for males were 1.4 times the rates for females, and among those 75 years of age and over, the visit rate for females was 1.3 times the rate for males.

ED injury visit rates for black males and females were higher than for white males and females, 23 and 17 per 100 persons compared with 16 and 12 per 100 persons. Rates for black males and females were higher than for white persons among children under 5 years of age and among persons 15–24 years, 25–44 years, and 45–64 years of age. Racial differences were larger for males ages 25–44 years and 45–64 years than for younger or older persons and were larger for females 25–44 years of age than for other groups. (Visit rates by ethnicity were not considered reliable.)

Patterns of Injury by Cause

Among children 1–14 years of age, motor vehicle traffic injuries were the leading cause of death in 1995. Among infants, suffocation was the leading cause of injury death. The five leading causes of injury death among infants and children under 15 years of age—motor vehicle traffic injuries, fires and burns, drowning, suffocation, and firearms—accounted for 80 percent of injury deaths. Among teenagers 15–19 years of age and young adults 20–24 years of age, motor vehicle traffic-related injuries and firearm-related injuries were the two leading causes of death in 1995. For older adults 65–74 years, motor vehicles and firearms were the two leading causes of injury deaths, accounting for one-half of injury mortality. At ages 75–84 years, motor vehicles and falls were the cause of close to one-half of all injury deaths. For those 85 years and over, falls caused one-third of injury deaths.

Hospital discharge rates for open wounds and for internal injuries for all males were 3 times the rates for all females. At ages 15–24 years the discharge rate for open wounds for males was 4.5 times the rate for females. On the other hand, discharge rates for poisoning for females 15–24 years and 45–64 years were 1.6 times the rates for males. In 1992–1994, three out of five injury hospitalizations among elderly persons 75 years of age and over were for fractures, and more than one-half of the fractures were to the hip. Hip fracture rates for elderly females were twice the rates for males.

Among young children and the elderly, falls were the most common cause of injury visits to the ED. For young persons 15–24 years, injuries resulting from being struck, from motor vehicle crashes, and from falls were most likely. The most common injury diagnoses among young children were open wounds and lacerations; for those 15–24 years, superficial injuries and sprains and strains resulted in ED visits, and among the elderly (and especially among females), fractures were the leading diagnosis.

Patterns of Occupational Injury

More than 125 million civilian workers are employed in the United States, with some risk of injury present in all jobs (NIOSH, 1996). In 1995, 6,210 fatal work injuries (5 per 100,000 workers) were reported in the Census of Fatal Occupational Injuries (BLS, 1996). Overall, transportation-related incidents are the leading cause (23 percent) of occupational injury deaths. Since 1980, homicide has been the second leading cause of occupational injury deaths, surpassing machine-related deaths (13 percent) (CDC, 1998). One in six occupational deaths in 1995 was a homicide, which was the leading cause of death for females in occupational settings, and accounted for 46 percent of fatal work injuries (Fingerhut and Warner, 1997). Occupations with the highest risk of fatal injury include truck drivers, fishermen, timber cutters, and airplane pilots.

Although information about nonfatal occupational injuries is not as comprehensive as that for deaths, they are estimated to number more than 13 million each year (Leigh et al., 1997). Nearly one-half (46 percent) of these injuries are disabling. Approximately one-third of nonfatal injuries are sustained by workers in eight industries (restaurants and bars, hospitals, nursing and personal care facilities, trucking and non-air courier services, grocery stores, department stores, motor vehicles and equipment, and hotels and motels), with the highest incidence rate (17.8 per 100 full-time workers) reported in persons employed in nursing and personal care facilities (BLS, 1997).

THE COST OF INJURY

The scope of the injury problem is measured primarily in terms of numbers and rates of death and in years of potential life lost (YPLL) due to premature death. It has become increasingly apparent over the past decade, however, that although death rates and YPLL are powerful indicators of the relative magnitude of the injury problem, they do not adequately measure the full burden of injuries on society. In 1996, unintentional injury was third in YPLL before age 75, following diseases of the heart and malignant neoplasms. In fact, all injury (including homicide and suicide) is the leading cause of YPLL before age 75 (Table 2.2) (NCHS, 1998). With few exceptions, the rank ordering of YPLL for injury follows the ordering for leading causes of injury death. Notably out of order, however, is the YPLL for fall-related deaths. Despite the fact that, overall, more injury deaths are attributed to falls than to suffocations, more YPLLs are associated with suffocations because they tend to occur at younger ages than deaths due to falls.

Totaling deaths and years of life lost, however, does not take into account the additional costs to federal, state, and local governments of public programs (e.g., Medicare, Medicaid, veterans' benefits); the costs to private insurance programs; and the costs accruing to injured individuals, their families, employers, and society in general. These are measured as both economic and quality-of-life factors of the cost of injury.

TABLE 2.2 Leading Causes of Years of Potential Life Lost (YPLL), Costs to Society, and Deaths

Disease or Condition	Age-Adjusted YPLL Before Age 75, 1996 (per 100,000 (population)[a]	Cost Estimate ($ billions, constant 1996 dollars)[b]	Number of Deaths (1996)[a]
Injury[c]	1,919.0	260[d]	147,126[e]
Cancer	1,554.2	115.4	539,533
Heart diseases	1,222.6	144.9	733,361
HIV infection and AIDS	401.9	NA	31,130
Stroke; cerebrovascular diseases	210.2	32.6	159,942
Chronic obstructive pulmonary diseases	161.1	31.8	106,027
Diabetes	153.5	102.7	61,767
Chronic liver disease and cirrhosis	145.7	4.8	25,047
Pneumonia and influenza	114.5	25.4	83,727

[a]SOURCE: NCHS (1998).

[b]These cost estimates were prepared by different authors, using different years as points of reference: heart disease (1991); cancer (1990); stroke (1993); pulmonary disease (1991); pneumonia (1991); diabetes (1992); liver disease (1985); and kidney disease (1985). All estimates (except injury) have been calculated to 1996 dollars and encompass both direct costs and indirect costs attributable to patient mortality (premature death), patient morbidity (reduced productivity), and other non-health care costs. NA = Not available. SOURCE: IOM (1998).

[c]Injury includes unintentional injuries, suicide, and homicide.

[d]The 1985 cost of injury in the United States estimates (Rice et al., 1989) were updated to 1995 separately by type of cost. Direct costs were inflated using the appropriate component of the Consumer Price Index (hospital and related services, physicians' services, prescription drugs, professional medical services, and medical care services). Indirect costs were inflated using the index of hourly compensation in the business sector.

[e]SOURCE: Peters et al. (1998).

Estimates of the economic cost of injury combine information on the incidence and impact of both fatal and nonfatal injuries into a single measure that is readily understandable by policy makers, employers, and the insurance industry. Using a cost-of-illness or human capital approach to valuing health, estimates of the cost of injury have been derived for several major categories (e.g., motor vehicles, firearms, falls, fires and burns, poisonings) of injury (Rice et al., 1989; Max and Rice, 1993; Miller et al., 1995; NSC, 1997; Blincoe, 1997; Leigh et al.,

1997).[4] These costs include (1) direct costs of medical care (both acute and long term) and other nonmedical goods and services related to the injury (e.g., costs for home modifications, vocational rehabilitation, administrative costs for delivering health and indemnity insurance); (2) indirect morbidity costs (i.e., the value of foregone productivity due to injury-related illness and disability); and (3) indirect mortality costs (i.e., the value of foregone productivity due to death at an early age). Also included in some analyses are costs associated with property damage, police and fire services, and legal fees related to compensation (Miller et al., 1995; Blincoe, 1997). These costs can add significantly to the overall cost of injuries from certain mechanisms such as motor vehicle crashes and fires or burns. Costs accrued to family members who lose time from work in order to take care of the injured can also contribute to the total lifetime costs, but these are difficult to determine (Chirikos, 1989).

One of the more comprehensive cost-of-illness studies on injury costs was published by Rice and colleagues (1989). In this study, estimates of the cost of injury were derived by age, gender, and six major injury mechanisms (motor vehicle, firearms, falls, fire or burns, poisonings, and drownings or near drownings). Total lifetime costs associated with both fatal and nonfatal injuries were estimated at $158 billion in 1985 and $182 billion in 1988 (Rice et al., 1989). When inflated to 1995 dollars, the total cost approaches $260 billion. The cost of fatalities represents a disproportionate share of total lifetime costs; while accounting for less than 1 percent of all injuries, fatal injuries contributed to 31 percent of the total calculated cost. An additional 51 percent of the costs accrue among persons with injuries resulting in hospitalization. Less than one-fifth of the total costs are associated with the overwhelming number of injuries that result in one or more days of restricted activity but do not require hospitalization (Rice et al., 1989). Direct medical-care and nonmedical-care expenditures account for an estimated 28 percent of the total costs of injury; approximately 55 percent of these direct costs are spent on hospital care (including both acute care and rehabilitation).

Miller and colleagues (1994) found that treatment of injuries and their long-term effects (excluding nursing home care and medical care for the institutionalized population) accounted for 12 percent of the total medical care spending in the United States, totaling an estimated $69 billion (in 1993 dollars). Injuries were identified as second only to cardiovascular disease ($80 billion) as a leading contributor to total health care costs. The authors further estimated that injuries account for 10 percent of all hospital inpatient expenditures, 46 percent of ED expenditures, and 16 percent of total outpatient and ambulatory care expenditures.

---

[4]Rice and colleagues (1989) estimate lifetime (incidence-based) costs and Miller and colleagues (1995) estimate annual prevalence costs. These are two different approaches, have different purposes, and may not produce similar results.

Although costs derived using the cost-of-illness or human capital approach provide some assessment of the economic impact of fatal and nonfatal injury, it is readily acknowledged that each is inadequate as a measure of the overall burden of injury, largely because they value life and health only in terms of foregone productivity and do not factor in pain, suffering, and reduced quality of life. Further, these estimates yield low values for the retired, the elderly, housewives, and children, since future earnings are typically discounted to present value and no monetary value is allowed for activities outside the marketplace. However, some critics of the human capital method claim that it overestimates true indirect costs because it does not take into account the possibility of substitution among workers when there is relatively high unemployment. These critics contend that indirect costs should be restricted to temporary production losses and to resources expended to recruit and train new employees. A variant on the human capital method—the friction cost method—attempts to account for the substitution of employees, although in practice it is difficult to apply because of a lack of good estimates of the friction period (i.e., time between the occurrence of the injury and the point at which previous production levels are restored; Koopmanshap and Rutten, 1994; van Beeck et al., 1997).

An alternative approach to valuing life and health involves a willingness-to-pay methodology. This method values human life according to the amount individuals are willing to pay (or in some instances actually do pay) for small changes such as reductions or increases in the probability of illness or death. It is a fundamentally different approach to estimating the burden of injury in terms of indirect costs, since it builds on the perspective of society as a population of consumers rather than producers. To derive willingness-to-pay estimates, individual preference values are obtained using one of two approaches. Using the revealed-preference method, a variety of data is used to reveal the trade-offs between dollars and risk of injury that people have actually made. These data have included wage premiums that compensate workers for risky jobs (an estimate of the price of increased risk), court awards for pain and suffering, and data on the actual consumption of goods that reduce the risk of injury (an estimate of the price of reduced risk), such as the costs of smoke detectors and extra safety features on cars (Drummond et al., 1997). The strength of the revealed-preference approach is that it is based on actual behavior; however, requisite data are often difficult to obtain.

An alternative approach to obtaining preferences is referred to as the stated-preference approach. Using this approach, preferences are obtained by asking people directly about their willingness to pay for changes that reduce the probability of death and/or disability (Drummond et al., 1997). The stated-preference approach, although theoretically appealing, is difficult to apply in practice because it assumes that people do indeed have well-formulated preferences about the value of nonmarket goods and, further, that they can articulate these preferences in a rational and consistent manner.

Regardless of the approach used, willingness-to-pay estimates of human costs are considerably higher than estimates of lost productivity obtained using a human capital approach. For example, based on a review of 47 technically sound studies, the willingness to pay to save one life ranges from $1 million to $3.8 million (average $2.3 million), whereas the human capital estimate of foregone productivity per injury death averaged across the age at death is only $334,849 (Rice et al., 1989; Miller, 1990).

The choice of a particular approach for computing the economic costs of injury will, in part, be dictated by the intended use of the derived estimates. The application of all methods discussed above is limited by our lack of understanding of these outcomes. For example, more research is needed to refine methodologies and evaluate the relative utility of alternative approaches, and all require better data on the long-term consequences of injury in terms of treatment needs, reduced productivity, and overall quality of life.

New and exciting approaches are being developed to quantify the burden of disease and injury in noneconomic terms. These methods typically involve the calculation of quality-adjusted life years (QALYs). The QALYs associated with a particular injury are calculated as the average number of years of life remaining after the occurrence of the injury, multiplied by a weight reflecting the quality of life during each of these years (Torrance and Feeny, 1989). The weights used to calculate QALYs should be based on the preferences people have for various health states and are expressed on an interval scale, with optimal health having a value of 1 and death having a value of 0. They have been derived using a variety of different health state classification systems, including the EuroQol (EuroQol Group, 1990), the Health Utilities Index (Feeny et al., 1995), and the Quality of Well-Being Scale (Kaplan and Anderson, 1988). These systems differ in the domains used to define various health states, the specific technique used to estimate preferences, and the fundamental assumptions made about the value of life when deriving estimates. Since substantial discrepancies may arise depending on the method used, it is important that standard approaches be developed (Gold et al., 1996). Extensive research is needed, however, before such a standard can be promulgated. Given the potential utility of QALYs as a composite measure of the burden of injury in noneconomic terms, the committee recommends that priority be given to the development and application of preference-based measures of quality of life that are valid across the broad spectrum by injury types and severities.

To date, there have been few applications of the QALY methodology for measuring the impact of injury (Holbrook et al., 1994; MacKenzie et al., 1996). Of some note, however, is the work recently completed by the World Health Organization in collaboration with the World Bank and Harvard University (Murray and Lopez, 1996), which has developed an internationally standard form of the QALY, referred to as the disability-adjusted life year (DALY). Although questions remain regarding the precise methods used in deriving DALY estimates, the effort represents a milestone in the development of new approaches for measuring the burden of disease in terms other than just the direct costs of mortality. This method results in the estimate that injuries account for 11 percent of the global burden of disease as measured by the number of DALYs experienced by the world's population. In projecting the future global burden of disease, it was found that road traffic injuries alone will rise from ninth place overall as a leading cause of disease burden to third place by the year 2020. Violence, which is currently in nineteenth place as a cause of disease burden is expected to rise to twelfth place and suicide from seventeenth place to fourteenth place (Murray and Lopez, 1996). These projections underscore the importance of injury as a major source of both death and disability now and in the future.

REFERENCES

Blincoe LJ. 1997. *Economic Costs of Motor Vehicle Crashes: 1994.* Washington, DC: National Highway Traffic Safety Administration.

BLS (Bureau of Labor Statistics). 1996. *BLS.* [World Wide Web document]. URL http://www.bls.gov.oshcftab.htm (accessed July 1998).

BLS (Bureau of Labor Statistics). 1997. *News Release: Workplace Injuries and Illnesses in 1995.* Washington, DC: U.S. Department of Labor. USDL 97-76.

CDC (Centers for Disease Control and Prevention). 1998. Fatal occupational injuries, United States, 1980–1994. *Morbidity and Mortality Weekly Report* 47(15):297–302.

Chirikos TN. 1989. Aggregate economic losses from disability in the United States: A preliminary assay. *Milbank Quarterly* 67:59–91.

Drummond MF, O'Brien B, Stoddart GL, Torrance GW. 1997. *Methods for the Economic Evaluation of Health Care Programs*, 2d edition. New York: Oxford University Press.

EuroQol Group. 1990. EuroQol: A new facility for the measurement of health-related quality of life. *Health Policy* 16:199.

Feeny D, Furlong W, Boyle M, Torrance GW. 1995. Multi-attribute health status classification systems: The Health Utilities Index. *PharmacoEconomics* 1:490–502.

Fingerhut LA, Warner M. 1997. *Injury Chartbook. Health, United States, 1996–97.* Hyattsville, MD: National Center for Health Statistics.

Gillum BS, Graves EJ, Wood E. 1998. *NHDS Annual Summary, 1995.* NCHS Vital Health Statistical Series. Hyattsville, MD: National Center for Health Statistics.

Gold MR, Siegel JE, Russell LB, Weinstein MC. 1996. Identifying and valuing outcomes. In: Gold MR, ed. *Cost-Effectiveness in Health and Medicine.* New York: Oxford University Press.

Holbrook TL, Hoyt DB, Anderson JP, Hollingsworth-Fridlund P, Shackford SR. 1994. Functional limitation after major trauma: A more sensitive assessment using the Quality of Well-Being scale. The trauma recovery pilot project. *Journal of Trauma* 36(1):74–78.

IOM (Institute of Medicine). 1998. *Scientific Opportunities and Public Needs: Improving Priority Setting and Public Input at the National Institutes of Health.* Washington, DC: National Academy Press.

Kaplan RM, Anderson JP. 1988. A general health policy model: Update and applications. *Health Service Research* 23:203–235.

Koopmanshap MA, Rutten FF. 1994. The impact of indirect costs on outcomes of health care programs. *Health Economics* 3(6):385–393.

Leigh JP, Markowitz SB, Fahs M, Shin C, Landrigan PJ. 1997. Occupational injury and illness in the United States. Estimates of costs, morbidity, and mortality. *Archives of Internal Medicine* 157(14):1557–1568.

MacKenzie EJ, Damiano A, Luchter S, Miller T. 1996. Development of the functional capacity index. *Journal of Trauma* 41:799–807.

Max W, Rice DP. 1993. Shooting in the dark: Estimating the cost of firearm injuries. *Health Affairs* 12(4):171–185.

Miller TR. 1990. The plausible range of the value of life: Red herrings among the mackerel. *Journal of Forensic Economics* 3(3):17–40.

Miller TR, Lestina DC, Galbraith MS, Viano DC. 1994. Medical-care spending, United States. *Morbidity and Mortality Weekly Report* 43(32):581–586.

Miller TR, Pindus NM, Douglass JB, Rossman SB. 1995. *Databook on Nonfatal Injury: Incidence, Costs and Consequences*. Washington, DC: Urban Institute Press.

Murray CJL, Lopez AD, eds. 1996. *The Global Burden of Disease*. Geneva: World Health Organization.

NCHS (National Center for Health Statistics). 1998. *Health, United States, 1998 with Socioeconomic Status and Health Chartbook*. Hyattsville, MD: NCHS. DHHS Publication No. (PHS) 98-1232.

NCIPC (National Center for Injury Prevention and Control). 1998. *Ten Leading Causes of Death by Age Group, 1995*. [World Wide Web Document]. URL http://www.cdc.gov/ncipc/images/10lc95.gif (accessed October 1998).

NHTSA (National Highway Traffic Safety Administration). 1998. *The Effect of Increased Speed Limits in the Post-NMSL Era*. Report to Congress. Washington, DC: Department of Transportation.

NIOSH (National Institute for Occupational Safety and Health). 1996. *National Occupational Research Agenda*. Washington, DC: NIOSH. DHHS (NIOSH) Publication No. 96-115.

NSC (National Safety Council). 1997. *Accident Facts*. Itasca, IL: National Safety Council.

Peters KD, Kochanek KD, Murphy SL. 1998. Deaths: Final data for 1996. *National Vital Statistics Reports* 47. Hyattsville, MD: National Center for Health Statistics.

Rice DP, MacKenzie EJ, Jones AS, Kaufman SR, deLissovoy GV, Max W, McLoughlin E, Miller TR, Robertson LS, Salkever DS, Smith GS. 1989. *Cost of Injury in the United States*. San Francisco, CA: Institute for Health and Aging, University of California and Injury Prevention Center, The Johns Hopkins University.

Torrance GW, Feeny D. 1989. Utilities and quality adjusted life years. *International Journal of Technology Assessment in Health Care* 5:559–575.

van Beeck EF, van Roijen L, Mackenbach JP. 1997. Medical costs and economic production losses due to injuries in the Netherlands. *Journal of Trauma* 42(6):1116–1123.

Ventura SJ, Anderson RN, Martin JA, Smith BL. 1998. Births and deaths: United States, preliminary data for 1997. *National Vital Statistics Reports* 47. Hyattsville, MD: National Center for Health Statistics.

3

Surveillance and Data

Surveillance may be defined as the systematic and ongoing collection of data. Surveillance serves at least four practical uses. First, surveillance describes the magnitude of a given type of injury relative to other types of injuries in the general population or in special populations. Thus, surveillance data may direct the priorities for injury research to the areas in greatest need of attention. Second, surveillance is used to monitor trends in specific areas of injury. Surveillance data may be analyzed to determine whether specific injury morbidity and mortality measures have increased, decreased, or remained stable over time. Surveillance systems are the primary means by which injury researchers and practitioners identify changes in the magnitude of a specific injury problem (see Fingerhut and Warner, 1997). Third, surveillance is used to identify new injury problems. Surveillance systems provide a means to identify injury risks that have been inadvertently created by the introduction of a new product or by a change in an existing product or process. For example, surveillance and follow-up investigations were instrumental in identifying the occupational hazards associated with skylights. The skylight itself was not dangerous; however, repair and installation presented a hazard because workers fell through the skylights and the openings cut in the roof for the skylight (NIOSH, 1989).

Fourth, surveillance is used as one way to evaluate injury prevention or intervention efforts. These can have differing outcomes: (1) a reduction in the incidence or severity of the target injury without resulting in an unintended adverse outcome; (2) a reduction in the incidence or severity of the target injury, but also resulting in an unintended adverse outcome; (3) little or no effect on the target injury and no unintended outcomes (other than the cost of implementation); or (4) little or no effect on the target injury, but an unintended adverse outcome. Two examples of the utility of surveillance data follow.

60

• Surveillance data played a critical role in the design and evaluation of a successful intervention to reduce burns and fatalities in residential fires in Oklahoma City. The city's surveillance system was used in designing the intervention, which consisted of providing homes with smoke detectors in neighborhoods with elevated rates of fires and then evaluating the intervention. Continued surveillance confirmed that the smoke detector program reduced the fire injury rate by 74 percent in areas targeted by the intervention, as compared with a small increase in the rest of the city. Additional information collected about each house and its occupants did not suggest any unexpected or undesirable outcomes as the result of the intervention (Mallonee et al., 1996).

• The mechanisms of airbag-associated deaths were elucidated through the Special Crash Investigation (SCI) program at the National Highway Traffic Safety Administration (NHTSA) (Winston and Reed, 1996). Through a voluntary national reporting network, the SCI program identified unusual crash circumstances in which minor- to moderate-severity collisions resulted in airbag-associated deaths. In-depth crash investigations were conducted in a timely manner across the United States, and the information was used by the automotive safety community to improve the performance of state-of-the-art safety systems. At the same time that data were collected regarding the role of airbags in fatal crashes, surveillance systems in trauma centers for the study of nonfatal injuries identified another unexpected outcome of the airbag intervention (Loo et al., 1996). In severe frontal crashes the occupants would survive but would sustain severe injuries to the lower feet, ankles, and lower legs. Although these types of injuries had always been present, they were of little consequence because the occupants usually died without the added protection of airbags.[1]

Surveillance data are needed at the national, state, and local (community) levels. National data are critical for drawing attention to the magnitude of an injury problem, for monitoring the impact of federal legislation, and for examining variations in injury rates by region of the country and by rural versus urban or suburban environments. They are also useful in aggregating sufficient numbers of rare cases of a particular type of injury to identify patterns of injury and mechanisms. State and local data better reflect injury problems in specific communities and are therefore more useful in setting program priorities and evaluating the impact of local policies and expenditures. Therefore, local data are usually needed to advocate effectively for the establishment of an injury-related policy or program at the local level.

As discussed in this chapter, significant strides over the past decade have greatly enhanced our understanding of the magnitude and impact of injury as a

---

[1] Despite these complications, analyses of surveillance data suggest that airbags reduce the risk of dying in a direct frontal crash by about 30 percent and had saved over 2,600 lives through November 1, 1997 (NHTSA, 1998a).

major public health problem (also see Chapter 2). As the availability, accessibility, and quality of the data have improved, they have played an increasingly important role in the development and evaluation of interventions at national, state, and local levels. However, significant impediments to effective injury surveillance remain, notably the high costs of development and maintenance of surveillance systems. Therefore, priority attention should be given to the improvement or expansion of existing data systems and to the development of efficient strategies for linking data across systems to gather additional and more complex information. Additionally, surveillance systems are dependent upon the quality of coded data. This chapter briefly discusses coding issues, and describes national, state, and local sources of injury data and points to areas where improvement is necessary.

CODING ISSUES

The World Health Organization's (WHO) International Classification of Diseases (ICD) is the most widely used system for coding and classifying the nature and external causes of injury (WHO, 1975). Originally developed in the late 1800s, the ICD is now in its tenth revision. Coding of U.S. mortality data will shift from ICD-9 to ICD-10 starting in 1999. To enhance the use of the ICD for coding nonfatal injury, the National Center for Health Statistics (NCHS) developed a clinical modification (CM) of the ninth revision of the ICD (ICD-9CM) that is the most commonly used classification system for morbidity reporting throughout the United States (U.S. DHHS, 1997). Work is currently under way to develop the clinical modification of ICD-10; its implementation is not expected until the year 2001. Use of the tenth revision of ICD and ICD-10CM will require major adjustments in the way nosologists and researchers approach data collection and analyses. In introducing ICD-10 and its clinical modification, it will be important to ensure that users are adequately trained to take full advantage of its added flexibility and specificity.

Coding the Nature of the Injury

The ICD-9 diagnostic codes characterize the nature of injury (e.g., open wounds and lacerations, fractures, sprains and strains, burns) as well as the affected region of the body. These codes are fewer in number than the codes in the ICD-9CM and historically have not been updated between revisions of the ICD. Consideration is being given for an updating process for ICD-10. For mortality, the nature of injury is considered to be a contributing rather than the underlying cause of death, which, by definition, is the external cause of the injury. Thus, to know the nature of the injuries contributing to the death, a researcher must have access to the multiple cause-of-death data tapes. At this time, routine data on contributing causes of injury death are not published.

For morbidity, the clinical modification of the ICD-10, currently under development, should improve its specificity regarding the extent and severity of the injury. These codes are widely used by health care providers throughout the United States, and are included in most administrative databases and registries. However, there has been little guidance from the injury field as to their optimal use in surveillance and research. The International Collaborative Effort for Injury Statistics (ICE) is currently developing recommendations for presenting injury morbidity data using the ICD nature-of-injury codes (L. Fingerhut, NCHS, personal communication, 1998).

Coding the Causes of Injury

The ICD-9 Supplementary Classification of External Causes of Injury and Poisoning (E codes) summarizes the circumstances causing the injury, including the intent (intentional and unintentional) and mechanism (e.g., falls, motor vehicle crashes, firearms) of the injury. For mortality data, coding guidelines indicate the use of an external cause-of-injury code as the underlying cause of death when the morbid condition is classifiable to an injury diagnosis.

For morbidity data, the 1990s have witnessed major advances in coding because of the increasing availability of external cause-of-injury codes in health systems data. In 1991, the National Committee on Vital and Health Statistics issued a series of recommendations regarding the use of E-codes. These included a recommendation that "whenever an injury is the principal diagnosis or directly related to the principal diagnosis for a hospitalized patient, there should be an external cause of injury recorded in the medical record" (NCHS, 1991).

Since 1992, the Emergency Department Component of the National Hospital Ambulatory Medical Care Survey (NHAMCS) has routinely included E-codes (Burt and Fingerhut, 1998). The National Ambulatory Medical Care Survey (NAMCS) added E-codes in 1995 and the format of the redesigned National Health Interview Survey (NHIS) in 1997 will facilitate the data being E-coded. Currently, 23 states have mandated that E-codes be included in their hospital discharge data systems; 9 states have mandated E-coding of all emergency department encounters (Annest et al., 1998). A new framework for presenting E-coded injury data promises to expedite comparisons of injury profiles across populations and regions (CDC, 1997).

Despite its usefulness for the general categorization of injuries by mechanism and intent, significant limitations of the ICD-9 E-code classification have been noted (Fingerhut and Cox, 1998; Smith and Langley, 1998). In response, the tenth revision of the ICD has made some notable improvements, including the addition of requisite codes for place of occurrence and activity in which the person was involved when injured. The addition of those codes should facilitate the identification of occupational-, residential-, and recreational-related injuries. Currently, further efforts are under way by the WHO Working Group on Injury Surveillance Methodology to develop a more detailed classification of external causes that would be compatible with the ICD classification. A draft of the International Classification for External Causes of Injuries (ICECI) was released for comment at the fourth World Conference on Injury Prevention and Control in 1998. Field testing of the system will begin later in the year. The committee endorses this development and suggests broad-based field testing of the ICECI, recognizing, however, that its success will depend largely on its compatibility with the ICD.

The effectiveness of external cause coding will be greatly enhanced by two additions to data bases: separate fields and free text. Without separate fields on discharge records, external cause codes may be dropped in preference to coding diagnoses, comorbidities, and complications. Allowance should be made for recording multiple codes, as a single code may be inadequate for describing the cause of injury. Free text, electronically accessible to searching, permits a fuller understanding of the circumstances surrounding an injury and can help identify specific injuries missed by conventional coding (Smith and Langley, 1998).

The committee recommends that a high priority be directed at ensuring uniform and reliable coding of both the external cause and the nature of the injury using the ICD on all health systems data, particularly on hospital and emergency department discharge records. Special efforts should be directed at training to ensure optimal use of the tenth revision of the ICD.

EXISTING DATA SOURCES

There are numerous national, state, and local surveillance systems. They vary in scope and in the extent to which they provide information on mechanism and intent, nature and severity, risk factors, health services use and costs, and health outcomes. A brief review of federal (national), state, and local data systems is presented below.

National Data Sources

There are 31 federally funded national data systems that collect data on injury mortality, morbidity, and risk factors (Annest et al., 1996). A summary of these data sources is included in Table 3.1. Eight of the systems provide data on work-related injuries. Approximately one-half are ongoing surveillance systems; the remainder are periodic surveys. Many of the systems report information on the location of injury occurrence, the external cause, and the nature of the injury.

Counts of all fatalities in the United States are available from vital statistics, although these data are often limited in the information they provide about the exact nature and circumstances of the injury. The National Vital Statistics System is used to describe the epidemiology of injury mortality. While most NCHS data systems are sample based, the National Vital Statistics System is universal in its coverage. For injury-related deaths, the U.S. Standard Certificate of Death has a number of items including the date and time of injury, whether the injury occurred at work, a description of how the injury occurred, the place of the injury, and the actual street location. Clearly, the death certificate is a potentially rich source of statistical information on injuries and could be made more useful by including directives about the acceptable level of detail when describing an injury-related death and by including additional information. For example, questions about the role of drug and alcohol involvement in a death due to injury and, in the case of motor vehicle crashes, specific questions about whether the decedent was a passenger or the driver and the type of vehicle involved. Directives about what information to provide might reduce the current limitation in the vital statistics, particularly with regard to motor vehicle injuries (Robertson, 1998). Specifically, there is a 38 percent underestimation of fatal injuries associated with motorcycle crashes when death certificates rather than police reports are used as the source of data (Lapidus et al., 1994). More detailed information about the nature and cause of death is generally available from a medical examiner's or coroner's investigation and report (see discussion later in chapter).

Uniform data on injuries resulting in hospitalization can be obtained from both the National Hospital Discharge Survey (NHDS) and the Health Care and Utilization Project (Version 3) (HCUP-3). HCUP-3 provides detailed information about the nature of injuries, treatment, and discharge disposition; however, both HCUP-3 and NHDS are limited in that not all states require external cause-of-injury coding on hospital discharge records. In 1994, only about half of the medical records for which an injury was the principal diagnosis had an accompanying E-code. This proportion has increased remarkably to 64 percent in 1996 as the number of states mandating external cause coding has increased. Although procedures exist for estimating distributions by mechanism and intent, given incomplete data, the lack of universal external cause coding of hospital discharges remains a significant impediment to the optimal use of these databases for studying the epidemiology of injury.

National data on nonfatal injuries resulting in a visit to an outpatient setting (e.g., emergency department, clinic, physician office) are available from the National Ambulatory Medical Care Survey (NAMCS), and more recently, the National Hospital Ambulatory Medical Care Survey (NHAMCS). Both the NAMCS and the NHAMCS consist of data abstracted from injury-related visits to hospital emergency departments, hospital outpatient departments, and/or physician offices, whereas the National Health Interview Survey (NHIS) relies on self-reports of injury events. National data on injuries that require medical atten-

TABLE 3.1 U.S. Federal Data Systems for Injury Surveillance, Research, and Prevention Activities

Data System	Federal Agency	Description
Census of Fatal Occupational Injuries (CFOI)	BLS	Compiles a count of work-related injury fatalities using multiple cross-referenced data sources.
Survey of Occupational Injuries and Illnesses (SOII)	BLS	Provides national and state data on work-related injuries and illnesses as reported by a sample of employers via an annual mail-out survey.
National Crime Victimization Survey (NCVS)	BJS	Measures the number, nature, and characteristics of specific types of crime and victims of crime. A sample of households is screened for victimization and then interviewed.
National Ambulatory Medical Care Survey (NAMCS)	NCHS	Collects data on visits by patients to nonfederal office-based physicians. Samples of surveys completed by a physician or staff are collected regarding patient visits and ambulatory care during a randomly assigned 7-day period per year.
National Hospital Ambulatory Medical Care Survey (NHAMCS)	NCHS	Collects data on visits to U.S. short-stay hospital emergency and outpatient departments from a set of primary sampling units.
National Hospital Discharge Survey (NHDS)	NCHS	Measures inpatient care and hospital utilization by data collected from NCHS or manually collected.
National Health Interview Survey (NHIS)	NCHS	Annual household interviews are conducted to measure the health status of the noninstitutionalized population. Supplemental questionnaires focus on specific health issues (HIV/AIDS, disability, etc.).
National Mortality Followback Survey—1993 (NMFS93)	NCHS	Data from personal interviews or medical records are used to examine socioeconomic differentials in mortality. Aims to evaluate risk factors, prevention, and effect of health care for individuals in their last year of life.

System	Agency	Description
National Vital Statistics System—Current Mortality Sample (NVSSS)	NCHS	Collects mortality data monthly on cause of death, race, age, location, and date from a sample of death certificates filed at state vital statistics offices.
National Vital Statistics System—Final Mortality Data (NVSSF)	NCHS	Compiles demographic and causal data on all death certificates filed in the United States.
Behavioral Risk Factor Surveillance System (BRFSS)	CDC	Monthly household phone surveys on behavioral risk factors are conducted and analyzed for reference when evaluating current and prospective public health programs.
Youth Risk Behavior Surveillance System (YRBSS)	CDC	School-based surveys are conducted every two years to monitor risk behaviors for pupils in grades 9–12 regarding causes of morbidity and mortality.
National Traumatic Occupational Fatality Surveillance System (NTOF)	NIOSH	Census of occupational injury death data for all workers in the United States.
National Electronic Injury Surveillance System (NEISS)	CPSC	Data regarding injuries associated with consumer products or recreational activities are collected from a sample of hospital emergency departments.
Law Enforcement Officers Killed and Assaulted (LEOKA)	FBI	Data from the FBI Uniform Crime Reporting (UCR) System is compiled to monitor law enforcement officer deaths and assaults.
National Incident Based Reporting System (NIBRS)	FBI	Compiles data from all crimes and arrests through the Uniform Crime Reporting System for use by law enforcement, legislators, criminologists, and the public.

Continued

TABLE 3.1 *Continued*

Data System	Federal Agency	Description
Nationwide Personal Transportation Survey (NPTS)	FHWA	Phone surveys are conducted to determine the amount of household travel within a year.
Health Care Financing (HCFA) Administration 5% Sample Standard Analysis File (SAF) and Medicare Provider Analysis and Review (MEDPAR) File	HCFA	Automated Medicare claims are gathered to provide Medicare claims data files for administrative and research purposes.
Indian Health Service—Ambulatory Care System (IHSACS)	IHS	Data from the IHS and tribally operated hospitals are compiled to reflect the ambulatory care issued to Native Americans by the IHS.
Indian Health Service—Inpatient Care System (IHSICS)	IHS	Data from the IHS and tribally operated hospitals are compiled to reflect the direct inpatient care provided to Native Americans by the IHS.
National Child Abuse and Neglect Data System (NCANDS)	DHHS	Data from automated state child abuse registries or the automated state child welfare social services information systems are compiled, analyzed, and made available as state child abuse and neglect reporting information.
National Incidence Study of Child Abuse and Neglect (NIS)	DHHS	Child protective services (CPS) agencies and non-CPS professionals submit data aimed at estimating the number of abused children and monitor changes.
Fatality Analysis Reporting System (FARS)	NHTSA	Details on motor vehicle crashes involving a fatality are collected within 30 days to provide a general measure of highway safety and problems.
National Automotive Sampling System—Crashworthiness Data System (NASSCDS)	NHTSA	Collects statistical data on motor-vehicle-related crashes, including police reports, medical records, physical evidence, and interviews.

National Automotive Sampling System—General Estimates System (NASSGES)	NHTSA	Samples from police department traffic crash reports are coded and used to estimate national characteristics of police-reported motor vehicle crashes.
National Occupant Protection Use Survey (NOPUS)	NHTSA	A sample of direct observations from observers is used to evaluate passenger vehicle occupant shoulder-belt use, motorcycle helmet use, and child occupant restraint use.
Monitoring the Future Study (MTFS)	NIDA	Surveys in schools are issued to assess the attitudes of youth in grades 8, 10, and 12 regarding drugs, alcohol, tobacco, and their relation to motor vehicle accidents, delinquency, and victimization.
Drug Abuse Warning Network (DAWN)	SAMHSA	Emergency department and medical examiner records regarding drug misuse are compiled in annual reports indicating the scope of substance abuse problems.
Census of Agriculture—1992 (BCCOA)	Bureau of the Census	Questionnaires are sent to all farm operators to gather data on injuries or deaths connected with farm or ranch work in 1992.
National Fire Incident Reporting System (NFIRS)	NFA	Local fire departments voluntarily report fire incidents and civilian and fire service casualties.
Health Care Cost and Utilization Project (HCUP)	DHHS	Compiles data from a sample of more than 900 hospitals regarding inpatient stays; detailing use and cost of medical services so as to better facilitate health services research and policy analysis nationwide.

NOTE: BJS = Bureau of Justice Statistics; BLS = Bureau of Labor Statistics; CDC = Centers for Disease Control and Prevention; CPSC = Consumer Product Safety Commission; DHHS = Department of Health and Human Services; FBI = Federal Bureau of Investigation; FHWA = Federal Highway Administration; HCFA = Health Care Financing Administration; IHS = Indian Health Service; NCHS = National Center for Health Statistics; NFA = National Fire Administration; NHTSA = National Highway Traffic Safety Administration; NIDA = National Institute on Drug Abuse; NIOSH = National Institute for Occupational Safety and Health; SAMHSA = Substance Abuse and Mental Health Services Administration. SOURCES: Annest et al. (1996); AHCPR (1998).

tion or restricted activity are available from the NHIS. Historically, however, the NHIS has not been a rich source of data on cause of injury because of the lack of detailed information on the mechanism and circumstances of the injury. Beginning in 1997, the core questions of NHIS were redesigned and an entire section on injury was added, including the narrative text of how the injury occurred. Additionally, the definition of injury was changed to include only those injuries that resulted in medical attention (either in person or via telephone). Data have yet to be released from these new questions, although they hold promise for enhancing our understanding of minor injuries. One of the advantages of the NHIS is the ability to link injury data with other kinds of health, social, and demographic information. Routine ICD external cause-of-injury coding on these health systems surveys now permit researchers to make national estimates of health care utilization for less severe injuries according to external cause of injury.

An important source of information on product-related injuries is the National Electronic Injury Surveillance System (NEISS) maintained for 25 years by the Consumer Product Safety Commission (CPSC). NEISS obtains statistical information through surveillance of 101 hospital emergency departments and through follow-up studies. Information collected from the NEISS database includes age and gender of the patient, nature of the injury, body part affected, disposition of the patient, product involved, and location of the incident. Also, the address and phone number of the injured person are included, permitting limited follow-up investigations about the nature and cause of the injury. CPSC uses the data for a variety of purposes, including national incidence estimates, priority setting, development and evaluation of product standards, and the identification of products to be banned or recalled. Although there are limitations to NEISS, from CPSC's perspective it provides the data necessary to carry out its mission.

Limitations of NEISS, as it is currently configured, include inadequate sampling of hospitals, because the current sampling system is so limited that the data cannot be used for state or even regional estimates; the lack of sufficient detail regarding the nature of the injury (ICD diagnostic codes are not incorporated); and the paucity of detailed data on circumstances surrounding the product's involvement (GAO, 1997). Despite these limitations, NEISS serves as one model for surveillance of injuries that do not necessarily result in death or hospitalization. For these reasons, the National Center for Injury Prevention and Control (NCIPC) recently collaborated with the CPSC in a pilot study to assess the feasibility of expanding NEISS to an all-injury data system. NEISS was expected to capture all causes and types of injuries treated in hospital emergency departments. Preliminary findings from the pilot study are encouraging. NEISS coders recorded about 80 percent of injury-related cases identified by an independent review of a representative sample of emergency department records from 6 of the 21 pilot hospitals. Additionally, about one-half of the 26 million trauma cases treated in emergency departments involved products under the jurisdiction of the CPSC. Other kinds of injury were also included, classified as due to automobiles (13 percent); work related (13 percent); intentional injuries, including firearms (6 percent); food and drugs (1 percent); and other (18 percent) (CPSC, personal communication, 1998).

National estimates of the number of injury-related emergency department visits, based on the pilot study, are comparable to those reported from other databases such as the NHAMCS. However, there has been some evidence to suggest that the sensitivity of case identification was somewhat lower for intentional injuries as opposed to unintentional injuries. This discrepancy needs to be addressed.

Based on the promising results of this pilot and discussions with staff at both the NCIPC and the CPSC, the committee recommends an expansion of NEISS data collection to include all injuries treated in emergency departments to increase knowledge of the causes and severity of nonfatal injuries. Furthermore, an expanded NEISS could greatly benefit the injury field because it would provide a new and important tool for gathering national estimates and monitoring national trends in injury morbidity, for identifying emerging problems, for evaluating interventions through follow-up studies, and for providing data for policy decisions. If NEISS is expanded to collect all injury data, the committee believes that the system should remain at CPSC since the system is vital to its mission. Additionally, this expansion will be more cost-effective if it remains at CPSC because the agency has already developed the hospital sampling frame, contracted with hospitals, established relationships with hospital personnel, trained hospital coders, and developed procedures for collecting data and for quality assurance. Thus, the work and cost of expanding the current system to all causes of injury would be minimized if CPSC continues to develop the NEISS.

The committee recommends that CPSC expand its NEISS system to gather nationally representative data on all injuries treated in emergency departments to increase knowledge of the causes and severity of nonfatal injuries.

To ensure the success of an expanded NEISS, the CPSC should convene a steering committee (with representation from CPSC, NCIPC, the Department of Justice, and other relevant federal and state agencies) to set policies and procedures for the expanded NEISS and its uses. Additionally, a comprehensive evaluation of the system's cost-effectiveness should be performed, by an independent body, to determine the utility and future of the effort. The committee stresses the need to ensure that the sampling frame is adequate for intentional injuries. Additionally, training sessions for hospital personnel and onsite NEISS coders will be important, not only in improving the information gathered related to the history of the injury, but also in identifying injuries related to violence since case identification appears to be lower for this type of injury. Finally, an independent evaluation of the expanded system should be conducted annually or biennially, to determine its utility to the field and its ultimate future.

In addition to NEISS, there exist several other sources of national data specific to a particular injury mechanism or intent. Examples include the Fatality Analysis Reporting System (FARS) and the National Automotive Sampling System (NASS) for motor vehicle-related injuries; the National Traumatic Occupational Fatality Surveillance System (NTOF), the Census of Fatal Occupational Injuries (CFOI), and the Survey of Occupational Injuries and Illnesses (SOII) for occupational injuries; the National Crime Victimization Survey (NCVS) and the Uniform Crime Reporting (UCR) System for intentional injuries associated with criminal conduct. These data systems are particularly useful for monitoring trends in injury rates specific to certain mechanisms and for identifying risk factors associated with their occurrence. This information, in turn, has been useful in setting national priorities for research and program implementation and in developing and evaluating national policies. For example, data from FARS was able to document the benefits of legislation that raised the minimum purchase age for alcoholic beverages (Chapter 5).

The committee considered the merits and feasibility of establishing a comprehensive fatal injury surveillance system that would collect detailed data on all fatal injuries not currently included in existing fatality surveillance systems and that would be coordinated with existing systems. However, the magnitude of that task would be enormous, given the approximately 140,000 injury deaths each year, of which approximately 42,000 are entered into the FARS database (NHTSA, 1998b) and approximately 6,200 are occupational fatalities (BLS, 1996). Therefore, the committee considered ways to accomplish that goal incrementally by identifying a subset of deaths (e.g., homicides and suicides).

The committee noted that an ongoing federally sponsored system of surveillance for all intentional injuries (homicides and suicides) is conspicuously absent from the array of data systems available on a national level. While the UCR System, maintained by the FBI, does provide some information on homicides, detailed information about the type of weapon involved is missing. Since the UCR is a voluntary reporting system, it tends to underestimate the actual incidence of homicide (as compared with the record of vital statistics). Moreover, suicides (which outnumber homicides) and unintentional firearm injury deaths are not included in the database.

Given the success of FARS, in monitoring motor vehicle fatalities, and the utility of occupational surveillance systems (e.g., CFOI), it seems reasonable to consider a system for recording detailed data on injury deaths that are ordinarily the subject of police investigations, such as suspected homicides and suicides. However, suicide is not a crime in all jurisdictions, and police do not necessarily investigate deaths that are clearly self-inflicted. Therefore, a system depending on police reports for case identification could miss a large proportion of the 31,000 suicides annually.

Injury researchers and practitioners have suggested the development of a firearm surveillance system (Teret et al., 1992). Firearms are the second leading mechanism, after motor vehicles, of injury deaths; better data on firearm deaths would be helpful in regulating firearm commerce and use. However, limiting a new system to firearms seem unnecessarily restrictive and would preclude a number of useful investigations involving other mechanisms on which surveillance data should be collected. It would also appear limiting because the same sources of information that would be tapped for a firearm surveillance system could provide information on homicides and suicides committed by other means, and they may all be amenable to appropriate and specific prevention interventions. Furthermore, a firearm-only system would preclude investigations into weapon substitution in homicides and suicides and provide an unrepresentative sample for investigations of crosscutting issues such as alcohol and other drug abuse.

In addition to police reports, medical examiner's and coroner's investigations and reports are another source of data about the nature and cause of death. The medical examiner and coroner systems vary among jurisdictions (whether state, county, district, or city). A medical examiner is usually a licensed physician, whereas a coroner need not be a physician and is often an elected official. A medical examiner system exists in 22 states, a coroner system exits in 11 states, and a "mixed" medical examiner–coroner system exists in 18 states (Combs et al., 1995).

Since the judgment of the medical examiner or coroner ultimately determines whether a death is a homicide, a suicide or an "accident" according to vital statistics, this system could be considered a potential starting point for a fatal intentional injury surveillance system. Medical examiner's and coroner's reports are particularly valuable when they include a full autopsy with blood screens for drugs and alcohol, and information from police reports and forensic scene investigation. However, the completeness of reports varies widely from jurisdiction to jurisdiction, as does the extent to which data are maintained in a centralized data system. Local funding for the medical examiner generally determines the degree of completeness and number of autopsies performed. In 1987, the CDC's National Center for Environmental Health (NCEH) established the Medical Examiner and Coroner Information Sharing Program, to improve the quality of data on death certificates and to increase the availability of those data for scientific research (NCEH, 1998).

The committee recommends the development of a fatal intentional injury surveillance system, modeled after FARS, for all homicides and suicides. The committee urges the CDC (specifically NCIPC, NCHS, and NCEH) in collaboration with the National Institute of Justice (NIJ) and NHTSA to conduct a feasibility study for estab-

lishing such a system as an extension of the medical examiner and coroner systems.

The study should examine the medical examiner and coroner system for ways to standardize, computerize, and centralize data; examine policies and practices of police investigations of both homicides and suicides to maximize the collection of pertinent data; and make realistic estimates of the costs in time and money to establish such a system.

The development of a fatal intentional injury surveillance system based on the medical examiner and coroner systems would have to address the variability in the completeness, quality, and reporting of death investigations and concerns about the underreporting of certain types of injury deaths in medical examiner reports (Dijkhuis et al., 1994). It would have to develop a centralized data system that would collect all the pertinent information on homicide and suicide cases from the medical examiner's and coroner's reports, information that often remains only in hard-copy form in the medical examiner's or coroner's office.

In an effort to develop as complete a picture as possible of each such event, the proposed system should, at a minimum, include information about (1) the time and place of the incident and of the actual death; (2) characteristics of the injury or wound; (3) characteristics of the victim and, if relevant, the perpetrator(s) and the relationship of the victim to the perpetrator; (4) the motivation and circumstances related to the death; (5) detailed characteristics of the mechanism or weapon; (6) key circumstances related to the death, including the possible role of alcohol and drugs; and (7) details on the location of the injury. Clearly, since much of this information will be supplied to the medical examiner or coroner by the police departments, it is essential that various offices within the Department of Justice and the NIJ participate fully in the development of this system. Unique challenges will be presented in the collection of data for this system, compared to the collection of data about motor vehicle crashes, because some of the desired information, particularly about the perpetrator, motivations, and weapons may not be known in every case.

The committee believes that the development of a fatal intentional injury surveillance system is essential for a nationwide effort in reducing fatal intentional injuries. It will identify common mechanisms and situations resulting in such deaths and will enable researchers to develop preventive interventions. Additionally, it will be a positive step in strengthening the medical examiner and coroner systems, which could ultimately lead to the goal of a comprehensive fatal injury surveillance system.

State and Local Sources of Injury Data

Although national data are useful in monitoring nationwide trends and evaluating national policies, they are often insufficient for identifying injury patterns or evaluating programs and policies specific to local areas. Indeed, all surveillance systems used to evaluate interventions must be relevant to the scope of the intervention in terms of the geography and the population involved. If the intervention is federally mandated (e.g., a driver's side airbag), then a national-level injury surveillance system is appropriate. If, however, an injury problem and its associated risk factors are initially identified by national-level surveillance but the intervention is conducted locally, then state and local data systems are needed to determine the effectiveness of an intervention. Use of local surveillance data, for instance, played a critical role in the design and evaluation of the intervention to reduce burns and fatalities from residential house fires in Oklahoma City (Mallonee et al., 1996). The type and availability of state and local data vary substantially by area and locale.

Vital statistics data are available for all injury-related deaths. As discussed above, however, these data are limited in the information they provide about the nature and circumstances of the injury and risk factors associated with the death, and potentially helpful medical examiner and coroner reports vary in their completeness and quality.

A potentially powerful source of data for states and local communities in identifying injury risks and priorities for prevention is routine review of selected deaths by multiagency teams of experts, generally referred to as death review teams. Multiagency review of unexplained deaths among children began in Los Angeles County in 1978. In the mid-1980s, in response to the increasing awareness of severe violence against children in the United States, more teams began to emerge across the country. By June 1997, there were multiagency state and/or local teams in every state and the District of Columbia.

A challenge facing many death review teams is the management of the data collected during review sessions, which are essential for establishing prevention goals and for future evaluation of the initiative. The Center on Children and the Law of the American Bar Association has provided leadership in developing guidelines and training modules for child death review teams. These guidelines should be reviewed as a possible basis for establishing similar programs for reviewing deaths other than those of children. Surveillance systems could be supplemented with the detailed data gathered from child death review teams and similar death review teams.

State and local data on injury hospitalizations are generally available from two principal sources: trauma registries and uniform hospital discharge data. The scope and quality of hospital-based trauma registries have improved significantly over the past several years, and nearly one-half of all states now maintain such registries on a statewide basis (Shapiro et al., 1994; Rutledge, 1995). They provide detailed information about the nature and severity of the injury, its treatment, and the status of the patient on discharge from the hospital. Although basic information about the cause of the injury is always included, most registries do not collect detailed information about the event or the circumstances surrounding the event. Although inclusion criteria vary from hospital to hospital and from state to state, most registries include only "major" trauma patients and generally exclude patients who survive and stay in the hospital less than three days. Further, some trauma registries do not include drowning, poisoning, and/or suffocation. Typically, however, deaths are included regardless of whether they occur in the emergency department or after admission to the hospital. Most statewide registries collect data only from trauma centers. The American College of Surgeons has developed a minimum data set recommended for use by all trauma centers in developing their registries. Efforts are also under way to establish a National Trauma Data Bank (NTDB) that will collate data from trauma centers and trauma systems across the country (G. Strauch, American College of Surgeons, personal communication, 1998). When fully operational, the NTDB, will be a valuable resource to injury researchers. In general, trauma registries can provide useful information, especially for continuous quality improvement initiatives and clinical research (Rutledge, 1995). However, it is important to remember that not all are population based, and some typically exclude data on "nonmajor" trauma and on trauma not treated at trauma centers; thus they are not as useful for evaluating the epidemiology of trauma or trauma systems evaluation (see Chapter 6). Perhaps the most limiting characteristic of most trauma registries is the lack of information about outcomes other than hospital morbidity and mortality. However, if registry data are kept for several years, over time, outcomes could be examined.

A recurrent theme of this report is that priority should be directed to the development of better information on the epidemiology, treatment, and outcomes of nonfatal injuries. As more lives are saved due to more effective prevention and regionalization of care, attention is shifting from a singular focus on survival as the criterion of success, to a detailed consideration of nonfatal outcomes as well. Extending the current concept of a trauma registry to include information on longer-term and nonfatal outcomes provides an excellent opportunity to begin developing this information for trauma patients. Considerable effort has been focused, over the past several years, on developing shorter, less time-consuming instruments to gather the necessary data. It will be important to evaluate these newer instruments for their sensitivity and responsiveness to a broad range of trauma patients. Further, effective and efficient systems for tracking patients are needed so that, at specified times following an injury, an assessment of outcomes can be made for patients who received or did not receive acute care. Guidelines for developing and maintaining these registries are critical and should include recommendations regarding specific outcome measures, supplementary data needed to interpret outcomes, methods for routinely tracking and assessing patients, the optimal timing of assessments, and approaches for summarizing and using data on outcomes. Information on long-term outcomes has to be uniformly collected. Attention to issues of data quality, privacy, and confidentiality must be carefully addressed.

The committee strongly urges extending the use of established trauma registries to monitor outcomes following injury. A consensus panel should be convened to develop the guidelines for collecting information on outcomes. The consensus panel, at a minimum, should include NCIPC and the Health Resources and Services Administration, in collaboration with the American College of Surgeons' Committee on Trauma, the American Academy of Physical Medicine and Rehabilitation, and the State and Territorial Injury Prevention Directors' Association (see Chapter 6).

Uniform hospital discharge data, currently maintained by 39 states (Annest et al., 1998), are another source of information about injuries resulting in hospitalization, and are most informative when external cause coding is appended to every discharge record. Hospital discharge data systems are particularly well suited for examining the epidemiology of injury-related hospitalizations and for system evaluation, because they maintain information on all hospitalizations regardless of where the patient is treated. Increasingly, they are being used to evaluate the performance of inclusive trauma systems (MacKenzie et al., 1990a; Mullins et al., 1994) and to examine the epidemiology of injury. However, to use these data to estimate the true incidence of injury resulting in hospitalization, one must avoid double counting those patients transferred from one facility to another and those admitted multiple times for treatment of the same injury. Although the percentage of patients transferred is generally low (e.g., less than 3 percent in Maryland), transferred patients represent an important subgroup (MacKenzie et al., 1990b). In most instances, a readmission should be assigned a principal diagnosis that reflects the complication or need for further treatment, with an additional code to indicate the late effect of a particular injury. Increasingly, databases are being constructed to facilitate the identification of readmissions either through the incorporation of an additional field for readmission data or by facilitating the ability to link information on multiple discharges referring to the same person. The committee strongly suggests that additional fields be added to hospital discharge systems to indicate that a patient transferred from another hospital; that the patient is being readmitted for a previous injury; and for the date of the injury.

Although statewide uniform hospital discharge data do not include information on injury deaths that occur in the field or during transport, they have become a valuable source of information for states and local communities. In particular, when linked to vital statistics or medical examiner data, they provide a complete picture of all trauma severe enough to result in death or hospitalization.

The epidemiology of less severe injuries requires data from emergency departments, hospital clinics, and physicians' offices. Nine state have recently established E-coded statewide emergency department record systems, an encouraging trend that can be assisted by the Data Elements for Emergency Department Systems, Release 1.0 (NCIPC, 1997). This new system contains uniform specifications for data entered in emergency department patient records, including external cause-of-injury coding, and incorporates national standards for electronic data interchange. Other state and local data that can be useful in studying the epidemiology of less severe injury include routinely collected information from emergency medical services, police and fire departments, and poison control centers.

DATA LINKAGES

The utility of existing data can be enhanced significantly by linkages across jurisdictions, which overcome the limitations of separate databases and go far in developing comprehensive information about an event, its circumstances, the occurrence and severity of the injury, the type and cost of treatment received, the outcome in terms of both mortality and morbidity, and the administrative or legal outcome. NHTSA has fostered development of linked databases by funding several states to develop Crash Outcome Data Evaluation Systems (CODES) (Johnson and Walker, 1996). CODES were initially designed to develop comprehensive data for determining the impact of safety-belt and motorcycle helmet use on the incidence and severity of injuries, health care costs, and outcome. The implementation of CODES required the linkage of police crash reports with death certificate or medical examiner data and health care data (including emergency medical services data, emergency department data, hospital discharge data, and occasionally data from the insurance claims). CODES databases are now being used to address a variety of motor vehicle injury research and evaluation questions at the local, state, and national levels. Similar linkages will be needed for other types of injuries.

Significant barriers exist to successful linkage, however, and are related to (1) limited access to databases (in some cases relevant data are collected but not computerized and, if computerized, are not readily available because of data release policies, concerns about confidentiality, and interagency politics); (2) high costs and limited resources for developing and maintaining databases; and (3) technical difficulties. When the databases to be linked use similar unique identifiers, linkage is relatively easy. However, for confidentiality reasons, most databases do not contain unique identifiers. Probabilistic matching software has been developed and used to link databases when unique identifiers are not available and to deal with inevitable discrepancies related to spelling, data entry errors, or similar problems (Johnson and Walker, 1996).

SUMMARY

In summary, although significant advances have been made in the development of effective strategies for injury surveillance, there is still much to be accomplished. The development of information to monitor trends in nonfatal injury (nationally and locally), to determine the place of occurrence of injuries, to determine trends and mechanisms for intentional injury deaths, to identify new or changing injury problems, and to evaluate promising new interventions will require a long-term funding commitment to develop new surveillance systems or to support and expand existing systems. Particularly promising efforts include (1) ensuring uniform and reliable coding with the ICD; (2) extending the current NEISS data system to include all injuries treated in the emergency department; (3) the development of a fatal intentional injury surveillance system, based on the successful FARS data system; (4) extending the use of trauma registries to monitor long-term outcome following injury; and (5) the further development and broader application of techniques for data linkage. All of these efforts require substantial coordination and cooperation among multiple agencies and professional groups. It will be important to identify and engage the relevant stakeholders early in the process to ensure successful implementation of each of these initiatives.

REFERENCES

AHCPR (Agency for Health Care Policy and Research). 1998. *Health Cost and Utilization Project.* [World Wide Web document]. URL http://www.ahcpr.gov/data/hcup-pkt.htm (accessed August 1998).

Annest JL, Conn JM, James SP. 1996. *Inventory of Federal Data Systems in the United States for Injury Surveillance, Research and Prevention Activities.* Atlanta, GA: National Center for Injury Prevention and Control.

Annest JL, Conn JM, McLoughlin E, Fingerhut LA, Pickett D, Gallagher S. 1998. *How States Are Collecting and Using Cause of Injury Data.* Report of the Data Committee of the Injury Control and Emergency Health Services Section of the American Public Health Association.

BLS (Bureau of Labor Statistics). 1996. *BLS* [World Wide Web document]. URL http://www.bls.gov.oshcftab.htm (accessed July 1998).

Burt CW, Fingerhut LA. 1998. Injury visits to hospital emergency departments: United States, 1992–95. *NCHS Vital Health Statistics* 13(131).

CDC (Centers for Disease Control and Prevention). 1997. Recommended framework for presenting injury mortality data. *MMWR Recommendations and Reports* 46(No. RR-14):1–32.

Combs DL, Parrish RG, Ing RT. 1995. *Death Investigation in the United States and Canada.* Atlanta, GA: Centers for Disease Control and Prevention.

Dijkhuis H, Zwerling C, Parrish G, Bennett T, Kemper HC. 1994. Medical examiner data in injury surveillance: A comparison with death certificates. *American Journal of Epidemiology* 139(6):637–642.

Fingerhut LA, Cox CS. 1998. Poisoning mortality 1985–1995. *Public Health Reports* 113(3):219–233.

Fingerhut LA, Warner M. 1997. *Injury Chartbook. Health, United States, 1996–97.* Hyattsville, MD: National Center for Health Statistics.

GAO (General Accounting Office). 1997. *Consumer Product Safety Commission: Better Data Needed to Help Identify and Analyze Potential Hazards.* Washington, DC: GAO. GAO/HEHS-97-147.

Johnson SW, Walker J. 1996. *NHTSA Technical Report: The Crash Outcome Evaluation System (CODES).* Washington, DC: NHTSA. DOT HS 808 338.

Lapidus GD, Braddock M, Schwartz R, Banco L, Jacobs L. 1994. Accuracy of fatal motorcycle-injury reporting on death certificates. *Accident Analysis and Prevention* 26(4):535–542.

Loo GT, Siegel JH, Dischinger PC, Rixen D, Burgess AR, Addis MD, O'Quinn T, McCammon L, Schmidhauser CB, Marsh P, Hodge PA, Bents F. 1996. Airbag protection versus compartment intrusion effect determines the pattern of injuries in multiple trauma motor vehicle crashes. *Journal of Trauma* 41(6):935–951.

MacKenzie EJ, Morris JA, Smith GS, Fahey M. 1990a. Acute hospital costs of trauma in the United States: Implications for regionalized systems of care. *Journal of Trauma* 30:1096–1103.

MacKenzie EJ, Steinwachs DM, Ramzy AI. 1990b. Evaluating performance of statewide regionalized systems of trauma care. *Journal of Trauma* 30(6):681–688.

Mallonee S, Istre GR, Rosenberg M, Reddish-Douglas M, Jordan F, Silverstein P, Tunell W. 1996. Surveillance and prevention of residential-fire injuries. *New England Journal of Medicine* 335(1):27–31.

Mullins RJ, Veum-Stone J, Helfand M, Zimmer-Gembeck M, Hedges JR, Southard PA, Trunkey DD. 1994. Outcome of hospitalized injured patients after institution of a trauma system in an urban area. *Journal of the American Medical Association* 271(24):1919–1924.

NCEH (National Center for Environmental Health). 1998. *CDC Medical Examiner and Coroner Information Sharing Program.* [World Wide Web document]. URL http://www.cdc.gov/nceh/programs/mec/mec.htm (accessed August 1998).

NCHS (National Center for Health Statistics). 1991. *Report on the Need to Collect External Cause of Injury Codes in Hospital Discharge Data.* Hyattsville, MD: NCHS. NCHS Working Paper Series No. 38.

NCIPC (National Center for Injury Prevention and Control). 1997. *Data Elements for Emergency Department Systems (DEEDS)* [World Wide Web document]. URL http://www.cdc.gov/ncipc/pub-res/deedspage.htm (accessed December 1997).

NHTSA (National Highway Traffic Safety Administration). 1998a. *Air Bags.* [World Wide Web document]. URL http://www.nhtsa.dot.gov/airbags (accessed August 1998).

NHTSA (National Highway Traffic Safety Administration). 1998b. *Traffic Safety Facts, 1997.* [World Wide Web document]. URL http://www.nhtsa.dot.gov/people/ncsa/pdf/Overview97.pdf (accessed August 1998).

NIOSH (National Institute for Occupational Safety and Health). 1989. *Preventing Worker Deaths and Injuries from Falls Through Skylights and Roof Openings.* Cincinnati, OH: NIOSH. DHHS (NIOSH) Publication No. 90-100.

Robertson LS. 1998. *Injury Epidemiology.* New York: Oxford University Press.

Rutledge R. 1995. The goals, development and use of trauma registries and trauma data sources in decision making in injury. *Surgical Clinics of North America* 75:305–326.

Shapiro MJ, Cole KE Jr, Keegan M, Prasad CN, Thompson RJ. 1994. National survey of state trauma registries, 1992. *Journal of Trauma* 37:835–840.

Smith GS, Langley JD. 1998. Drowning surveillance: How well do E codes identify submersion fatalities. *Injury Prevention* 4:135–139.

Teret SP, Wintemuite GJ, Beilenson PL. 1992. The firearm fatality reporting system: A proposal. *Journal of the American Medical Association* 267:3073–3074.

U.S. DHHS (Department of Health and Human Services), Public Health Service, Health Care Financing Administration. 1997. *International Classification of Diseases, 9th Revision, Clinical Modification, 6th Edition.* Washington, DC: U.S. Government Printing Office. DHHS Publication PHS 96-1260.

WHO (World Health Organization). 1975. *Manual of the International Statistical Classification of Diseases, Injuries, and Causes of Death, 9th Revision.* Vol. 1. Geneva: WHO.

Winston FK, Reed R. 1996. Airbags and children: Results of a National Highway Traffic Safety Administration special investigation into actual crashes. In: *40th Stapp Car Crash Conference Proceedings.* Albuquerque, NM: Society of Automotive Engineers. SAE Publication 962438. Pp. 383–389.

4

Prevention Research

This chapter addresses research on injury prevention, a paramount goal of the injury field. The value of prevention research lies in its contribution to the design and implementation of interventions that successfully reduce injuries or ameliorate their consequences. Over the past quarter century, research has contributed in this way to actual reductions in injury mortality rates (Baker et al., 1992), most clearly in relation to motor vehicle injuries (see Chapter 5). Additionally, injury research has documented the effectiveness of many interventions (i.e., programs and policies) designed to reduce injury. Research also makes an important contribution when it demonstrates that interventions do not achieve the desired results or have unintended consequences. Such research helps to refine and improve interventions and to enhance the conceptual foundation for prevention.

A formal scientific approach to injury prevention calls for interventions to be designed, evaluated, and then implemented based on a research-driven process of surveillance, hazard identification, risk assessment and analysis, intervention design and evaluation, and transfer of successful interventions into widespread practice. However, the actual practice of developing interventions is not always so neatly ordered. Many interventions are undertaken based on intuition, advocacy, or legal considerations rather than on scientific evidence, and many interventions are unevaluated (IOM, 1998). Moreover, many successful injury prevention interventions are serendipitous since they occur as a result of actions undertaken for other reasons. The imposition in 1975 of a federal maximum speed limit of 55 miles per hour, a policy that saved hundreds to thousands of lives per year, was instituted as a fuel conservation measure rather than as a safety measure (TRB, 1984; National Committee, 1989).

This chapter outlines the challenges ahead for prevention research, which include strengthening the multidisciplinary nature of injury research, developing and evaluating a wide range of prevention interventions, training a highly skilled cadre of injury prevention researchers, and undertaking the research needed to guide the effective prevention of unintentional and intentional injuries. This chapter refers to, but does not concentrate on, treatment research (e.g., acute care and rehabilitation) because treatment research priorities have been addressed by several recent landmark reports, including the *NIH Task Force on Trauma Research* (NIH, 1994), *Disability in America: Toward a National Agenda for Prevention* (IOM, 1991), and *Enabling America* (IOM, 1997). As in other areas of clinical practice, the need to demonstrate the relationship between the quality of acute care and rehabilitation, costs, and outcome has never been more critical (see also Chapter 6).

RESEARCH ACCOMPLISHMENTS

Prevention research has garnered numerous accomplishments over the past 30 years in terms of understanding risk factors, injury mechanisms, and effective ways to reduce injuries. The greatest research progress has been made with motor vehicle and traffic safety, an area with the longest period of sustained federal support for research and prevention programs (see Chapter 5). The same has not been true for other types of unintentional injuries or for intentional injuries (i.e., suicide and violence). These areas have not received sustained support of sufficient magnitude (Chapter 8).

Unintentional Injury Prevention

Unintentional injuries, as a group, represent the most common cause of injury death. There were a total of 90,402 unintentional injury deaths in 1995 (Fingerhut and Warner, 1997). A strong research base on motor vehicle and highway safety has contributed to the increased crashworthiness of vehicles, and increased use of safety belts, and to decreases in drinking and driving. Certainly, other factors are involved, such as increased public awareness and consumer demand for safe products; federal, state, and local programs; improved medical care; and legislation and enforcement activities. Separating the contribution of research and these other factors is rarely possible in any area of injury prevention, in part because the factors are so interrelated. Research and surveillance, for instance, are used to galvanize public opinion, to justify legislation, and to evaluate legislative impact. Research forms an essential underpinning to a comprehensive approach to tackling the problem of injury.

One of the most impressive research and programmatic accomplishments in the history of injury prevention occurred in the area of childhood poisonings from consumer products. In 1970, 226 poisoning deaths among children under age 5 occurred in the United States, whereas in 1985, only 55 such deaths occurred (CDC, 1985). Aspirin poisoning—the single leading cause of childhood poisoning death in the 1960s and early 1970s—had virtually disappeared by 1985. This accomplishment was due, in large measure, to a body of research on the epidemiology of childhood poisoning; ongoing surveillance of childhood poisoning through the nation's poison control centers; and innovative work on the development of environmental and legislative approaches to keep hazardous substances, particularly baby aspirin, out of the hands and mouths of young children. The final vehicle for this success was passage of the Poison Prevention Packaging Act of 1970 that required the use of special childproof containers and limited the number of pills of baby aspirin to 30 per bottle. Subsequent research investigated compliance with the legislation (Dole et al., 1986). A recent study by Rodgers (1996) found that child-resistant packaging of prescription drugs was associated with a 45 percent reduction in mortality rates involving children younger than 5 from 1974–1992, resulting in 460 fewer child deaths over this period than otherwise projected. This study controlled for long-term safety trends and changes in consumption of prescription drugs. The overall strategy of combining regulation and community-based intervention through poison control centers has been used as a case study of effective injury prevention (National Committee, 1989).

Falls are the most common cause of nonfatal injuries and among the most common causes of injury deaths. They are an especially serious problem for the elderly and for children (Chapter 2). Falls occur annually in about 30 percent of elderly persons living in the community (NCIPC, 1996). Research has provided the scientific foundation for interventions (e.g., hormone replacement therapy, vitamin supplements, exercise, protective hip pads) that can prevent or protect the elderly from hip fractures, the most serious consequence of falls in this group (Paganini-Hill et al., 1991; Grady et al., 1992; Lauritzen et al., 1993; Tinetti et al., 1993, 1994; Meunier et al., 1994; Province et al., 1995).

Research has established that many population-based injury prevention strategies are inexpensive and easily integrated into existing systems or practice. For example, counseling by physicians has been found to prevent or alleviate many types of unintentional injuries, including certain traffic-related injuries and injuries related to falls and burns (Christophersen and Sullivan, 1982; Berger et al., 1984; Katcher et al., 1989; Persson and Magnusson, 1989; Bien et al., 1993; Miller and Galbraith, 1995). The installation of smoke alarms in high-risk homes in a community-wide program in Oklahoma City was found to achieve a 74 percent decrease in fatal and nonfatal injuries from residential fires (Mallonee et al., 1996). In a randomized controlled trial of low-income women and children, home visits by nurses during the pregnancy of the women and for two years after the birth were found to significantly reduce childhood injuries (Kitzman et al., 1997).

One of the most effective prevention strategies is the use of helmets by bicyclists and motorcyclists (Elliott and Rodriguez, 1996). Helmets prevent traumatic brain injury, the foremost cause of death in cycle-related injuries (Rivara et al., 1997a,b). A population-based, case-control study found the use of bicycle helmets to reduce the risk of head injury by 85 percent and the risk of brain injury by 88 percent (Thompson et al., 1989). Bicycle helmets also reduce the risk of injury to the upper and middle face (Thompson et al., 1996b). As a result of sustaining less severe injuries, helmeted cyclists have shorter lengths of stay in hospitals and intensive care units and lower overall hospital costs (Elliott and Rodriguez, 1996). Research has contributed to the enactment of legislation in many states mandating helmet use and the support by many public and private agencies of helmet education programs.

These examples illustrate the pivotal value of research in many established interventions that avert unintentional injuries (see Table 4.1, Box 4.1). Yet, although there has been much progress in research, more is needed. The 12 percent decline in unintentional injury deaths from 1985–1995 while encouraging, was driven by the decline in motor vehicle fatalities (Fingerhut and Warner, 1997). The overall decline thus obscures the continued need to reduce unintentional injury fatalities related to falls, poisonings, drownings, suffocations, and fires and burns, particularly in special populations such as children and the elderly.

BOX 4.1
Harlem Hospital Injury Prevention Program

A program in New York City is a model injury prevention program whose creation epitomizes many of the aspects of prevention research described in this chapter. The Harlem Hospital Injury Prevention Program was created in 1988 as a result of surveillance revealing that the injury rate to Harlem children was twice the national rate. With the aid of community coalitions and public agencies, a broad-based, surveillance-driven prevention program was established to create a safe community for children (Laraque et al., 1995). The program was geared to reduce injuries from violence, motor vehicles, and recreational activities. A surveillance system was established—the Northern Manhattan Injury Surveillance System—to provide population-based injury data by zip code. This system allowed the program to focus and evaluate interventions by neighborhoods. The Harlem Hospital Pediatric Trauma Registry also provided social data on children admitted to the hospital for injury and carefully evaluated the injury event. The community was surveyed and photographed to document dangers in children's play spaces, propelling a risk-factor analysis of unsafe conditions. Interventions, which served more than 10,000 children, included educational projects, renovation of playgrounds, safe activities, and other social changes. For example, intensive educational programs were established for traffic safety and violence prevention. Twenty safe playgrounds were built at community schools, and parks were refurbished. Bicycle helmets were distributed at reasonable cost. Safe activities were developed by the program or supported in the community to keep children engaged in supervised

Continued

BOX 4.1 *Continued*

activities that also provided mentoring and role models. Drug activity at the new play sites was controlled by the district attorney's community outreach project. Following the implementation of these interventions, the Northern Manhattan Injury Surveillance System found a 46 percent decrease in injury due to guns and assaults (Durkin et al., 1996) and about a 50 percent reduction in traffic injury (Davidson et al., 1994; Laraque et al., 1995). The incidence of pediatric neurological trauma, the leading cause of death and disability from injury, was reduced by 44 percent in the intervention cohort (Durkin et al., 1998).

Intentional Injury Prevention

Suicide Prevention

The overall suicide rate has remained relatively stable for the past decade, as it has over much of the past 50 years (Baker et al., 1992; Kachur et al., 1995). This stability masks some disturbing trends among such subgroups as adolescents, young adults, and the elderly. From 1980 to 1992, the suicide rate increased by 121 percent for children ages 10–14, by 27 percent for adolescents ages 15–19, and by more than 10 percent for the elderly ages 70 and older (Kachur et al., 1995). The highest suicide rate is among persons ages 80–84, for whom the rate increased 36 percent over this time frame (Kachur et al., 1995). The increase in suicide among the very old is thought to be related, in part, to longer yet poorer quality of life, for which better palliative care is needed (GAO, 1998).

The majority of suicides (60 percent) in 1992 were committed with a firearm, and firearm suicides accounted for most of the increase in age-specific suicide rates during the 1980s (Kachur et al., 1995). Case-control injury studies have shown that the risk of suicide is up to five times higher for persons living in a home where firearms are present (Brent et al., 1991, 1993; Kellermann et al., 1992). Access to firearms raises suicide risk among teens without a psychiatric disorder (Brent et al., 1993), supporting the view that restrictions on firearm access can curtail suicides among teens who, as a group, are often more prone than older adults to suicide as an impulsive act.

Mental disorders constitute the most important risk factors for suicide. Many suicide victims have affective, substance abuse, personality, or other mental disorders (U.S. Preventive Services Task Force, 1996). Research also has identified environmental and social risk factors, including access to firearms, problems of social adjustment, serious medical illness, living alone, recent bereavement, family history of completed suicide, and others (Shaffer et al., 1988; U.S. Preventive Services Task Force, 1996).

TABLE 4.1 Examples of Effective Unintentional Injury Prevention Interventions

Injury Problem	Interventions	Evaluation Studies
Bicycle injuries	Bicycle helmet use; mandatory helmet laws	Maimaris et al. (1994); Thompson et al. (1996a,b); Ni et al. (1997)
Choking and suffocation	Legislation and product design changes (e.g., refrigerator disposal, warning labels on thin plastic bags)	Kraus (1985)
Falls in older adults	Weight-bearing exercise; multimodal programs (home visits by nurses, exercise programs, elimination of hazards, etc.); protective hip pads	Lauritzen et al. (1993); Tinetti et al. (1993, 1994)
Fires and burns	Smoke detectors; legislation regulating flammability of children's clothing; legislation requiring safe preset temperatures for water heaters	McLoughlin et al. (1977, 1982); Erdmann et al. (1991); Runyan et al. (1992); Mallonce et al. (1996)
Motor vehicle crashes	Safety belts; air bags; child safety seats; sobriety checkpoints; minimum legal drinking age laws	Baker-Dickman (1987); Womble (1988); Henry et al. (1996); NHTSA (1996)
Sports injuries	Mouthguards; equipment modification (e.g., breakaway bases); protective equipment (e.g., knee and elbow pads, helmets, wrist pads for inline skating)	Janda et al. (1988); Schieber et al. (1996)

SOURCE: National Committee (1989); Rivara et al. (1997a,b).

Research has helped to fuel awareness that some deaths from suicide are preventable through social and environmental changes. Different lines of evidence converge to suggest that broad-based public health approaches that seek to modify social and environmental risk factors may be enlisted for prevention purposes. Epidemiologic research has highlighted the need for interventions to prevent the presence of youth suicide "clusters." Clusters are the occurrence of several suicides in the same community or vicinity, apparently triggered by one suicide (Gould et al., 1990). Furthermore, research has found that many adolescent suicide victims do not meet the clinical criteria for depression or other treatable mental disorders (Shaffer et al., 1988). Finally, research has found that reducing access to a means of suicide can lower the suicide rate. Studies from Great Britain in the 1970s found that as the carbon monoxide content of cooking gas was lowered (for reasons unrelated to suicide prevention), the overall suicide rate declined. Not only was the most common method of suicide (i.e., inhalation of cooking gas) less effective, but individuals did not resort to other means (Kreitman, 1976; Brown, 1979).

Much of the subsequent progress in suicide prevention research has been made in identifying risk factors for suicide, as this is one of the first steps toward prevention. Less progress has been made in the design and evaluation of programs to prevent suicides. The major challenge for research is the development and testing of new interventions to prevent suicide. The task ahead is formidable even for the most skillful researchers. Evaluation of prevention efforts has been fraught with methodological problems, including definitions of suicidal behavior, the validity and reliability of assessment instruments, the relative rarity of suicide, and the need for large samples and lengthy follow-up (Meehan et al., 1992; U.S. Preventive Services Task Force, 1996; NIMH, 1998). For example, although teen cluster suicides are seen as preventable, they have proved difficult to study because of definitional and methodological complexities.

Research on the prevention of suicide clearly warrants higher priority from the Department of Health and Human Services, which houses virtually all federal suicide prevention programs. The committee applauds the U.S. Surgeon General's recognition of inadequate attention to suicide and his initiation of various measures to prevent suicide, including the first National Suicide Prevention Conference in October 1998. Research must be expanded, as described in Chapter 8.

Violence Prevention

There can be no doubt that violence exacts a grievous toll on the nation's health (Chapter 2). The toll encompasses death, injuries, long-term disabilities, and strain on the trauma care system (Chapter 6). The homicide rate in 1995 was 8.6 per 100,000 population, a rate that overshadows that of all other industrialized nations (Fingerhut and Warner, 1997; Ventura et al., 1997). The impact is greatest on young people, especially minorities. Homicide is the foremost cause of death for African-American males ages 15–34 and the second most important cause of death for young people of all races ages 15–24 (NCIPC, 1996). The magnitude of nonfatal assaultive injuries—defined as physical harm occurring during the course of an assault, robbery, or rape between strangers, acquaintances, or family members—is much higher than that of homicides but is more difficult to capture because of problems in reporting, especially family violence. According to the National Crime Victimization Survey, assault injuries among those age 12 and older occurred at a rate of 12.7 per 1,000 people in 1994 (CDC, 1996; BJS, 1997).

The fields of criminal justice and public health bring different perspectives and strengths to bear on the violence problem. The criminal justice system—the police, courts, and corrections system—works to prevent violence primarily through arrests and incarceration, which act to deter, incapacitate, and rehabilitate criminals (Moore, 1993). Deterrence is seen as working either on potential offenders in the community or on incarcerated offenders in relation to the commission of future crimes. More recently, there has been an increased emphasis on crime prevention via community policing and other means to prevent crime and violence. A major impetus was the passage of the federal Violent Crime Control and Law Enforcement Act of 1994, which provided funds to state and local governments for new prevention programs.

The recognition of the growing health consequences of violence propelled the public health community, beginning in the 1970s, to consider violence as a public health problem (National Committee, 1989). In 1985, the Surgeon General's Workshop on Violence and Public Health signaled the entry of public health into what traditionally had been the domain of the criminal justice system (U.S. DHHS, 1986; Mercy et al., 1993). Viewing violence prevention as a public health goal calls attention to the measurable health consequences of assaultive injuries, highlights the role of the health sector in identifying and reducing the violence embedded in situations and relationships, and highlights the potential utility of epidemiologic tools in identifying risk factors and designing interventions that lie outside the usual sphere of crime prevention and control. In this way the perspective and methods of public health usefully complement the perspective and methods of criminal justice in understanding and responding to violence.

Recognizing the validity and benefits of both public health and criminal justice perspectives, Moore and colleagues (1993) argued for a synthesis. In their view, "to deal effectively with what can now be seen as a far more complex problem of violence and its consequences, there is urgent need for an effective collaboration between the two communities." The committee agrees with this assessment and urges continued and expanded collaboration to bring the resources and creative approaches of the criminal justice and public health communities to violence prevention.

Although numerous factors enhance the risk of violence, research has determined that some of these factors appear to be salient as proximate causes of potentially lethal violence (i.e., the subset of violent events that present a risk of serious injury or death). These include the use of firearms, the use of alcohol and illicit drugs, the interaction of mental disorders and substance abuse, and the developmental and contextual features of adolescence in urban America that accentuate all other risk factors for violence (NRC, 1993, 1994; IOM, 1996; Zimring and Hawkins, 1997).

A number of NRC reports have summarized the accumulating body of knowledge on the causes of violence (NRC, 1993, 1994, 1996, 1998). Progress has been less pronounced in developing and evaluating prevention programs, in large part, because of the time lag between understanding causation and translating this understanding into programs, the complexity of the problem, and the imperfections of current surveillance systems.

The NRC report *Violence in Families* (NRC, 1998) examined the research literature on evaluations of interventions for child maltreatment, domestic violence, and elder abuse. Although it identified 114 evaluation studies in these areas, it found most to be "not yet mature enough to guide policy and program development." Only one area, home visitation programs for child maltreatment (see Olds et al. [1997]), was recommended as policy for first-time parents living in social settings with high reported rates of child maltreatment.

Evaluation research is needed for a number of prevention interventions, including peer mediation, social skills training, comprehensive community initiatives, shelter programs and other services for victims of domestic violence, child fatality review panels, mental health and counseling services for child maltreatment and domestic violence, child witness to violence prevention and treatment programs, and elder abuse services (NRC, 1998). Finally, the committee believes that, from the perspective of violence research, a high priority is to strengthen the health system databases for monitoring nonfatal injuries. Accurate measures of violence can be achieved only by establishing reliable health-based surveillance systems. Strengthening these databases will advance the field of violence research whether it is conducted by criminologists or public health specialists, and whatever the source of funding.

Violence prevention research is the purview of multiple federal agencies, including the Office of Justice Programs of the Department of Justice and the following agencies of the Department of Health and Human Services: the National Center for Injury Prevention and Control (NCIPC), the National Institute of Mental Health, the Maternal and Child Health Bureau, the National Institute on Alcohol Abuse and Alcoholism, and the National Institute on Drug Abuse. Many of these federal programs are discussed at greater length in Chapter 8, where the committee makes several recommendations. In addition, the committee urges that the research recommendations of previous NRC reports be implemented to promote effective violence interventions.

Prevention Interventions

Injury prevention encompasses a vast array of programs and policies aimed at reducing the frequency or severity of injuries. Although these interventions can be categorized in a variety of ways, the committee elected to group them as follows: (1) interventions for changing individual behavior; (2) interventions for modifying products or agents of injury; (3) interventions for modifying the physical environment; and (4) interventions for modifying the sociocultural and economic environment. These categories are adapted from those originally proposed by William Haddon more than three decades ago (Haddon et al., 1964).

Research on injury interventions often begins with estimating their efficacy, effectiveness, and cost-effectiveness. Factors that are considered include feasibility; potential mortality and morbidity reduction; economic impact; ethical, social, and political considerations; and likely acceptance by the target population. Through this predevelopment analysis, proposed interventions can be categorized and prioritized according to their potential impact. Those interventions with the greatest potential can be targeted for further development and pilot-tested for identification of unexpected consequences and efficacy. What follows is a summary of recent developments, including a few key research areas that appear to be ripe for further advances.

Individual Behavior

Behavioral research has demonstrated that many injury interventions require changes in human behavior, either to reduce the exposure or vulnerability of potential victims to injury-causing events or to reduce the risk that one person will become the agent or instrument of harm to another. Behavior change can be achieved by incentives and deterrence, education, and persuasion. Research has shown that beneficial behavioral changes rarely occur through education or persuasion alone. Some of the factors that influence the success or failure of education programs are known (including education levels, timing of educational approaches, e.g., child safety information for expectant parents), but focused research on the specification of these factors is needed. As research continues to increase our knowledge of efficacious strategies, promotion of these strategies has to be emphasized.

Incentives and deterrence. One of the most significant developments in the injury prevention field over the past two decades has been to include the fruits of behavioral and criminologic research in developing behavioral incentives and disincentives, including threats of legal sanctions (deterrence) (Bonnie, 1986). Incentives are often financial. In the consumer arena, discounts in homeowner and automobile insurance premiums can be used as incentives to promote precautionary behavior, such as installing smoke detectors or purchasing cars with airbags, respectively. In the occupational arena, discounts in workers' compensation premiums are being used as incentives for promoting safe work practices.

Deterrence through criminal punishment has been the backbone of the nation's policy for reducing assaultive behavior, and there is a growing body of literature on the preventive effects of criminal sanctions in general and of specific statutory provisions, such as mandatory jail terms for using a weapon in criminal activity (McDowall et al., 1992). Two of the most thorough investigations of deterrence have been in the area of highway safety. Over the past 20 years, a large body of research has been developed on the differential impact of various punishment schemes for drunk driving, including mandatory jail terms and administrative license suspension (Jacobs, 1989; Ross, 1993). More recently, a significant body of knowledge has emerged on the efficacy of laws mandating child restraint and safety belt use, demonstrating that enactment of these laws has significantly increased the rate of restraint use (Graham, 1993). In both cases, public education efforts have accompanied and spurred enactment of this legislation, transmitted knowledge about the provisions and penalties of laws to promote compliance, and generated public support for law enforcement programs.

Self-protection. Another key development has been increased attention to the ways in which potential victims can reduce their own vulnerability or exposure to injury. Research on promoting helmet use by cyclists and safety belt use by motorists and passengers is a natural extension of medical research on the logic of immunization or prophylaxis. When extended to assaultive injuries, self-protection takes the form of bulletproof vests for police officers and other forms of personal security aiming to reduce exposure or vulnerability (NRC, 1993). Avoiding intoxication is another way that potential victims can protect themselves (Room et al., 1995). Increased scientific attention to the opportunities for precautionary behavior reflects an enriched appreciation of the ways in which changing the behavior of potential victims can reduce the risk of injury. It should be acknowledged, however, that one of the potential pitfalls of efforts to promote self-protection is the tendency to blame victims for failing to take precautions if injury does occur. This concern highlights the interaction of attitudes toward prevention and personal responsibility in an overall injury prevention strategy.

High-risk groups. Another area requiring systematic research is in understanding and developing strategies for reaching high-risk groups. Although many interventions are appropriately aimed at the general population, research is needed on prevention interventions aimed specifically at groups with above-average risk. However, proper targeting is a first step. For example, most infants and young children traveling in passenger vehicles are in child safety seats. Yet there is an important but relatively neglected subgroup (an estimated 35 percent of children ages 4 and under) that travels without such restraints and has twice the risk of death and injury as those who use safety seats (SAFE KIDS, 1998). Research on protecting children who travel without restraints may be more useful than cataloging all the forms of misuse. Additionally, research has shown the promise of reducing injuries through home visitation for high-risk first-time mothers (Kitzman et al., 1997; Olds et al., 1997).

Research demonstrates that at-risk populations do not necessarily have to be addressed directly in order to change their behavior. For example, there has been some success with peer intervention training in high schools as a means of getting students to intervene in the drinking and driving of their associates (McKnight and McPherson, 1986). Others who have some influence over at-risk individuals—for example, sellers and servers of alcohol—can be targeted, and server intervention programs have shown some success in reducing excessive alcohol consumption (McKnight and Streff, 1994).

Agent

The agent of injury is often a product obtained by a consumer in the marketplace (including motor vehicles, firearms, or other consumer products). Many of the great successes of injury prevention have involved research demonstrating that product alterations may reduce the risk of an injury-causing event or ameliorate its effects. Research on pre-event interventions resulted in the development of center high-mounted brake lights on automobiles that assist in preventing rear-end collisions by giving drivers that follow a quicker warning of deceleration (Rausch et al., 1982; Kahane, 1989; McKnight et al., 1989); childproof caps to keep medicine, that can cause poisonings from being opened (discussed earlier); and safety locks on firearms (see Chapter 5).

Prevention of fire-related injuries encompasses a wide range of opportunities for modifying the vector of thermal energy to reduce the risk that the energy will escape from control. For example, research has demonstrated the feasibility of safer designs for cigarettes (to make them self-extinguish more quickly) and lighters (to make them less likely to be ignited by a child). This research has led to product liability litigation against manufacturers of cigarettes and lighters, and has also provided the scientific basis for a 1994 Consumer Product Safety Commission regulation requiring cigarette lighters to be child-resistant. Research has also demonstrated the feasibility of making mattresses and upholstered furniture less flammable and, accordingly, less likely to be ignited by cigarettes, leading to the implementation of industry safety standards.

Research on the safety features of these products is conducted primarily by manufacturers, regulatory agencies, or watchdog consumer organizations. From the perspective of "intervention research," research questions concern the incentives for developing and implementing product safety designs that arise in the market (through which manufacturers respond to consumer preferences for safety); the efficacy of "interventions" designed to modify these incentives through direct regulation by authorized agencies (through standard setting or remedial action); or the indirect regulatory effects of bad publicity and tort liability. Surprisingly few researchers have explored empirically the operation of the market for safety, the effects of tort liability, and the effects of regulatory action. This area of research is in need of greater attention, particularly the safety effects of tort liability; here, public health proponents typically assume that expansive liability rules are safety enhancing, whereas skeptics believe that the existing liability scheme tends to reduce safety by retarding innovation or inducing override behavior (Sugarman, 1990; Rose-Ackerman, 1991; Viscusi, 1992; Viscusi and Magat, 1995; Dewees et al., 1996).

Physical Environment

Research has shown that some of the most successfully engineered safety interventions are often unnoticed factors in the environment. Everyday examples are roadway modifications that help drivers stay on the road rather than going off the road at curves or other hazardous locations (TRB, 1990), guard railings on upper-level terraces, and window guards to prevent childhood falls (Spiegel and Lindaman, 1977; Barlow et al., 1983). Through research, safety engineers and injury specialists have been able to modify building codes and change engineering designs to build in these safety features.

In recent years, increasing attention has been paid to preventing assaultive injuries through changes in environmental design. Examples of environmental changes include improved lighting in parking lots, the addition of police call-boxes, installing plexiglass shields for lone employees who need to handle cash transactions especially at night, and locating automatic teller machines in well-lit, high-traffic areas. Creative environmental interventions include efforts to reduce the incentives for committing robbery by using exact fare systems on public transport (Chaiken et al., 1974).

Socioeconomic Environment

Any planned intervention designed to reduce injuries occurs in the context of broad economic and social forces, such as employment rates, wealth distribution, social norms about health and safety, and population demography, that also fundamentally shape injury rates. Economic conditions, social practices, and cultural understandings constitute the context for of all these other factors and the prospect of altering them. Death rates are high in low-income areas for most types of unintentional injuries and for homicide; however, for suicide, there is little relationship between injury death rate and per capita income (Baker et al., 1992). Racial disparities in childhood unintentional injury rates are associated more with living in impoverished environments that with ethnicity (Singh and Yu, 1996; SAFE KIDS, 1998).

An example of the impact of the socioeconomic environment is seen in the increases in the rate of highway fatalities during economic upturns and the decreases during recessions (Graham, 1993). People tend to drive more during boom times, and the fatality rate per mile also increases (relative to long-term trends) as the economy expands, probably because more miles are driven by more high-risk drivers such as teenagers and people who have been drinking. This example illustrates two points. First, researchers studying the effects of planned injury prevention interventions on injury rates must always be alert to the effects of these background socioeconomic trends and conditions. Second, some types of public policies can be utilized explicitly as levers of injury prevention, even though they are not ordinarily seen from this perspective. A good example is the excise tax on alcohol, which is largely considered as a means to raise public revenues. In recent years, studies have demonstrated that raising the alcohol excise tax reduces the highway fatality rate and the rate of violent crime (Cook and Moore, 1993). Policies to increase alcohol excise taxes deserve to be viewed in terms of both revenue enhancement and injury prevention.

Studies of recent safety interventions have highlighted the possibility of modifying social norms and expectations about safety. Changes in attitudes toward alcohol-impaired driving have been associated with changes in driver behavior and with consequent reductions in injury rates. Increased parental use of child occupant restraints as well as increased rates of safety belt use among motor vehicle drivers and passengers has also called attention to the "declarative" role played by legal norms in reinforcing, stimulating, accelerating, or symbolizing changes in public attitudes or expectations about socially desirable behavior (Wagenaar and Webster, 1986; CDC, 1991). One of the interesting challenges faced by researchers investigating the effects of legal prohibitions or requirements is to distinguish between behavioral effects attributable to classical deterrence (behavior modified in response to threatened sanctions) and those attributable to the "declarative" effects of the law, which affect behavior indirectly by changing attitudes (Bonnie, 1986). Further attention to this issue will help policy makers design the most promising ways of deploying legal changes together with educational messages to promote safe behavior, such as safe storage of firearms and other dangerous articles.

RESEARCH OPPORTUNITIES

Broadening the Scope of Prevention Research

Once an injury problem is identified through surveillance or other means, research is brought to bear to identify causes, circumstances, and risk factors, as well as to develop and evaluate interventions. Evaluating interventions encompasses assessments of feasibility, efficacy, effectiveness, and cost-effectiveness. Outcome measures include changes in attitudes, knowledge, behavior, mortality, morbidity and disability reduction, and economic cost.

Prevention research is accomplished through a burgeoning variety of disciplines. Disciplines at the core of injury prevention research—epidemiology, behavioral science, biomedicine, and biomechanics—continue to be critical to the advancement of the field. Other disciplines are playing increasingly important roles, including economics, criminology, sociology, engineering, law, and molecular biology. As the scope of injury prevention is broadened to incorporate concepts and methodologies from many diverse fields, there is the potential for the development and testing of a far-reaching variety of new and better interventions and a fuller, multipronged approach to reducing the incidence and consequences of injury. For example, in the aviation industry, a broad array of interventions—including pilot training, air traffic control, aircraft design, and the use of safety belts—has been institutionalized to reduce passenger fatalities on U.S. commercial aircraft in 1996 to 1.8 per million passenger enplanements (NTSB, 1998). Such integration of approaches from multiple disciplines is crucial to injury prevention research.

Injury Biomechanics

Injury biomechanics has been a fundamental discipline in experimental studies of injury, especially injury causation. Experimental biomechanics reproduces the circumstances of injury under well-controlled laboratory conditions and examines structural and biologic responses. The work of Hugh DeHaven and William Haddon defined the field of injury biomechanics by describing the implications of abrupt dissipation of mechanical energy (see also Chapter 1 and Baker et al. [1992]). Injury biomechanics research uses the principles of mechanics to explore the physical and physiologic responses to impact, including penetrating and nonpenetrating blows to the body (NRC, 1985). Classically, injury biomechanics research has focused on injuries in their acute phase, establishing the causative forces or motions that provoke the injury, allowing countermeasures to be designed and tested. Yet, biomechanics has many applications in injury research, including testing the efficacy of interventions involving product design. Currently, the field of biomechanics includes investigators studying robotics, physical therapy, orthopedics, physical and sports medicine, exercise science, limb prosthetics, orthotics, and tissue engineering. This multidisciplinary science promises to provide the scientific and technical knowledge to develop strategies that will prevent injury or assist impaired neuromuscular systems (IOM, 1997).

Biomechanics research has established injury tolerance levels for many types of body tissue and has elucidated many of the biological processes that affect the injury process. The most complete picture of injury tolerances, pathophysiology, and reparative processes involves adult bone and connective tissue (McElhaney et al., 1976; Nahum and Melvin, 1993). Yet, despite significant strides in the past decade, the biomechanical properties of the brain and the biologic response of the brain to injury are not as well characterized. This variability in the knowledge base of injury biomechanics is also evident in the sophistication of interventions available. Techniques for the prevention and treatment of orthopedic injury are vast, ranging from hormonal supplementation to strengthen bone in order to prevent fracture (Folsom et al., 1995) to successful treatment for the nonunion of fractures by electrical stimulation (Esterhai et al., 1986). The options available to the clinician treating traumatic brain injury are essentially limited to minimizing secondary injuries due to brain swelling or hemorrhage (Chesnut, 1997).

Although the development of head injury tolerances began over 40 years ago and made use of a broad range of innovative experimental techniques, including human volunteer and cadaver tests and animal experiments, conducted by John Stapp and other pioneers in the field (Stapp, 1955), continued progress has been slow. The tests and experiments were extremely useful in developing an understanding of biodynamic responses under well-controlled crash situations. Denny-Brown and Russell (1941) conducted a series of animal experiments to study concussion. As a result of their work, estimates were developed regarding the amount of pressure in head impact that causes concussion. Researchers replicated those pressure levels in head impact tests on human cadavers, and determined average head accelerations required to cause injury across different impact durations (Viano et al., 1989; King et al., 1995). Subsequent analyses showed that mathematical relationships, known as the Severity Index and the Head Injury Criterion (HIC), could be developed from head acceleration data to establish a threshold for life-threatening injury. This elegant evolutionary process in the development of head impact protection stopped, however, when the HIC was adopted as one of the standards for evaluating motor vehicle safety performance. However, research on brain injury mechanisms have shown that HIC may not be appropriate for predicting specific forms of injury, notably diffuse brain injuries (Margulies and Thibault, 1992). Unfortunately, this work has been inadequately funded and restrictions on the use of animal and cadaver surrogates have impeded further progress.

Although there are other areas of biomechanics research (e.g., severe maxillofacial, thoracic, abdominal, and internal organ injuries), neurotrauma to the head resulting in traumatic brain injury continues to be a critical area. In the United States, someone suffers a head injury every 15 seconds. Every 5 minutes, one of those individuals dies and another becomes permanently disabled. There are 75,000 deaths from head injuries every year, and another 70,000 to 90,000 suffer permanent disability. Furthermore, 5,000 of those individuals develop epilepsy and another 2,000 remain in a chronic vegetative state. Traumatic brain injury is primarily a disability of the young, and the economic costs alone approach $25 billion annually (U.S. DHHS, 1992). Thus, research on neurotrauma to the head remains a priority area for biomechanics researchers.

To date, limited funding (Chapter 8) and difficulties in conducting animal and human cadaver research remain significant impediments to biomechanics research. Animal and cadaver use has greatly enhanced our understanding of injuries to specific areas of the body. Unfortunately, societal stigma and institutional policies limit the availability of animals and cadavers for research, particularly on pediatric injury. As a result, most knowledge of injury biomechanics is based on average-sized adults, and child injury (as well as injury to small women) assessment reference values are actually scaled-down estimates based on tests on adults, despite uncertainty regarding the accuracy of the scaling assumptions. There is also limited knowledge of the biomechanics of whiplash-associated disorders, even though neck strains and sprains result in significant numbers of claims made to insurance companies each year (Insurance Research Council, 1994).

Despite such obstacles, the field of injury biomechanics has made progress; for example, an advanced frontal crash test dummy has been developed that incorporates improved biofidelic features and expanded instrumentation. The new dummy potentially represents an effective tool for whole-body trauma assessment. Additionally, the clarification of design and performance specifications for child crash dummies will be useful for evaluating children's responses and injury potential in automobile crashes (NHTSA, 1998). Other advances are clearly demonstrated by the development of computerized models of injury. The revolution in computer and information technology in the past decade has led to the development of biofidelic models (i.e., realistic computer-based models of human anatomy and physiology). In many instances, anatomically accurate models that only five years ago were considered impractical are now examined routinely by biomechanics researchers. In addition, the decreasing cost of computer technology has allowed more research groups to develop and test computational models for studying injury mechanisms and tolerance.

Nevertheless, the utility of the models is dependent on the use of animals and cadavers for validation. Further, computer models are often developed in parallel with research on animals and cadavers; for example, a computer model of the neck under compressive loading is developed and validated with data from similar experiments on cadavers. Three principal benefits occur when such a parallel approach is used: (1) the computational models are more consistent, since they are validated with experimental data; (2) computational simulations, when exercised over a broad range of mechanical conditions, can highlight important new areas of investigation for the experimental models; and (3) the models are more easily extended to different segments of the human population, thereby increasing their impact. In all, the parallel approach can yield new insights, as well as new research directions, for investigators in injury prevention.

In the future, the role of modeling will continue to grow as an important tool for understanding injury causation and may also represent an effective proactive prevention tool by identifying harmful environments, harmful products, or at-risk populations before injuries occur. However, animal and cadaver research will continue to be an important component because it will be needed to establish the fidelity of computer models and to provide accurate measures of response to injury in children and small adults. Inasmuch as current support for both cadaver and animal experiments is inadequate, research support must be expanded.

The committee recommends the continued development of physical, mathematical, cellular, and biofidelic models of injury, particularly for high-risk populations (such as children and small women), while continuing to use animals and cadavers to validate biomechanical models of injury.

Biological Sciences

The application of molecular and cellular biology, neurobiology, and pharmacology to the study of injury has shed new light on the pathophysiology and treatment of injury. As an example, study of the role of calcium as a mediator of cell death following brain injury has provided hope that pharmacologic interventions can inhibit this process (Saatman et al., 1996). The exchange of information from other fields has further enhanced the body of knowledge in injury pathophysiology. For example, injury researchers have drawn on cancer biology to study apoptosis, the process of programmed cell death, in relation to injury (Rink et al., 1995; Liu et al., 1997). The application of knowledge regarding apoptosis to the study of populations of cells that die after brain or spinal cord injury has resulted in more sophisticated thinking about a cascade of biochemical events triggered by injury. Knowledge of a greater number of biochemical steps in the process of cell death results in more possibilities for intervention. Promoting the exchange of information and techniques from other areas of research can increase the resources and talent available to solve the complex problems of injury etiology and prevention.

Additionally, there are new and promising developments in the study of the relationship between injury and disease. For example, clinical data have suggested that an episode of trauma to the musculoskeletal system can lead to osteoarthritis many years after the event. Recent biomechanics research has shown that nondebilitating trauma to the knee can cause long-term osteoarthritis in the knee joint (Haut et al., 1995; Newberry et al., 1997). Similarly, clinical data have shown that neuropathological changes in brain-injured patients exhibit striking parallels to brains of Alzheimer's patients (Graham et al., 1995, 1996). The relationship between neurodegenerative diseases and traumatic brain injury is even more convincing in experimental models of brain injury (Roberts et al., 1994) and suggests both a new direction for brain injury prevention and treatment research and the need to extend studies on injury outcomes to include debilitating neurodegenerative disorders.

The committee recommends an investment in research on the pathophysiology and reparative processes necessary to further the understanding of nonfatal injury causes and consequences, in particular, those that result in long-term disability.

Behavioral Sciences

The importance of behavioral research to injury prevention was highlighted more than three decades ago by William Haddon in his early publications on preventing motor vehicle injuries (Haddon et al., 1964). The behavioral sciences contribute to injury research by developing knowledge about psychosocial determinants of human behavior, guiding the measurement of these determinants, and shaping the development and measurement of interventions for reducing injuries (National Committee, 1989). It is abundantly clear that injury rates vary according to gender, age, and ethnicity (Chapter 2). Adolescent males, for example, represent one of the groups at greatest risk of injury, especially for motor vehicle and firearm injuries (Fingerhut and Warner, 1997). Behavioral sciences, using a combination of empirical and theoretical approaches, help to explain why gender, developmental age, and ethnicity are important. They examine the influence not only of social and cultural norms, but also of individual and family characteristics that predispose to injury (Irwin et al., 1992; Robertson, 1992). Better understanding of the psychosocial determinants of behavior helps to focus efforts to intervene to change behavior in order to reduce injury risk.

Behavioral research has led to growing awareness of how individuals perceive risk (Kahneman et al., 1982) and how their perception of risk influences their risk-taking behavior (e.g., substance use, recreational vehicle use) that leads to injury (Irwin et al., 1992; Zuckerman, 1993). Risk perception is guided by individuals' understanding of the magnitude of a given risk and also by value judgments about its attributes, such as its familiarity and controllability (Slovic et al., 1982; NRC, 1989). Risk perception and risk decision making are also closely tied to age (Reyna and Ellis, 1992) and gender (Flynn et al., 1994; Barke et al., 1997). This information has helped to explain why facts alone are often insufficient to induce behavioral change for prevention purposes. For example, it is all too clear from the mixed results with HIV (human immunodeficiency virus) prevention efforts that psychosocial determinants, including risk perception and risk-taking behavior, must be taken into account in the design of interventions that strive for enduring behavioral change (IOM, 1994).

Behavioral researchers have also investigated the possibility that people will alter their behavior in response to safety improvements in products or in the environment so as to reduce the safety benefits of these changes. That is, people may increase their level of risk, thereby offsetting some or all of the anticipated safety benefits. It is clear that people behave differently when the risks they perceive change; for example, people walk more carefully when barefoot, drive with greater caution when roads are icy. In similar fashion, consumers are likely to respond in some way to safety-enhanced technology or environmental changes of which they are aware. It may even be that each person has a target level of risk that he or she wishes to maintain, so that, for example, if cars are made safer and the cost of risky driving is lowered, then the driver compensates by taking greater risks. Research seeks to clarify the conditions under which offsetting behavior is likely to occur and to what extent.

Most of the literature on this topic deals with motor vehicle injuries. Evans (1991) outlined some general patterns as to how consumers react to safety-related changes. "If the safety change affects vehicle performance, it is likely to be used to increase mobility. Thus, improved braking or handling characteristics are likely to lead to increased speeds, closer following, and faster cornering.

Safety may also increase, but by less than if there had been no behavioral re-sponse. When safety changes are largely invisible to the user, there is no evi-dence of any measurable human behavioral feedback. Likewise, when measures affect only the outcome of crashes, rather than their probability, no user re-sponses have been measured." Lund and O'Neill (1986) reached similar conclu-sions. These conclusions based on studies involving motor vehicles are likely to apply to other injury areas (e.g., falls, firearms) when changes in products or the environment alter perceived risks, but relevant studies are not available. One area that has received attention is child-resistant packaging. Concern was ex-pressed that child-resistant packaging would not decrease poisonings because, for example, parents would be prone to leave the bottles more accessible to children (Viscusi, 1984), but there is definitive evidence that child-resistant packaging does reduce child poisonings (Rodgers, 1996). Behavioral adaptation to safety improvements is an important area for future behavioral research.

The behavioral sciences also contribute to methodological advances in the study of injury causation and intervention effectiveness. They emphasize the importance of developing reliable, valid, and quantitative outcome measures related to attitudes, knowledge, and behaviors. This is extremely important for assessing the effectiveness of educational and regulatory interventions designed to induce behavioral change. They have also contributed to the refinement of study designs widely used in injury research, particularly by epidemiologists (see following section). A more prominent role for behavioral scientists in suicide and violence research is warranted, given the need for increasing methodological rigor in these areas of injury research (see NRC [1993, 1994, 1996, 1998]). Finally, behavioral research has cultivated new research tools, such as qualitative research. By using observation, in-depth interviews, and focus groups, qualita-tive research strives to make sense of, or interpret, a particular behavioral or clinical issue (Greenhalgh and Taylor, 1997). However, because it lacks quanti-tative rigor, qualitative research is best used to describe new phenomena and generate research questions and hypotheses (Poses and Isen, 1998).

The committee recommends intensified research on differences in risk perception, risk taking, and behavioral responses to safety im-provements among different segments of the population, particu-larly among those groups at highest risk of injury.

Epidemiology

The tools of epidemiology may be used to design studies to elucidate the nature or cause of injury and to determine the effectiveness of interventions. Over the past decade, epidemiologic studies have advanced the injury field by quantifying the relationship between risk factors and injury. Risk-factor identifi-cation ranges from identification of risky behavior and at-risk populations to proximate physical causes of energy exchange (e.g., contact points in vehicle interiors). As the injury field matures, research has to move away from a reliance on descriptive case studies and toward more rigorous analytical methodologies.

Randomized controlled trials (RCTs) are considered the gold standard in evaluating the effectiveness of interventions. Randomization maximizes the comparability of intervention and nonintervention groups with respect to factors that may influence the outcome of the trial. Through randomization to intervention and control groups, RCTs are designed to adjust for a variety of potential confounding factors. In addition, the investigator can control the conditions under which the trial is conducted to ensure that standardized procedures are followed. Although RCTs are expensive, time-consuming, and not always feasible, they are the standard in other fields of research and should be in injury research as well.

Cohort studies are used to compare the rate of injury of individuals exposed to a suspected risk factor with the rate of injury among individuals unexposed to the risk factor (Lilienfeld and Stolley, 1994). One major difficulty is that large numbers of individuals may have to be followed in order to capture a sufficient number of injuries for meaningful analysis of risk. The other major difficulty is the need to follow individuals over time. Together, these often make cohort studies expensive and logistically problematic. Increased attention should be devoted to the development of multi-institutional cooperation to maximize generalizability and spread the burden of subject follow-up. Better ways to ascertain exposure are needed for use in cohort studies of injury. Cost-efficient data collection methods that maintain data quality also are required.

Case-control studies compare injured individuals (cases) with those who are not injured (controls) in order to determine what characteristics are associated with the injury (e.g., lack of safety belt use in severe motor vehicle crashes). Case-control studies are especially useful in the identification of risk factors for rare events. To conduct studies over reasonable periods of time, it is often necessary for investigators at multiple sites to collaborate in order to accrue sufficient numbers of injuries for study. The limitations of case-control studies include vulnerability to recall bias, the possibility of confounding by unidentified factors, and the inability to definitively establish causality.

Recent variants of the case-control design have been used in injury research, including studies that compare persons with specified types of injuries to persons with other types of injuries and studies in which the site of death or injury is compared with a site where an injurious event did not occur (Wright and Robertson, 1976). Studies of the efficacy of helmets have compared bicyclists with head injuries to those with injuries to other regions of the body (McDermott et al., 1993; Thompson et al., 1996a). Another variant is a case-crossover study, which uses study participants as their own controls. This type of study compares behavior during the event (e.g., a crash or injury) with that preceding the event to determine whether participants were exposed to the factor of interest. For example, a case-crossover study was used to determine the risk associated with the use of cellular telephones in automobile crashes (Redelmeier and Tibshirani, 1997). Case-crossover studies control for variability in individual characteristics and are uniquely capable of identifying transient risk factors.

Researchers also employ ecologic study designs in which the investigator does not assign the exposure and in which the unit of analysis is a group rather than the individual subject. Injury epidemiologists frequently utilize ecologic designs to evaluate laws and regulations. These natural experiments allow comparisons of jurisdictions with a law to those without it, for example, comparing firearm fatality rates in two cities with different firearm laws (e.g., Sloan et al. [1988]); other times, a single jurisdiction after a law has taken effect is compared to the same jurisdiction before the law (time-series design). Time-series designs may use simple before-and-after comparisons, such as comparing fatal motor vehicle crash rates among young people before and after the passage of a law lowering the legal blood alcohol level for young drivers (e.g., Hingson et al. [1994]), but can also incorporate approaches that account for background secular trends. Interpretation of ecologic studies is difficult because, in addition to controlling all the normal sources of bias, researchers must also deal with ecologic bias and the failure of ecologic analyses to account for the distribution of confounders at the individual level.

Finally, case studies are a traditional research design that have yielded important advances in understanding causes of injury but frequently are misused. Case studies are vital when attempting to elucidate the physical mechanisms for excessive energy transmission. For example, the mechanisms by which occupants are injured during motor vehicle crashes were determined by thorough case investigations. However, case studies can be used only to ascertain directly observable proximate causes of injury. One common misuse of case studies is for study of risk factors for injury that are not directly observable, particularly indirect human factors such as fatigue or alcohol. Studies with comparison groups are the only scientifically valid method of quantifying the extent to which indirect risk factors contribute to injury causation.

The committee strongly recommends the utilization of rigorous analytical methods in injury research. Collaborations between research centers are critical for assembling populations and cohort groups necessary for conducting large-scale randomized controlled trials, cohort studies, and case-control studies.

Training and Research Funding

There is a dearth of funding for research training in injury prevention, except for occupational injuries. Although the latter is supported by the National Institute for Occupational Safety and Health (NIOSH), a unit of the Centers for Disease Control and Prevention with a long-standing commitment to pre- and postdoctoral training (see Chapter 8), there is no comparable training program anywhere in the federal government for injury prevention in a non-occupational setting. Such training has to emphasize the same interdisciplinary orientation that underlies the research described earlier in this chapter. Training should include epidemiology, biostatistics, program evaluation, engineering, ergonomics, economics, biomechanics, law, and behavioral sciences, all of which form the backbone of injury prevention. Recommendations for training in non-occupational prevention research have been made repeatedly by the National Research Council and the Institute of Medicine (NRC, 1985, 1988), but funding has not been forthcoming.

The lack of research training is a major barrier to the development of the field of injury prevention. Training attracts young people to a field and equips them for a lifelong commitment to research and education. A cadre of talented young researchers ensures the growth, innovation, and continuity of a field. Training programs are supported in every major field of public health, with the exception of injury prevention. (Treatment of trauma is supported by training programs of the National Institutes of Health; see Chapter 8.)

In addition to funds for training, the maintenance of a vital extramural research community will require adequate funding for investigator-initiated, peer-reviewed research grants. It is necessary to ensure viable careers for the country's best young researchers and to sustain experienced investigators. Investigator-initiated research should be encouraged to ensure the emergence of innovative approaches to injury research. To ensure the scientific rigor of this research, proposed projects should be peer-reviewed by scientists outside the sponsoring federal agencies. These points and the need for sustained federal research support are addressed further in Chapter 8.

Public health agencies need not be the only sources of research funding. There also are opportunities to recruit employers and health care payers as partners in funding prevention research. These organizations have strong economic incentives to support research that can lead to injury reductions. Injury reductions can yield cost savings, in terms of lower health care costs, workers' compensation costs, and indemnity costs. Moreover, the cost savings to payers can be realized almost immediately after the successful introduction of an intervention program. In contrast, cost savings from disease-oriented prevention programs take longer to realize because of the time lag between intervention and health outcome (e.g., reductions in stroke or heart attack). The immediacy of cost savings should be especially tantalizing for employers, because the total number of fatal and nonfatal job-related injuries is far higher (more than 13 million annually) than that for job-related illnesses (Leigh et al., 1997).

The committee recommends the expansion of research training opportunities by the relevant federal agencies (e.g., NCIPC, NIOSH, and the National Highway Traffic Safety Administration [NHTSA]). This includes an increase in the number of individual

and institutional training grants for injury prevention; research grant proposals should have independent peer review. Adequate federal funding must be forthcoming to sustain careers in the injury field.

Communicating Results

The scientific foundation of injury prevention has grown considerably over the past decade, having been cultivated by many different disciplines. As noted, researchers come from a variety of disparate disciplines. This has been a source of strength for the field and also at times an impediment in terms of scientific communication. The injury field lacks established channels of communication. This is illustrated in a variety of ways. One fundamental problem is that the terminology varies, depending on the discipline represented, for concepts related to risk perception, behavioral change, and prevention measures.

Another illustration of the problem is that the scientific literature in injury prevention is indexed in many different government and private-sector databases. No one database contains all of the injury literature. Assembling published research on motor vehicle safety presents a case in point. Articles are separated between the epidemiologic and the engineering research literature. Epidemiologists publish predominantly in the medical literature that is accessible through the National Library of Medicine's (NLM's) MEDLINE database. Automotive safety engineers publish predominantly in Society of Automotive Engineers (SAE) publications that are indexed and accessible only through a subscription to SAE databases. Additionally, NHTSA research publications are often not published in the peer-reviewed literature and can be located only through the National Technical Information Service's database of government reports. Other databases that index scientific literature relevant to the injury field include PsychLIT, Sociological Abstracts, Criminal Justice Periodical Index, National Criminal Justice Reference Service, EMBASE, and Transportation Research Information Services. To date, the field of injury research has generated little interest among those working in medical informatics. There are notable exceptions—for example, the focus on computer applications that support decision making in trauma care (Clarke et al., 1994; Ogunyemi et al., 1995, 1997).

Long-term consideration should be given to the opportunities that medical informatics and the Internet can offer. The NLM, in conjunction with relevant federal agencies, could explore the potential of linking injury-related databases by applying online metathesauri (e.g., NLM's Unified Medical Language System Metathesaurus). These approaches integrate diverse vocabularies by linking terms on the basis of conceptual, semantic, and lexical connections (Schuyler and Hole, 1993). Additionally, links could be explored on the Internet to the multiple databases that house the injury field's scientific literature. Although there are proprietary and search-fee considerations for some of these databases, at a minimum, links to the databases have to be forged.

Problems in the communication of research significantly inhibit opportunities for cross-fertilization, collaboration, and growth of the field. The committee encourages the creation of an organization of injury prevention researchers, analogous to scientific organizations that have emerged in other interdisciplinary areas (e.g., College of Problems of Drug Dependence). Such an organization could sponsor annual research conferences, where injury researchers would present the results of new and encouraging research, and could support the development of an injury prevention research journal and electronic networks and work to solve the problems associated with database linkages. A new organization would have far-reaching effects in mobilizing injury prevention researchers.

SUMMARY

Scientific inquiry has transformed our notions of injury from accidental, unavoidable occurrences to events that are predictable and amenable to prevention. The development of future prevention interventions to address injury and the evaluation of the success of these interventions require a national commitment to expanding the scientific foundation for injury prevention. Support for injury prevention research should be commensurate with the enormous toll of injury on society. In particular, biomechanics, residential and recreational injuries, suicide, and violence are areas of research in need of higher priority. A national, long-term commitment to the expansion of interdisciplinary research and training in injury prevention is essential to public health. Without this commitment, injury research will not achieve the sophistication necessary for effective intervention development; talented new researchers will not be attracted to the field; and existing injury researchers may be forced to leave the field. In short, without a national commitment, the field of injury science will stagnate and the unnecessary toll of injury will persist.

REFERENCES

Baker SP, O'Neill B, Ginsburg MJ, Li G. 1992. *The Injury Fact Book*. New York: Oxford University Press.

Baker-Dickman F. 1987. *Sobriety Checkpoints for DWI Enforcement: A Review of Current Research*. Washington, DC: National Highway Traffic Safety Administration.

Barke RP, Jenkins-Smith H, Slovic P. 1997. Risk perceptions of men and women scientists. *Social Science Quarterly* 78(1):167–176.

Barlow B, Niemirska M, Gandhi RP, Leblanc W. 1983. Ten years of experience with falls from a height in children. *Journal of Pediatric Surgery* 18:509–511.

Berger LR, Saunders S, Armitage K, Schauer L. 1984. Promoting the use of car safety devices for infants: An intensive health education approach. *Pediatrics* 74:16–19.

Bien TH, Miller WR, Tonigan JS. 1993. Brief interventions for alcohol problems: A review. *Addiction* 88:315–335.

BJS (Bureau of Justice Statistics). 1997. *Criminal Victimization in the United States, 1994.* Washington, DC: BJS. NCJ162126. [World Wide Web document]. URL http://www.ojp.usdoj.gov/bjs/abstract/cvius94.htm (accessed August 1998).

Bonnie R. 1986. The efficacy of law as a paternalistic instrument. In: Melton G, ed. *Nebraska Symposium on Human Motivation, 1985: The Law as a Behavioral Instrument.* Lincoln, NE: University of Nebraska Press. Pp. 131–211.

Brent DA, Perper JA, Allman CJ, Moritz GM, Wartella ME, Zelenak JP. 1991. The presence and accessibility of firearms in the homes of adolescent suicides. *Journal of the American Medical Association* 266(21):2989–2995.

Brent DA, Perper JA, Moritz G, Baugher M, Schweers, Roth C. 1993. Firearms and adolescent suicide: A community case-control study. *American Journal of Diseases of Children* 147:1066–1071.

Brown JH. 1979. Suicide in Britain. *Archives of General Psychiatry* 36:1119–1124.

CDC (Centers for Disease Control and Prevention). 1985. Update: Childhood poisonings—United States. *Morbidity and Mortality Weekly Report* 34(9):26 27.

CDC (Centers for Disease Control and Prevention). 1991. Child passenger restraint use and motor-vehicle-related fatalities among children, United States, 1982 1990. *Morbidity and Mortality Weekly Report* 40(34):600–602.

CDC (Centers for Disease Control and Prevention). 1996. *Healthy People 2000: Violent and Abusive Behavior Progress Review, 1996.* Atlanta, GA: CDC.

Chaiken JM, Lawless MW, Stevenson KA. 1974. The impact of police activity on subway crime. *Urban Analysis* 3:173–205.

Chesnut RM. 1997. The management of severe traumatic brain injury. *Emergency Medicine Clinics of North America* 15(3):581–604.

Christophersen ER, Sullivan MA. 1982. Increasing the protection of newborn infants in cars. *Pediatrics* 70:21–25.

Clarke JR, Webber BL, Gertner A, Kaye J, Rymon R. 1994. On-line decision support for emergency trauma management. *Proceedings of the Annual Symposium on Computer Applications in Medical Care.* P. 1028.

Cook PJ, Moore MJ. 1993. Taxation of alcoholic beverages. In: Hilton ME, Bloss G, eds. *Economics and the Prevention of Alcohol-Related Problems.* Rockville, MD: National Institute on Alcohol Abuse and Alcoholism. Research Monograph No. 25. NIH Publication No. 93-3513.

Davidson LL, Durkin MS, Kuhn L, O'Connor P, Barlow B, Heagarty MC. 1994. The impact of the Safe Kids/Healthy Neighborhoods Injury Prevention Program in Harlem, 1988 through 1991. *American Journal of Public Health* 84(4):580–586.

Denny-Brown DE, Russell WR. 1941. Experimental cerebral concussion. *Brain* 64:93–164.

Dewees DN, David D, Trebilcock MJ. 1996. *Exploring the Domain of Accident Law: Taking the Facts Seriously.* New York: Oxford University Press.

Dole EJ, Czajka PA, Rivara FP. 1986. Evaluation of pharmacists' compliance with the Poison Prevention Act. *American Journal of Public Health* 76:1335–1336.

Durkin MS, Kuhn L, Davidson LL, Laraque D, Barlow B. 1996. Epidemiology and prevention of severe assault and gun injuries to children in an urban community. *Journal of Trauma* 41(4):667–673.

Durkin MS, Olsen S, Barlow B, Virella A, Connolly ES. 1998. The epidemiology of urban pediatric neurological trauma: Evaluation of, and implications for, injury prevention programs. *Neurosurgery* 42(2):300–310.

Elliott DC, Rodriguez A. 1996. Cost effectiveness in trauma care. *Surgical Clinics of North America* 76(1):47–62.

Erdmann TC, Feldman KW, Rivara FP, Heimbach DM, Wall HA. 1991. Tap water burn prevention: The effect of legislation. *Pediatrics* 88(3):572–577.

Esterhai JL Jr, Brighton CT, Heppenstall RB, Thrower A. 1986. Nonunion of the humerus. Clinical, roentgenographic, scintigraphic, and response characteristics to treatment with constant direct current stimulation of osteogenesis. *Clinical Orthopaedics and Related Research* 211:228–234.

Evans L. 1991. *Traffic Safety and the Driver.* New York: Van Nostrand Reinhold.

Fingerhut LA, Warner M. 1997. *Injury Chartbook. Health, United States, 1996–97.* Hyattsville, MD: National Center for Health Statistics.

Flynn J, Slovic P, Mertz CK. 1994. Gender, race, and perception of environmental health risks. *Risk Analysis* 14(6):1101–1108.

Folsom AR, Mink PJ, Sellars TA, Hong CP, Zheng W, Potter JD. 1995. Hormonal replacement therapy and morbidity and mortality in a prospective study of postmenopausal women. *American Journal of Public Health* 85(8 Pt 1):1128–1132.

GAO (General Accounting Office). 1998. *Suicide Prevention: Efforts to Increase Research and Education in Palliative Care.* Washington, DC: GAO. GAO/HEHS-98-128.

Gould MS, Wallenstein S, Kleinman MH, O'Carroll P, Mercy J. 1990. Suicide clusters: An examination of age-specific effects. *American Journal of Public Health* 80(2):211–212.

Grady D, Rubin SM, Petitti DB, Fox CS, Black D, Ettinger B, Ernster VL, Cummings SR. 1992. Hormone therapy to prevent disease and prolong life in postmenopausal women. *Annals of Internal Medicine* 117:1016–1037.

Graham DI, Gentleman SM, Lynch A, Roberts GW. 1995. Distribution of beta-amyloid protein in the brain following severe head injury. *Neuropathology and Applied Neurobiology* 21(1):27–34.

Graham DI, Gentleman SM, Nicoll JA, Royston MC, McKenzie JE, Roberts GW, Griffin WS. 1996. Altered beta-APP metabolism after head injury and its relationship to the aetiology of Alzheimer's disease. *Acta Neurochirurgica—Supplementum (Wien)* 66:96–102.

Graham JD. 1993. Injuries from traffic crashes: Meeting the challenge. *Annual Review of Public Health* 14:515–543.

Greenhalgh T, Taylor R. 1997. How to read a paper: Papers that go beyond numbers (qualitative research). *British Medical Journal* 315:740–743.

Haddon W Jr, Sussman EA, Klein D. 1964. *Accident Research: Methods and Approaches.* New York: Harper and Row.

Haut R, Ide T, Decamp C. 1995. Mechanical responses of the rabbit patello-femoral joint to blunt impact. *Journal of Biomechanical Engineering* 117:402–408.

Henry MC, Hollander JE, Alicandro JM, Cassara G, O'Malley S, Thode HC. 1996. Prospective countywide evaluation of the effects of motor vehicle safety device use on hospital resource use and injury severity. *Annals of Emergency Medicine* 28:627–634.

Hingson R, Heeren T, Winter M. 1994. Lower legal blood alcohol limits for young drivers. *Public Health Reports* 109:738–744.

Insurance Research Council. 1994. *Auto Injuries: Claiming Behavior and Its Impact on Insurance Costs*. Oak Brook, IL: Insurance Research Council.

IOM (Institute of Medicine). 1991. *Disability in America: Toward a National Agenda for Prevention*. Washington, DC: National Academy Press.

IOM (Institute of Medicine). 1994. *AIDS and Behavior: An Integrated Approach*. Washington, DC: National Academy Press.

IOM (Institute of Medicine). 1996. *Pathways of Addiction: Opportunities in Drug Abuse Research*. Washington, DC: National Academy Press.

IOM (Institute of Medicine). 1997. *Enabling America: Assessing the Role of Rehabilitation Science and Engineering*. Washington, DC: National Academy Press.

IOM (Institute of Medicine). 1998. *Scientific Opportunities and Public Needs: Improving Priority Setting and Public Input at the National Institutes of Health*. Washington, DC: National Academy Press.

Irwin CE, Cataldo MF, Matheny AP, Peterson L. 1992. Health consequences of behaviors: Injury as a model. *Pediatrics* 90(5):798–807.

Jacobs JB. 1989. *Drunk Driving: An American Dilemma*. Chicago: University of Chicago Press.

Janda DH, Wojtys EM, Hankin FM, Benedict ME. 1988. Softball sliding injuries: A prospective study comparing standard and modified bases. *Journal of the American Medical Association* 259(12):1848–1850.

Kachur SP, Potter LB, James SP, Powell KE. 1995. *Suicide in the United States, 1980–1992*. Atlanta, GA: National Center for Injury Prevention and Control. Violence Surveillance Summary Series, No. 1.

Kahane CJ. 1989. *An Evaluation of Center-Mounted Stop Lamps Based on 1987 Data*. Washington, DC: National Highway Traffic Safety Administration. Report DOT-HS-807-442.

Kahneman D, Slovic P, Tversky A. 1982. *Judgment Under Uncertainty: Heuristics and Biases*. Cambridge, England: Cambridge University Press.

Katcher ML, Landry GL, Shapiro MM. 1989. Liquid-crystal thermometer use in pediatric office counseling about tap water burn prevention. *Pediatrics* 83:766–771.

Kellerman AL, Rivara FP, Somes G, Reay DT, Francisco J, Banton JG, Prodzinski J, Fligner C, Hackman BB. 1992. Suicide in the home in relation to gun ownership. *New England Journal of Medicine* 327(7):467–472.

King AI, Ruan JS, Zhou C, Hardy WN, Khalil TB. 1995. Recent advances in biomechanics of brain injury research: A review. *Journal of Neurotrauma* 12(4):651–658.

Kitzman H, Olds DL, Henderson CR Jr, Hanks C, Cole R, Tatelbaum R, McConnochie KM, Sidora K, Luckey DW, Shaver D, Engelhardt K, James D, Barnard K. 1997. Effect of prenatal and infancy home visitation by nurses on pregnancy outcomes, childhood injuries and repeated childbearing. A randomized control trial. *Journal of the American Medical Association* 278(8):644–652.

Kraus JF. 1985. Effectiveness of measures to prevent unintentional deaths of infants and children from suffocation and strangulation. *Public Health Reports* 100(2):231–240.

Kreitman N. 1976. The coal gas story: United Kingdom suicide rates, 1960–1971. *British Journal of Preventive and Social Medicine* 30:89–93.

Laraque D, Barlow B, Durkin M, Heagarty M. 1995. Injury prevention in an urban setting: Challenges and successes. *Bulletin of the New York Academy of Medicine* 72:16–30.

Lauritzen JB, Petersen MM, Lund B. 1993. Effect of external hip protectors on hip fractures. *Lancet* 341:11–13.

Leigh JP, Markowitz SB, Fahs M, Shin C, Landrigan PJ. 1997. Occupational injury and illness in the United States: Estimates of costs, morbidity, and mortality. *Archives of Internal Medicine* 157(14):1557–1568.

Lilienfeld DE, Stolley PD. 1994. *Foundation of Epidemiology*, 3rd edition. New York: Oxford University Press.

Liu XZ, Xu XM, Hu R, Du C, Zhang SX, McDonald JW, Dong HX, Wu YJ, Fan GS, Jacquin MF, Hsu CY, Choi DW. 1997. Neuronal and glial cell apoptosis after traumatic spinal cord injury. *Journal of Neuroscience* 17(14):5395–5406.

Lund AK, O'Neill B. 1986. Perceived risks and driving behavior. *Accident Analysis and Prevention* 18(5):367–370.

Maimaris C, Summers CL, Browning C, Palmer CR. 1994. Injury patterns in cyclists attending an accident and emergency department: A comparison of helmet wearers and non-wearers. *British Medical Journal* 308(6943):1537–1540.

Mallonee S, Istre GR, Rosenberg M, Reddish-Douglas M, Jordan F, Silverstein P, Tunell W. 1996. Surveillance and prevention of residential-fire injuries. *New England Journal of Medicine* 335(1):27–31.

Margulies SS, Thibault LE. 1992. A proposed tolerance criterion for diffuse axonal injury in man. *Journal of Biomechanics* 25(8):917–923.

McDermott FT, Lane JC, Brazenor GA, Debney EA. 1993. The effectiveness of bicyclist helmets: A study of 1710 casualties. *Journal of Trauma* 34(6):834–844.

McDowall D, Loftin C, Wiersma D. 1992. A comparative study of the preventive effects of mandatory sentencing laws for gun crimes. *Journal of Criminal Law and Criminology* 83(2):378–394.

McElhaney JH, Roberts VL, Hilyard JF. 1976. *Handbook of Human Tolerance*. Tokyo: Automobile Research Institute, Inc.

McKnight AJ, McPherson K. 1986. Evaluation of peer intervention training for high school alcohol safety education. *Accident Analysis and Prevention* 18(4):339–347.

McKnight AJ, Streff FM. 1994. The effect of enforcement upon service of alcohol to intoxicated patrons of bars and restaurants. *Accident Analysis and Prevention* 26(1):79–88.

McKnight AJ, Shinar D, Reizes A. 1989. *The Effects of Center High-Mounted Stop Lamp on Vans and Trucks*. Washington, DC: National Highway Traffic Safety Administration. Report DOT-HS-807-506.

McLoughlin E, Clarke N, Stahl K, Crawford JD. 1977. One pediatric burn unit's experience with sleepwear-related injuries. *Pediatrics* 60(4):405–409.

McLoughlin E, Vince C, Lee A, Crawford JD. 1982. Project Burn Prevention: Outcome and implications. *American Journal of Public Health* 72(3):241–247.

Meehan PJ, Lamb JA, Saltzman LE, O'Carroll PW. 1992. Attempted suicide among young adults: Progress toward a meaningful estimate of prevalence. *American Journal of Psychiatry* 149:41–44.

Mercy JA, Rosenberg ML, Powell KE, Broome CV, Roper WL. 1993. Public health policy for preventing violence. *Health Affairs* 12(4):7–29.

Meunier PJ, Chapuy MC, Arlot ME, Delmas PD, Duboeuf F. 1994. Can we stop bone loss and prevent hip fractures in the elderly. *Osteoporosis International* 4(Suppl. 1): 71–76.

Miller TR, Galbraith M. 1995. Injury prevention counseling by pediatricians: A benefit-cost comparison. *Pediatrics* 96:1–4.

Moore MH. 1993. Violence prevention: Criminal justice or public health. *Health Affairs* 12(4):34–45.

Moore MH, Prothrow-Stith D, Guyer B, Spivak H. 1993. Violence and intentional injuries: Criminal justice and public health perspectives on an urgent national problem. In: *Understanding and Preventing Violence, Vol. 3.* Washington, DC: National Academy Press.

Nahum AM, Melvin JW. 1993. *Accidental Injury: Biomechanics and Prevention.* New York: Springer-Verlag.

National Committee (National Committee for Injury Prevention and Control). 1989. *Injury Prevention: Meeting the Challenge.* New York: Oxford University Press. Published as a supplement to the *American Journal of Preventive Medicine* 5(3).

NCIPC (National Center for Injury Prevention and Control). 1996. *1996 Fact Book.* Atlanta, GA: Centers for Disease Control and Prevention.

Newberry W, Zukosky D, Haut R. 1997. Subfracture insult to a knee joint causes alterations in bone and in the functional stiffness of overlying cartilage. *Journal of Orthopaedic Research* 15:450–455.

NHTSA (National Highway Traffic Safety Administration). 1996. *Effectiveness of Occupant Protection Systems and Their Use: Third Report to Congress.* Washington, DC: NHTSA.

NHTSA (National Highway Traffic Safety Administration. 1998. *NHTSA Proposes New Child Crash Dummy.* [World Wide Web document]. URL http:www.dot.gov/affairs/nhtsa3398.htm (accessed September 1998).

Ni H, Sacks JJ, Curtis L, Cieslak PR, Hedberg K. 1997. Evaluation of a statewide bicycle helmet law via multiple measures of helmet use. *Archives of Pediatric and Adolescent Medicine* 151:59–65.

NIH (National Institutes of Health). 1994. *NIH Task Force on Trauma Research.* Bethesda, MD: NIH.

NIMH (National Institute of Mental Health). 1998. Suicide research program. [World Wide Web document]. URL http://www.nimh.gov/research/suicide.htm (accessed May 1998).

NRC (National Research Council). 1985. *Injury in America: A Continuing Public Health Problem.* Washington, DC: National Academy Press.

NRC (National Research Council). 1988. *Injury Control: A Review of the Status and Progress of the Injury Control Program at the Centers for Disease Control.* Washington, DC: National Academy Press.

NRC (National Research Council). 1989. *Improving Risk Communication.* Washington, DC: National Academy Press.

NRC (National Research Council). 1993. *Understanding and Preventing Violence.* Washington, DC: National Academy Press.

NRC (National Research Council) and the John F. Kennedy School of Government, Harvard University. 1994. *Violence in Urban America: Mobilizing a Response.* Washington, DC: National Academy Press.

NRC (National Research Council). 1996. *Understanding Violence Against Women.* Washington, DC: National Academy Press.

NRC (National Research Council). 1998. *Violence in Families: Assessing Prevention and Treatment Programs.* Washington, DC: National Academy Press.

NTSB (National Transportation Safety Board). 1998. *Aviation Accident Statistics.* [World Wide Web document]. URL http://www.ntsb.gov/aviation/Stats.htm (accessed September 1998).

Ogunyemi O, Kaye J, Webber B, Clarke JR. 1995. Generating penetration path hypotheses for decision support in multiple trauma. *Proceedings of the Annual Symposium on Computer Applications in Medical Care.* Pp. 42–46.

Ogunyemi O, Webber B, Clarke JR. 1997. Probabilistic predictions of penetrating injury to anatomic structures. *Proceeding of the AMIA Annual Fall Symposium.* Pp. 714–718.

Olds DL, Eckenrode J, Henderson CR Jr, Kitzman H, Powers J, Cole R, Sidora K, Morris P, Pettitt LM, Luckey D. 1997. Long-term effects of home visitation on maternal life course and child abuse and neglect. *Journal of the American Medical Association* 278(8):637–643.

Paganini-Hill A, Chao A, Ross RK, Henderson BE. 1991. Exercise and other risk factors in the prevention of hip fracture: The Leisure World study. *Epidemiology* 2(1):16–25.

Persson J, Magnusson PH. 1989. Early interventions in patients with excessive consumption of alcohol: A controlled study. *Alcohol* 6:403–408.

Poses RM, Isen AM. 1998. Qualitative research in medicine and health care: Questions and controversy. *Journal of General Internal Medicine* 13:32–38.

Province MA, Hadley EC, Hornbrook EC, Lipsitz LA, Miller JP, Mulrow CD, Ory MG, Sattin RW, Tinetti ME, Wolf SL. 1995. The effects of exercise on falls in elderly patients: A preplanned meta-analysis of the FICSIT Trials: Fraility and Injuries: Cooperative Studies of Intervention Techniques. *Journal of the American Medical Association* 273:1341–1347.

Rausch A, Wong J, Kirkpatrick M. 1982. A field test of two single center high mounted brake light systems. *Accident Analysis and Prevention* 14(4):287–291.

Redelmeier DA, Tibshirani RJ. 1997. Association between cellular-telephone calls and motor vehicle collisions. *New England Journal of Medicine* 336(7):453–458.

Reyna VF, Ellis SC. 1992. Fuzzy-trace theory and framing effect in children's risky decision making. *Psychological Science* 5(5):275–279.

Rink A, Fung KM, Trojanowski JQ, Lee VM, Neugebauer E, McIntosh TK. 1995. Evidence of apoptotic cell death after experimental traumatic brain injury in the rat. *American Journal of Pathology* 147(6):1575–1583.

Rivara FP, Grossman DC, Cummings P. 1997a. Injury prevention. First of two parts. *New England Journal of Medicine* 337(8):543–548.

Rivara FP, Grossman DC, Cummings P. 1997b. Injury prevention. Second of two parts. *New England Journal of Medicine* 337(9):613–618.

Roberts GW, Gentleman SM, Lynch A, Murray L, Landon M, Graham DI. 1994. Beta amyloid protein deposition in the brain after severe head injury: Implications for the pathogenesis of Alzheimer's disease. *Journal of Neurology, Neurosurgery, and Psychiatry* 57(4):419–425.

Robertson L. 1992. *Injury Epidemiology.* New York: Oxford University Press.

Rodgers GB. 1996. The safety effects of child-resistant packaging for oral prescription drugs. Two decades of experience. *Journal of the American Medical Association* 275(21):1661–1665.

Room R, Bondy SJ, Ferris, J. 1995. The risk of harm to oneself from drinking, Canada 1989. *Addiction* 90(4):499–513.

Rose-Ackerman S. 1991. Tort law in the regulatory state. In: Schuck PH, ed. *Tort Law and the Public Interest.* New York: Norton. Pp. 105–126.

Ross HL. 1993. Punishment as a factor is preventing alcohol-related accidents. *Addiction* 88:997–1002.

Runyan CW, Bangdiwala SI, Linzer MA, Sacks JJ, Butts J. 1992. Risk factors for fatal residential fires. *New England Journal of Medicine* 37(12):859–863.

Saatman KE, Murai H, Bartus RT, Smith DH, Hayward NJ, Perri BR, McIntosh TK. 1996. Calpain inhibitor AK295 attenuates motor and cognitive deficits following experimental brain injury in the rat. *Proceedings of the National Academy of Sciences (USA)* 93(8):3428–3433.

SAFE KIDS (National SAFE KIDS Campaign). 1998. *Safe Kids at Home, at Play, and on the Way: A Report to the Nation on Unintentional Childhood Injury.* Washington, DC: National SAFE KIDS Campaign.

Schieber RA, Branche-Dorsey CM, Ryan GW, Rutherford GW, Stevens JA, O'Neil J. 1996. Risk factors for injuries from in-line skating and the effectiveness of safety gear. *New England Journal of Medicine* 335:1630–1635.

Schuyler PL, Hole WT. 1993. The UMLS Metathesaurus: Representing different views of biomedical concepts. *Bulletin of the Medical Library Association* 81(2):217–221.

Shaffer D, Garland A, Fisher P, Trautman P. 1988. Preventing teenage suicide: A critical review. *Journal of the American Academy of Child and Adolescent Psychiatry* 27:675–687.

Singh GK, Yu SM. 1996. U.S. childhood mortality, 1950 through 1993: Trends and socioeconomic differentials. *American Journal of Public Health* 86(4):505–512.

Sloan JH, Kellermann AL, Reay DT, Ferris JA, Koepsell T, Rivara FP, Rice C, Gray LG, LoGerfo J. 1988. Handgun regulations, crime, assaults, and homicide: A tale of two cities. *New England Journal of Medicine* 319:1256–1262.

Slovic P, Fischhoff B, Lichtenstein S. 1982. Facts and fears: Understanding perceived risk. In: Kahneman D, Slovic P, Tversky A, eds. *Judgment Under Uncertainty: Heuristics and Biases.* Cambridge, England: Cambridge University Press. Pp. 181–216.

Spiegel CN, Lindaman FC. 1977. Children can't fly: A program to prevent childhood morbidity and mortality from window falls. *American Journal of Public Health* 76:1143–1147.

Stapp JP. 1955. Effects of mechanical force on living tissue: I. Abrupt deceleration and windblast. *Journal of Aviation Medicine* 26:268–288.

Sugarman SD. 1990. The need to reform personal injury law leaving scientific disputes to scientists. *Science* 249(4957):823–827.

Thompson DC, Rivara FP, Thompson RS. 1996a. Effectiveness of bicycle safety helmets in preventing head injuries: A case-control study. *Journal of the American Medical Association* 276(24):1968–1973.

Thompson DC, Nunn ME, Thompson RS, Rivara FP. 1996b. Effectiveness of bicycle safety helmets in preventing serious facial injury. *Journal of the American Medical Association* 276(24):1974–1975.

Thompson RS, Rivara FP, Thompson DC. 1989. A case-control study on the effectiveness of bicycle safety helmets. *New England Journal of Medicine* 320(21):1361–1367.

Tinetti ME, Baker DI, Garrett PA, Gottschalk M, Koch ML, Horwitz RI. 1993. Yale FICSIT: Risk factor abatement strategy for fall prevention. *Journal of the American Geriatric Society* 41:315–320.

Tinetti ME, Baker DI, McAvay G, Claus EB, Garrett P, Gottschalk M, Koch ML, Trainor K, Horwitz RI. 1994. A multifactorial intervention to reduce the risk of falling among elderly people living in the community. *New England Journal of Medicine* 331:821–827.

TRB (Transportation Research Board, National Research Council). 1984. *55: A Decade of Experience*. Washington, DC: TRB. Special Report 204.

TRB (Transportation Research Board, National Research Council). 1990. *Safety Research for a Changing Highway Environment*. Washington, DC: TRB.

U.S. DHHS (U.S. Department of Health and Human Services). 1986. *Surgeon General's Workshop on Violence and Public Health*. October 27–29, 1985. DHHS Publication No. HRS-D-MC 86-1.

U.S. DHHS (U.S. Department of Health and Human Services). 1992. *Position Papers from the Third National Injury Conference, Setting the National Agenda for Injury Control in the 1990s, April 22–25, 1991, Denver, CO.* Washington, DC: DHHS.

U.S. Preventive Services Task Force. 1996. *Guide to Clinical Preventive Services*, 2d edition. Baltimore: Williams and Wilkins.

Ventura SJ, Peters KD, Martin JA, Maurer JD. 1997. Births and deaths: United States, 1996. *Monthly Vital Statistics Report* 46(1 Suppl. 2):1-40.

Viano DC, King AI, Melvin JW, Weber K. 1989. Injury biomechanics research: An essential element in the prevention of trauma. *Journal of Biomechanics* 22(5):403–417.

Viscusi WK. 1984. The lulling effect: The impact of child resistant packaging on aspirin and analgesic ingestions. *American Economic Review* 74(2):324–327.

Viscusi WK. 1992. *Fatal Tradeoffs*. New York: Oxford University Press.

Viscusi WK, Magat WA. 1995. *Informational Approaches to Regulation*. Cambridge, MA: MIT Press.

Wagenaar AC, Webster DW. 1986. Preventing injuries to children through compulsory automobile safety seat use. *Pediatrics* 78(4):662–672.

Womble KB. 1988. *The Impact of Minimum Drinking Age Laws on Fatal Crash Involvements: An Update of the NHTSA Analysis*. Washington, DC: NHTSA.

Wright PH, Robertson LS. 1976. Priorities for roadside hazard modification: A study of 300 fatal roadside object crashes. In: *Proceedings of the Twentieth Conference of the American Association for Automotive Medicine*. Arlington Heights, IL: American Association for Automotive Medicine. Pp. 114–127.

Zimring FE, Hawkins G. 1997. *Crime Is Not the Problem: Lethal Violence in America*. New York: Oxford University Press.

Zuckerman M. 1993. P-impulsive sensation seeking and its behavioral, psychophysiological and biochemical correlates. *Neuropsychobiology* 28(1–2):30–36.

5

Case Studies on Prevention

The two leading mechanisms causing fatal injury in the United States are motor vehicles and firearms; in 1995, 42,452 people died from motor vehicle traffic injuries and 35,957 people died as a result of firearm injuries (Fingerhut and Warner, 1997). Over the past three decades, dramatic progress has been made in reducing motor vehicle injuries by understanding the factors that increase the risk of injury, designing interventions to reduce these risks, implementing and evaluating a wide array of interventions and assessing their benefits and costs, and providing a scientific foundation for individual and business choices and public policy judgments. However, a similar comprehensive multidisciplinary approach has not been taken in relation to firearm injuries. The goal of this chapter is to explore the comprehensive approach that has been utilized successfully to promote motor vehicle safety and to recommend steps that could be taken to implement a similar effort to reduce firearm injuries.

MOTOR VEHICLE INJURIES

Although motor vehicle crashes remain the single largest cause of injury deaths in the United States, rates of motor vehicle deaths have declined substantially over the past 25 years, especially when the increasing numbers of drivers and the number of miles traveled are taken into account (Figure 5.1). Yearly fluctuations in the numbers of motor vehicle deaths (reaching a high of 56,278 in 1972) have taken place against a backdrop of increasing levels of exposure, including an increase in the number of licensed drivers and an increase in motor vehicle travel (NSC, 1997). In 1930, the number of miles driven in the United States was 206 billion, and the death rate was 15.97 per 100 million miles; in 1972, 1,268 billion

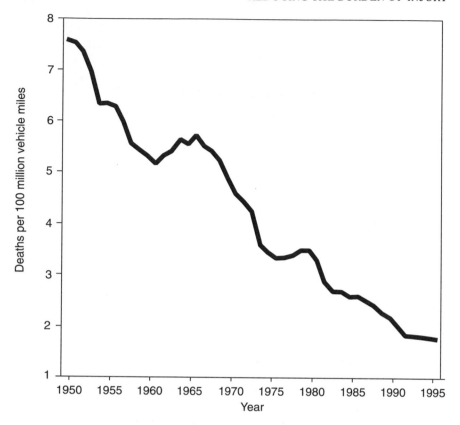

FIGURE 5.1 Motor vehicle traffic injury deaths per 100 million vehicle miles in the United States, 1950–1996. SOURCE: National Safety Council, 1997.

miles were driven, with a death rate of 4.43; and in 1996, the figure was 2,467 billion miles driven, with a death rate of 1.76 per 100 million miles. Had the mileage death rate of 1972 prevailed in 1996, the number of deaths would have been almost 110,000 rather than 43,399. It has been estimated that between 1966 and 1990, 243,400 lives were saved as a result of federal highway, traffic, and motor vehicle safety programs (NHTSA and FHWA, 1991).

Reasons for Progress: A Comprehensive Approach

For the first six decades of motor vehicle traffic on the highways, the federal and state governments worked primarily on building and improving highways and roads, while state and local governments regulated who could drive and how; vehicle design was left to the marketplace. In most respects during those years the focus on reducing motor vehicle injury was on improving drivers' skills (Waller, 1994). Although the vehicles offered for sale in the 1950s were safer in many respects than those of earlier decades, the technology for protecting occupants in a crash had developed still further and offered potential gains in safety that were not being put into production (DeHaven, 1942; Stapp, 1957).

In recent years, an increasingly sophisticated and comprehensive approach to the motor vehicle injury problem has developed that addresses safety issues for the driver, occupant, vehicle, and highway system (CDC, 1994). The conceptualization of this approach has been based largely on the work of William Haddon, who developed models for the systematic exploration of countermeasures to reduce or prevent injuries involving components of the causal sequence leading to injury—pre-crash, crash, and post-crash events (see Chapter 1 for a fuller description of the Haddon matrix; Haddon [1972, 1980]). When applied to motor vehicle safety, this approach involves addressing issues concerning the host (driver and passenger), agent (vehicle), and environment (roads and highways). The effort to reduce motor vehicle injuries has been both sustained and multipronged, involving surveillance systems; regulatory measures; behavioral, biomedical, and engineering research; state and local programs; and public support. This comprehensive, data-driven approach has been supported by stable federal funding and involves efforts at the federal, state, local, and private-sector levels.

Surveillance

National data systems have been instrumental in allowing trends in motor vehicle injuries to be tracked and injury patterns identified and in assessing the outcomes of prevention interventions. Data systems include the National Vital Statistics System, with information on deaths in the United States; the Fatality Analysis Reporting System (FARS), an in-depth collection of data on all fatal motor vehicle crashes on public roads; and the National Automotive Sampling System, which consists of the Crashworthiness Data System that collects detailed data through crash investigations and hospital injury data and the General Estimates System, a national probability sample of police-reported crashes. The federal government has also made major efforts to improve the quality and consistency of state data systems and has fostered linkages of data systems (e.g., police crash reports and hospital data). These data systems have been used both to identify research questions of importance and to address such questions with high-quality data.

Surveillance data were essential for the enactment and assessment of legislation establishing the minimum age for the purchase of alcoholic beverages. In the early 1970s, about half of the states lowered their minimum age for alcohol purchase, from 21 to 18 in most cases. Beginning in 1976, states reversed course and began to raise the minimum age, a trend that continued into the early 1980s. Multistate research based on FARS and vital statistics data showed the beneficial effects of this reversal on a national level (Cook and Tauchen, 1984; GAO, 1987). Without these data, it would have been necessary to try to obtain data for a large number of states and determine which data elements were comparable, a difficult task, or to rely on the accumulation of single-state studies, which by themselves are often unreliable because of small sample sizes. The research findings were instrumental in leading to federal legislation that influenced states to establish 21 as the minimum age for purchase of alcohol or to lose federal highway funds (Wagenaar, 1993). This policy is now in effect in all states and is credited with having saved 16,513 lives from 1975 through 1996 (NHTSA, 1996).

Regulation and Legislation

In 1966, legislation was enacted that marked a significant change in the nation's approach to reducing motor vehicle injuries. The National Highway Traffic and Motor Vehicle Safety Act authorized the federal government to set safety standards for new vehicles and equipment, and the Highway Safety Act of 1966 authorized the federal government to develop a coordinated national highway safety program. The two acts legislated, for the first time, a comprehensive national program addressing the human, vehicular, and environmental factors that lead to motor vehicle injuries. They allowed for the development of safety standards for new vehicles and equipment and also targeted human factors (e.g., driver fatigue, effects of alcohol on driving). In 1967, the National Highway Safety Bureau issued highway program standards that were to be adopted by the states, including requirements for driver education, driver licensing, alcohol countermeasures, school bus safety, and motorcycle safety laws. States had to report on annual progress and could be penalized by the withholding of federal highway funds if the programs were not implemented. Thus, many states enacted new safety programs and legislation to meet federal requirements.

The passage of the Highway Safety Act of 1970 established the National Highway Traffic Safety Administration (NHTSA) as the successor to the National Highway Safety Bureau. NHTSA was charged with the responsibility of reducing deaths, injuries, and economic losses resulting from motor vehicle crashes and had regulatory, surveillance, research, and programmatic responsibilities, a mission and charges that it continues to implement. Additionally, the Federal Highway Administration works to improve highway safety and has regulatory jurisdiction over the safety performance of interstate commercial motor carriers and those carriers transporting hazardous materials. The federal regulatory program is designed to raise vehicle and highway safety standards and, despite legal impediments (Mashaw and Harfst, 1990), has led to a vehicle fleet that is far more crashworthy than 30 years ago. Initial resistance to federal regulation of vehicles has gradually subsided, so that there is currently a more cooperative relationship between federal regulatory agencies and industry.

In addition to federal regulation, states and local governments have extensive regulatory and administrative responsibilities for highway safety, including driver licensing, driver education programs, motor vehicle inspections, setting speed limits, highway and road design and maintenance upgrades, and legislation and enforcement of traffic safety laws including those on alcohol-impaired driving, safety belt use, and use of child safety seats.

The national objective of reducing motor vehicle injuries has been pursued under the constraint that regulations were to be aimed at improving safety per vehicle mile, without attempting to influence the amount that people drive. Policies such as improved public transportation, higher gas taxes, mixed-use zoning (access to goods and services available within residential areas), and others have been advocated at various times and places, but usually not in the context of the nation's effort to improve highway safety.

Research

There has been a significant federal, state, and private-sector investment in highway and traffic safety research. This multidisciplinary effort has focused on each of the four principal elements affecting motor vehicle safety—the human (driver and occupant), the vehicle, the roadway, and the socioeconomic environment. Increasingly sophisticated research has enriched the empirical foundation for informed policy debate and has led to improved safety features and effective prevention programs. Biomechanics research has provided information on injury mechanisms and human tolerances to trauma that has been used in testing vehicle crashworthiness and improving safety measures. Interventions to reduce alcohol-impaired driving and other human factors that affect highway safety have been developed and evaluated through extensive behavioral research. Engineering, highway planning, and other disciplines have contributed to improved vehicle and highway design and to the development of safety-enhancing features such as center high-mounted rear brake lights, improved tire and brake performance, breakaway sign and light poles, protective guardrails, and work-zone safety measures (TRB, 1990). Research by emergency medical services (EMS) and trauma care professionals has improved trauma services and trauma care, and rehabilitation specialists have focused research efforts on improving outcomes for individuals with traumatic brain injury or spinal cord injury due to motor vehicle crashes.

Several federal agencies fund motor vehicle safety research. NHTSA funds research primarily on human factors and vehicle safety, while the Federal Highway Administration funds research on improving highway safety. Additionally, other federal agencies have focused on topic-specific transportation safety research. For example, the National Institute on Aging funds some research on the effects of aging on driving performance; the National Institute on Alcohol Abuse and Alcoholism has funded some research on the effect of alcohol on motor vehicle injury and on adolescent alcohol use and high-risk driving behaviors; the National Institute for Occupational Safety and Health (NIOSH) studies work-related vehicle safety issues; and the Health Resources and Services Administration and the National Center for Injury Prevention and Control (NCIPC) have funded EMS and trauma systems development and evaluation research. Further, there has been a significant private-sector investment in research through the automobile manufacturers, the Insurance Institute for Highway Safety (funded by more than 75 insurance companies), and nonprofit consumer groups.

State and Local Programs

The Highway Safety Act of 1966 created a partnership among federal, state, and local governments to improve and expand the nation's highway safety activities by establishing the State and Community Highway Safety Grant Program (the Section 402 program) (NAGHSR, 1998). This program's funding has provided for the establishment of a highway safety office in every state, headed by a Governor's Highway Safety Representative, and has enabled a state-level focus for coordinating traffic safety efforts. State offices of highway safety often work closely with driver licensing, driver education, state police, public health departments, and state highway departments, and provide a coordinating function across state agencies that have some responsibility for highway safety. Examples of effective use of 402 funding include evaluation of the effectiveness of motorcycle helmet laws, innovative programs to increase safety belt use, design and implementation of improved driver license examinations for different classes of vehicles, child safety seat programs, and evaluation of effects of changes in speed limits. The 402 programs enable states to serve as laboratories to test new highway safety programs; successful programs are adopted nationwide.

Public Support

Public support for motor vehicle safety has also played a role in the progress achieved, through the burgeoning interest in vehicle safety and consumer movements. A remarkable surge in interest in vehicle safety has occurred in the past decade with the maturation of the "baby boom" generation. This increased interest has, in turn, provided overall support for highway safety initiatives, particularly child safety, and has influenced automakers to provide and emphasize safety features and to compete in a safety marketplace.

Additionally, citizen activist groups such as Mothers Against Drunk Driving and Remove Intoxicated Drivers have been influential in improving highway safety. These groups elevate the visibility of the families of victims who died as a result of drunk driving and influence the public agenda, bringing pressure to bear on policy makers.

Ongoing Controversies

Although substantial areas of consensus have emerged in highway safety regulation, several controversies continue, primarily related to the proper balance between safety, mobility, and individual freedom.

Safety Versus Mobility

Motor vehicle injuries are part of the price paid for enhanced mobility. It might be possible to eliminate serious motor vehicle injuries almost completely by disallowing motor vehicles that can exceed 25 miles per hour (mph). In practice, there is a balance between mobility and safety, although where the balance is best struck can be quite controversial. The setting of speed limits has been an area of ongoing discussion and changing legislation. It has been estimated that raising the speed limit on rural interstate highways in the late 1980s resulted in about 400 additional deaths annually (Baum et al., 1991) and that in the 32 states that raised speed limits in 1996,[1] about 350 more deaths occurred in the subsequent year than would have been expected based on historical trends (NHTSA, 1998).

Active Versus Passive Protection

Passive measures, including most vehicle modifications, are those that protect individuals automatically without cooperation or action on their part, for example, motorcycle headlights that are automatically turned on by the ignition key to increase daytime visibility of the motorcycle. In contrast, active measures require individual action by the person to be protected, for example, relying on motorcyclists to remember to turn on their headlights each time they ride during daylight hours. The advantage of passive measures is that, once in place, they protect virtually everyone. Active measures must be implemented by each person on each occasion to provide protection. The effect of requiring all vehicles to be equipped with so-called passive protections is to make the benefit-cost or mobility-safety trade-offs at the societal level rather than the individual level.

Clearly there are instances (as in the motorcycle headlight example above) in which passive measures are preferable, but in most cases such a clear-cut either/or situation does not exist. The overriding considerations in countermeasure choice are efficacy, effectiveness, acceptability, and cost. In reality, a combination of active and passive strategies is usually called for, and both have contributed to reductions in motor vehicle injuries.

---

[1] The National Highway System Designation Act of 1995 (P.L. 104-59) eliminated the federally mandated national maximum speed limit of 55 mph.

Risk Compensation

There is ongoing study of the extent to which individuals respond to safety-enhanced technology or environmental changes of which they are aware. Some drivers may compensate for, and thus offset, the safety gains of an improved or safety-enhanced product by reducing precautions or taking greater risks. For example, improved braking or handling can lead to increased speeds, closer following, and faster cornering (Evans, 1991). However, when the risk of injury is reduced in ways not apparent to the user, which is the case with most forms of automatic or passive protection, behavioral adaptation is unlikely to occur (Lund and O'Neill, 1986; Evans, 1991).

Mandatory Requirements and Primary Enforcement

The proper scope of mandatory or compulsory requirements for self-protection has long been an issue in the ethical literature on paternalism and public health (Cole, 1995). No one questions the legitimacy of informing people about the benefits of wearing safety belts or motorcycle and bicycle helmets, taking steps to persuade people to wear them, or using incentives to encourage safe behavior. However, it has proved difficult in many cases to change driver behavior through educational or persuasive techniques alone. Laws, such as those requiring safety belt use and wearing of helmets, have been successful, particularly when augmented by highly publicized enforcement programs and focused educational programs (Williams et al., 1996; Lacey et al., 1997).

In recent years an important shift in public attitudes appears to have occurred, increasing the level of support for mandatory safety belt laws. The residual debate concerns the benefits and costs of increasing the level of enforcement. To what extent, and at what cost, would allowing primary enforcement[2] increase the level of compliance and reduce injuries? Evidence indicates that, for a given level of enforcement, primary belt-use laws result in higher rates of usage (Campbell, 1988; NHTSA, 1995; Ulmer et al., 1995). Thus, states with secondary laws are not realizing the benefits that could be gained for the enforcement they are already supporting. Even so, there is concern among minorities that primary, or standard, enforcement could lead to police harassment. Additionally, mandatory motorcycle helmet laws remain controversial, although the evidence of effectiveness in preventing death and brain injury is well documented (Kraus et al., 1994; Kraus and Peek, 1995).

---

[2]Primary, or standard, enforcement refers to the stipulation in the law allowing law enforcement officers to stop a driver on the basis of a safety belt use violation.

Access and Licensing Issues

Screening and licensing are tools for regulating access to driving. In the United States, the courts have made a clear distinction between driving for financial gain (commercial driving) and driving for one's own personal purposes. In the latter case, the courts have ruled that the license is more than a privilege and cannot be denied or revoked without due process (Reese, 1965). Because mobility is recognized as so important in our society, states must be reasonably justified in restricting licensure (e.g., using licensing restrictions, suspensions, and revocations as methods to limit driving by individuals convicted of drunk driving) (Jacobs, 1989).

Current controversies relate to restrictive licensing of teenagers and to age-based requirements for elderly drivers. Night-time driving restrictions for young beginning drivers reduce injuries (Williams and Preusser, 1997) but are debated in terms of fairness, and the needs and desires for mobility during adolescence on the part of teens and their families. Although cognitive, perceptual, and motor abilities are known to decrease with increasing age, these changes are highly individual, and screening for licensing restrictions is difficult.

Opportunities for Further Progress

Although significant progress has been made in reducing motor vehicle injuries, not all developments have been positive, and there are important opportunities for further gains. Numbers of motor vehicle deaths have risen slightly in recent years, although the decline in the mileage-based death rate has continued (NSC, 1997). Even though 49 states now have laws regarding safety belt use, national belt use is at a relatively low 61 percent (NHTSA, 1997). States have been reluctant to allow primary enforcement of safety belt laws or to institute strong enforcement programs of the type that has enabled Canadian provinces to achieve belt-use rates in excess of 90 percent (Transport Canada, 1998). Many states have raised speed limits in recent years, after Congress allowed states to do so without sanctions in 1995, and as a result, fatalities have increased (Farmer et al., 1997; NHTSA, 1998).

Research is needed to continue to improve both the design and the use of safety features. Additionally, although airbags are effective in reducing injuries overall, further research is needed to prevent airbag-related deaths of children and others. The lack of injury reduction associated with antilock brakes—a highly touted safety feature—has been disappointing. A newly emerging issue concerns vehicle design mismatch between sport-utility vehicles and passenger cars.

Opportunities for further progress include continued improvement of public transport systems and wider application of safety-related highway and traffic countermeasures that are known—on the basis of competent research—to be effective. For this to happen, increased public and political support is needed.

Additionally, with 50 separate legislatures, developing consistent countermeasures at the state level has proved difficult. The conditional funding mechanism for states to adopt federally endorsed injury prevention legislation has been effective when used, as in the case of the minimum age for the purchase of alcohol. Opportunities to increase use of this mechanism, rather than restrict its use, will be important to furthering progress.

FIREARM INJURIES

Firearm discharges kill almost as many people each year in the United States as motor vehicle crashes, yet the response to this threat to public safety has been quite different from the response to motor vehicle crashes. In the case of motor vehicles, the public and policy makers have demanded safer vehicles, better highways, and more stringent regulation and law enforcement directed at drivers. Together with improved trauma care, these measures have been effective over several decades in reducing the fatality rate per occupant mile. Unfortunately, there has not been a similar comprehensive response—or similar progress—in reducing firearm injuries.

From 1962 to 1994, 992,388 people in the United States died from firearm-related injuries (Ikeda et al., 1997). Firearm deaths and death rates in the United States reached a 30-year high in 1993 (39,595 deaths) and declined in 1994 and 1995 (Fingerhut and Warner, 1997; Ikeda et al., 1997). Although a major cause of morbidity and mortality throughout the life span, firearm deaths particularly affect teens and young adults (mainly homicides) and the elderly (mainly suicides). In 1995, 35,957 people died as a result of firearm injuries; over half of these fatalities (18,003 deaths) were of persons 15–34 years old (Fingerhut and Warner, 1997). In 1995, a greater percentage of firearm deaths were due to suicide (51 percent) than homicide (43 percent) (Fingerhut and Warner, 1997). There were 1,225 unintentional firearm deaths in 1995 (3 percent of all firearm deaths) (Fingerhut and Warner, 1997). An international comparison of 26 industrialized countries found that the firearm death rate for U.S. children younger than 15 years was nearly 12 times higher than among children in the other 25 countries combined (CDC, 1997).

There are similarities in the high degree of lethality of both motor vehicles and firearms. Each product has the potential to produce serious injury or death in a matter of seconds. However, whereas most motor vehicle injuries are unintentional, most firearm injuries are intentional. This difference in intentionality creates complexities in dealing with the emotional, psychological, and behavioral antecedents and consequences of firearm injury. However, this further challenge does not preclude—but rather emphasizes—the need for a concerted effort to focus the full breadth of scientific expertise on preventing and reducing the health consequences of firearm injury.

Current Overview and Future Opportunities

The comprehensive scientific approach that has been fully implemented to address motor vehicle injuries is, by comparison, only a fledgling effort with regard to firearm injuries. Over the long term, an effective national policy directed at reducing the risk and severity of firearm-related injury requires a strong federal presence. The multipronged approach used to develop federal motor vehicle safety policy—surveillance, regulatory action, multidisciplinary research, support for state and local prevention initiatives, and public support—provides a useful model. The following section describes progress to date and focuses on future opportunities.

Surveillance

A number of national surveillance systems provide some data on firearm injuries (see Chapter 3 for additional information); however, there is no national surveillance system that provides detailed information on specific products and incidents—data that are needed to develop effective interventions to prevent and reduce firearm injuries.

The Federal Bureau of Investigation's Uniform Crime Reporting (UCR) System is a voluntary system based on reports from law enforcement agencies. The Supplementary Homicide Report to the UCR System collects information on homicide incidents. Since 1973, the National Institute of Justice has conducted an annual National Crime Victimization Survey, in which cohorts of individuals ages 12 and older are queried semiannually about their experiences related to crime, including crimes involving guns. The Bureau of Alcohol, Tobacco, and Firearms' (ATF) Project LEAD (Law Enforcement Agency Data) includes an automated system that collects information gathered during traces of crime-related firearms. The Consumer Product Safety Commission's (CPSC's) National Electronic Injury Surveillance System (NEISS)—a sample of emergency room admissions—routinely includes information on nonpowder firearm injuries. A recent study performed by the Centers for Disease Control and Prevention (CDC) used NEISS to estimate all nonfatal firearm injuries in the United States (Annest et al., 1995). Vital statistics data compiled by the National Center for Health Statistics include information on suicide and unintentional injury as well as homicide deaths related to firearms (Fingerhut et al., 1992). In 1994, NCIPC funded seven state health departments to support the development, implementation, and evaluation of state-based firearm injury surveillance systems. These programs were three-year cooperative agreements with funding ending in 1997.

Although these systems do provide some data, more complete surveillance systems are needed to monitor firearm injuries over time, to add detail that can guide prevention efforts, and to assess the effectiveness of interventions. The data collected should include geographic, sociodemographic, and product-specific information in addition to information on key causal sequence factors such as alcohol and drug use, perpetrator–victim relationship, and any crime involvement. Complete counting of deaths and sampling of nonfatal injuries is recommended for firearm injuries, as for all other types of injuries, with routine state and national reporting (see Chapter 3).

Regulation and Legislation

The United States has in place a complex regulatory structure for keeping firearms out of the hands of people who are deemed likely to make criminal or irresponsible use of guns (e.g., convicted felons, illegal immigrants, individuals under indictment, people involuntarily committed to mental institutions). Additionally, there are federal oversight of gun commerce (particularly interstate firearm sales) and limits or bans on the sale or possession of certain types of firearms or ammunition. Federal law has also established a minimum age for firearm purchase. Federal regulations on firearms have resulted from the passage of a number of laws that have frequently been initiated in response to violent historical events (e.g., gangland violence in the 1930s, assassination of political leaders in the 1960s, the assassination attempt on President Reagan; see Box 5.1).

The U.S. Department of Justice has the authority to enforce federal laws related to firearms, including interstate commerce. ATF is responsible for federal licensure of firearm dealers. This authority is exercised via regulations that establish specific procedures for documenting the sale of firearms at the wholesale and retail levels. ATF also has responsibility for criminal investigations of interstate gunrunning by those who lack the appropriate license. Funding limitations, however, have curtailed ATF's enforcement efforts.

However, in contrast to motor vehicles and most other consumer products, no federal agency has regulatory jurisdiction over gun design (firearms are specifically exempted from the jurisdiction of the CPSC). Issues include specifying product safety standards and regulating or banning products that can be shown to be dangerous in relation to alternative designs. Thus, it seems reasonable to recommend that Congress establish a regulatory structure, with suitable criteria, to govern the design of firearms, ammunition, and safety devices. Although formulating the regulatory criteria will require difficult judgments regarding the best ways to preserve the utility of firearms for legitimate purposes while reducing risks of unintentional injuries and unlawful uses, the committee encourages the Congress to undertake this important challenge. Whether regulatory authority should be conferred on the CPSC or on a new regulatory agency in the Department of Justice, also requires further study. In either case, the agency should be empowered to set safety and performance standards for firearms, ammunition, and safety devices in accordance with the criteria prescribed by statute. Such legislation would rectify the anomalous exclusion of one of the most lethal consumer products from the jurisdiction of all federal regulatory agencies.

BOX 5.1
Brief Overview of Federal Firearm Laws and Regulations

1919   War Revenue Act imposed a federal excise tax on firearms.

1927   Firearms in U.S. mails, banned interstate mailing of firearms through the U.S. Postal Service.

1934   National Firearms Act regulated the sale of fully automatic weapons, silencers, sawed-off shotguns, and other "gangster-type weapons."

1938   Legislation mandated the licensing of dealers and manufacturers involved in interstate transactions and prohibited firearm sales to people convicted of certain crimes.

1958   Legislation required serial numbers on all guns except .22 caliber rifles.

1968   Gun Control Act placed additional restrictions on who could own guns, established minimum ages for purchase of long guns (18 years of age) and handguns (21 years of age), set minimum standards for imported firearms, established the federal firearm licensing system administered by ATF.

1986   Firearm Owner Protection Act banned further manufacture of automatic weapons and legalized interstate sale of long guns under specified conditions.

1900   Undetectable Firearms Act required plastic guns to be visible by x-ray or to trigger metal detectors.

1994   Brady Handgun Violence Prevention Act established federal requirements for a maximum five-day waiting period for handgun purchases in order to perform criminal background checks and increased the Federal Firearms License fee for gun dealers.

1994   Violent Crime Control and Law Enforcement Act banned manufacture and sale of any ammunition magazines with a capacity in excess of 10 rounds and banned manufacture and sale of semiautomatic rifles and handguns with specific characteristics.

1996   Domestic Violence Offenders Gun Ban prohibited gun purchase by individuals convicted of a domestic violence misdemeanor.

SOURCES: National Committee (1989), Karlson and Hargarten (1997).

Recent regulatory trends at the state level include laws to deter and punish criminal use of firearms, gun safe-storage laws that hold the gun owner responsible if children gain access to the weapon (Cummings et al., 1997), limits on handgun purchases to one per month (Weil and Knox, 1996), and the issuing of licenses for carrying concealed weapons. In contrast to highway and traffic safety, no federal leverage has been used that could encourage the development, application, or evaluation of stringent state legislative approaches to reduce the accessibility of firearms in situations in which they are likely to lead to death and injury or to implement well-evaluated educational programs or licensing arrangements for gun purchasers.

Research

There are numerous unanswered research questions concerning the role of firearms in injury occurrence and the optimal interventions for reducing firearm injury. The nation's recent focus on the larger issue of violence has increased research and program funding for violence prevention at the Department of Justice. Additionally, other federal agencies are conducting research on violence-related issues, including a focus on violence in the workplace by NIOSH and a focus on the biological and behavioral correlates of violence at the National Institute of Mental Health. The National Science Foundation has recently funded a university-based National Consortium on Violence Research. Federally sponsored research that is specifically focused on firearm injury has been funded primarily through the Office of Justice Programs. Additionally, the NCIPC has funded epidemiologic research and state surveillance efforts. The remainder of this section outlines some of the research questions and issues that should be considered in framing a comprehensive research agenda with the goal of reducing firearm injury.

To design interventions that may protect particular high-risk groups identified by surveillance mechanisms—such as teens, inner-city dwellers, domestic violence victims, or the elderly—more information is needed on common causal sequences; victim and perpetrator attitudes toward guns, gun storage, and potential alternative self-protection devices; prevalence of gun use in various settings; and environmental and behavioral risk factors for gun misuse. Although most domestic violence fatalities are caused by guns, the role of guns in relationships that involve domestic violence—for example, in intimidation, self-protection, and other roles—has not yet been well studied. Patterns of mental stress related to prevalent or intimate exposure to gun injuries and death remain to be fully elucidated; such research is needed in multiple sociodemographic settings. Rigorous studies are required of the efficacy and effectiveness of interventions designed to reduce the risk of firearm injury.

Research should be expanded on gun markets to elucidate the flow of firearms from the legitimate sector to the hands of minors and criminals, and how this flow might effectively be interdicted. The main "leakages" from legal gun commerce include theft from private vehicles and homes (more than half a million per year), casual transfers by friends and family, and illegal sales by licensed dealers (Cook and Ludwig, 1996). In some cities, interstate gun-running is also an important source of guns in crime. Developing effective countermeasures that will limit illegal gun commerce requires improved understanding of the economics of the relevant "black" and "gray" markets.

Research is also needed on the ways in which individuals of varying ages, sizes, and strengths use guns, locking devices, and bullets; the resulting information can guide product design toward measures that may reduce the risk of injury and death. Recent engineering innovations designed to increase safety include magazine interlocks that prevent firing when a pistol's magazine is removed but a bullet remains in the firing chamber, and multiple approaches to gun personalization that would limit firing to one person (Robinson et al., 1996). Evolving approaches to the design of guns, such as personalization and increasingly sophisticated automatic safety locks, require real-world testing to allow an understanding of the net effects that these will have on gun ownership, storage, misuse, and injury morbidity and mortality incidence and severity patterns. The biomechanics of gun injuries has been well studied in war situations but should be studied as well in civilian settings that involve wider variations in the age of victims, types of weapons and bullets, and social crowding contexts. Research is also needed on alternative personal protection devices and their risks and benefits, individual perception of the risk of injury from firearms, assessment of various approaches to risk communication, and the effective ways to convey safety information.

Studies are necessary on the effectiveness of current acute medical treatments and on ways to improve such treatment so as to reduce death and permanent disability due to firearm injuries. The role of EMS personnel in clarifying injury circumstances and initiating psychosocial—as well as cardiorespiratory—treatment remains to be fully explored.

One of the puzzles still to be solved in firearm research is the identity of the most informative measure of exposure. For example, one possible analogue of vehicle-miles traveled would be time in the presence of a person with access to a firearm (as compared with time in the presence of people), but such a measure is not empirically feasible. In the aggregate, number of licensed drivers and number of licensed firearm owners would be functionally equivalent exposure measures if licenses were required of gun owners (and if possession of a firearm without a license were as rare as driving a vehicle without a license), but this is not now the case. Presence of a firearm in the home has been used as an exposure measure, but its usefulness is limited to incidents in the home. It is conceivable that no single exposure measure can be utilized for firearm injuries in all locations and contexts. For unintentional injuries, presence of a gun in the home may be a suitable measure, but this does not work as well for intentional injuries. For assaultive injuries, including firearm injuries, one possible measure of exposure would be violent interactions, occurrences that are theoretically measurable through survey interviews. In the committee's view, further attention to this problem, both conceptually and empirically, is needed.

This is a robust multidisciplinary research agenda that must be developed and implemented to identify optimal interventions for the reduction of firearm injuries. Two of the most pertinent lessons from motor vehicle safety research that can be applied to firearm safety research are that a comprehensive approach offers hope for the reduction of firearm morbidity and mortality and that many disciplines have important contributions to make. The strength of integrating work from varied disciplines is evident when the multidisciplinary approach is tried (OJJDP, 1996; Rand, 1997). Research by criminologists is needed to explain the economic, sociocultural, and psychological factors that affect the firearm-related criminal behavior of youths. Research by economists is needed to understand the flow of firearms in and between licit and illicit markets. Epidemiologic research is needed to clarify risks and risk factors and to explore the causal sequences of firearm injury. Biomechanical and clinical research is needed to explicate the acute and chronic effects of gunshot injuries. Mental health and substance abuse researchers can contribute to an understanding of the behavioral and biologic contributors to violence.

Multidisciplinary collaboration on violence research has begun to emerge. Examples include the interdisciplinary Homicide Research Working Group, based in the American Society for Criminology, and the National Consortium on Violence Research. The committee believes that sustained advances in applied research bearing on prevention of firearm violence and other firearm injuries requires such collaborative efforts, including criminologists, economists, psychologists, bioengineers, epidemiologists, and clinicians, working within the comprehensive model of prevention that now shapes research on highway safety.

State and Local Programs

The federal government is involved in a growing number of criminal justice efforts to stem juvenile gun crime, and there are a number of local and private-sector initiatives to this end (OJJDP, 1996). However, there is no federal program, similar to NHTSA's Section 402 program, that would fund firearm injury prevention efforts in each state. Further, the federal government has not used federal revenue streams as leverage for the adoption of firearm injury prevention measures as it has for prevention of motor vehicle injuries.

There are opportunities for encouraging states to improve data systems and implement programs with the goal of reducing firearm injuries. Congress should consider a two-step strategy for encouraging state and local governments to implement and evaluate strategies and programs for reducing firearm injuries, especially involving children and adolescents. First, program funds should be made available to support well-designed state or local program initiatives— encompassing the full range of interventions, including legislation—conditioned upon sound evaluation. Second, when specific programs and legislative approaches have been shown to reduce firearm injuries, Congress should make crime prevention funding through the Office of Justice Programs contingent upon the adoption and implementation of these successful approaches.

The committee recommends the implementation of a comprehensive approach for preventing and reducing firearm injuries that includes firearm surveillance, firearm safety regulation, multidisciplinary research, enforcement of existing restrictions on access by minors and other unlawful purchasers, prevention programs at the state and local levels, and mobilization of public support.

Ongoing Controversies

The firearms debate is often contentious and polarized. In contrast to highway safety policy, no consensus has emerged among policy makers regarding many aspects of firearms policy. Although recent public opinion surveys reveal a large area of agreement on many policy issues (Teret et al., 1998), agreement is lacking among policy makers about the goals of national policy, or indeed whether there should be a national policy in this area; about the benefits and costs of restrictions on ownership, availability, and use of firearms; and about the balance that should be struck between safety-enhancing regulation and individual freedom. Some of these ongoing controversies are briefly described below.

Issues of Individual Freedom

There is ongoing debate over balancing the rights of individuals to own firearms for self-protection (and the security of loved ones) or for recreational use (e.g., hunting, target shooting) against societal concerns about the risk of harm in other contexts. There is general acceptance of the concept that individuals have legitimate rights to engage in recreational hunting or target shooting and to protect themselves and their families and friends, as well as ample evidence that handgun ownership provides a sense of greater security (Cook and Ludwig, 1996). The policy issue is how to balance the values of individual autonomy with the community's interest in reducing the risk of firearm fatalities and injuries.

Instrumentality and Availability

One of the issues examined in ongoing studies is the extent to which guns are instrumental in increasing the risk of death or injury, independent of other factors. The type of weapon used in any violent act, including suicide, may be an important determinant of whether the victim survives and of the risk of disability. Studies of this issue focus on the lethality of various types of weapons; the extent to which the intent of the assailant, rather than the weapon, determines the injury outcome; and the extent to which an individual's choice of weapon is calculated to ensure injury or death or is a matter of chance or access.

Additionally, there is ongoing discussion and study of the extent to which gun ownership, gun availability, or the expense and time required to acquire a firearm influences the likelihood that it will be used in a violent or suicidal act. Issues of access include studies on the effects of the presence of a firearm in a specific location (e.g., home or vehicle); gun commerce, including black markets for firearm purchase; and the effects of regulations on carrying concealed weapons.

Child and Adolescent Vulnerability

Another important issue involves the relative importance of child and adolescent vulnerability on the one hand and adult freedom on the other. Because they live in environments that are generally controlled by adults, children and adolescents are vulnerable to risks that result from adult decisions, including decisions to keep and use guns and decisions on gun storage, particularly in the home. When children and adolescents encounter a gun, they have a reduced capacity to make safe decisions because of their lack of experience, immaturity of judgment, and impulsivity. Their decisions can result in increased risk of injury related to play, assault, or suicidal behavior.

Goals and Priorities for Action

As noted above, a workable political consensus has not yet developed on the balance that should be struck between the prerogatives of firearm ownership and the reduction of firearm-related injuries, especially in a social context in which about 192 million firearms, including 65 million handguns, are in circulation (Cook and Ludwig, 1996). In the committee's view, a workable consensus is most likely to emerge if the discussion is focused less on ownership issues and more on the steps that can be taken to reduce the adverse health consequences of firearm use and to strengthen the scientific basis of policy making. In short, the points of departure for national firearms policy should be harm reduction and better science.

Within the overall framework, initial priority should be given to measures that reduce the risk of harm to the most vulnerable segments of the population, particularly children and adolescents and that curtail the risk of firearm injury caused by children and adolescents. Even in the absence of a broad consensus about the aims of national policy, few people are likely to contest the ethical legitimacy of aggressive measures designed to reduce gun-related injuries to and by youths.

In 1995, firearms were the second leading cause of death among children ages 10–14 years (48 percent of those deaths were homicides; Fingerhut and Warner [1997]). In 1994, 185 children, ages 0–14 years, and 327 adolescents, ages 15–19 years, died from unintentional firearm injuries (Ikeda et al., 1997).

Children and adolescents accounted for 23 percent of the arrests for weapons offenses in 1993. Between 1985 and 1993, the number of juvenile arrests for weapons offenses rose from under 30,000 arrests to more than 61,000 (Greenfeld and Zawitz, 1995). In what has been described as an "age-related" epidemic of juvenile firearm use (Zimring, 1996), firearm homicides committed by youths under 18 increased 229 percent between 1985 and 1992 (Blumstein and Cork, 1996).

A youth-centered injury prevention strategy is needed that would have several components: reducing the number of locations in which youth have access to guns, restricting their ability to gain access to the guns and ammunition in these settings, building features into guns that will reduce the risk of accidental or unauthorized use if the gun does get into the hands of youth, and building community coalitions to make youth environments safer.

All reasonable steps should be taken to prevent access to, and possession of, guns and ammunition by children and adolescents (other than in supervised target shooting or appropriate hunting situations). Although recent federal legislation makes youth handgun sale and possession federal offenses, primary responsibility for enforcing such prohibitions lies with state and local governments. Enforcement efforts should be grounded in systematic research on firearm distribution patterns, focused on revealing the paths by which firearms find their way from initial adult purchase into the hands of children and adolescents. Legislation and judicial rulings punishing gun owners who fail to properly store and secure their weapons, or holding them liable for harm caused by people who have gained access to negligently stored or secured weapons, merit careful consideration and evaluation.

Technologies and practices are now rapidly evolving that promise to make it easier to better secure weapons in the home and community, so that even if guns are obtained by youths or intruders, they will not be usable. Some of these approaches utilize trigger guards and other add-on locking systems (whose performance has not yet been well evaluated). Over a very long term, personalization of guns would be expected to have major benefits in reducing firearm injuries. If personalized firearms replace other weapons in home and community environments, they should eliminate child play injuries and shut down the firearm resale market and its pipeline to youth and criminals. Of course, even if all new weapons are personalized, it will take many years for personalized weapons to displace the existing supply of nonpersonalized ones. Reducing firearm injuries requires a long-term perspective. Perfecting the technology and stimulating the market for safer firearms are important goals for today, even though the full payoff will not occur for decades to come.

Recent experience with tobacco control and alcohol-impaired driving suggests that strong community coalitions can stimulate public support and organize effective action around a powerful youth-centered public health theme. Local communities that want to keep guns out of the hands of children and adolescents now have access to strategic advice and technical assistance from many national resource centers and professional organizations, which can enable them to work out means to affect various steps in the gun distribution chain. Community coalitions can bring together law enforcement, public health, child protective services, and numerous citizen groups to develop, implement, and monitor a local plan to reduce youth gun access. Such a plan might include a wide variety of interventions, such as police enforcement strategies designed to disrupt local gun markets and to keep guns off the streets and out of schools; interventions focused on altering the "ecology of danger" (Wilkinson and Fagan, 1996) and changing norms relating to gun carrying and violence among urban youths; public education regarding the risks of gun ownership and the responsibility of adults for their firearms; and public education and legal measures promoting secure storage of weapons in the home.

> **The committee recommends the development of a national policy on the prevention of firearm injuries directed toward the reduction of morbidity and mortality associated with unintended or unlawful uses of firearms. An immediate priority should be a strategic focus on reduction of firearm injuries caused by children and adolescents.**

To ensure the success of a youth-centered prevention initiative, Congress and relevant federal agencies (e.g., the Departments of Health and Human Services and Justice) should set national goals for reducing assaultive injuries, suicide, and unintentional injuries by young people using firearms. As a long-term commitment to this goal, consideration should be given to appointing a high-level task force for implementing and evaluating such an initiative.

SUMMARY

A comprehensive approach to reducing firearm injuries is necessary. Strengthened firearm and firearm injury surveillance efforts and multidisciplinary research initiatives can bring the depth and breadth of scientific and engineering expertise that is needed to develop and evaluate innovative firearm injury prevention measures. Designation of a federal agency to have regulatory jurisdiction over firearm safety issues, enforcement of current regulations, particularly on access to guns by children and adolescents, and expansion of state and local prevention programs are all necessary components of an effective comprehensive approach. The federal role should not involve the establishment of new bureaucracies but rather should be to provide national leadership and coordination to leverage the related programs at state and local levels, to generate new knowledge, and to promote the application of new findings. The committee believes that progress can be made in preventing and reducing the adverse health consequences of firearm injury if the U.S. government will lead a concerted and sustained effort to address this major national problem.

REFERENCES

Annest JL, Mercy JA, Gibson DR, Ryan GW. 1995. National estimates of nonfatal firearm-related injuries: Beyond the tip of the iceberg. *Journal of the American Medical Association* 273:1749–1754.

Baum HM, Wells JK, Lund AK. 1991. The fatality consequences of the 65 mph speed limits. *Journal of Safety Research* 22:171–177.

Blumstein A, Cork D. 1996. Linking gun availability to youth gun violence. *Law and Contemporary Problems* 59(1):5–24.

Campbell BJ. 1988. Highway safety in 2010: Compromising among values. In: Stammer ME, ed. *Highway Safety at the Crossroads*. New York: American Society of Civil Engineers. Pp. 279–289.

CDC (Centers for Disease Control and Prevention). 1994. Deaths resulting from firearm- and motor-vehicle-related injuries—United States, 1968–1991. *Morbidity and Mortality Weekly Report* 43(3):37–42.

CDC (Centers for Disease Control and Prevention). 1997. Rates of homicide, suicide, and firearm-related death among children—26 industrialized countries. *Morbidity and Mortality Weekly Report* 46(5);101–105.

Cole P. 1995. The moral bases for public health interventions. *Epidemiology* 6(1):78–83.

Cook PJ, Ludwig J. 1996. *Guns in America: Results of a Comprehensive National Survey on Firearms Ownership and Use*. Washington, DC: Police Foundation.

Cook PJ, Tauchen G. 1984. The effect of minimum drinking age legislation on youthful auto fatalities. *Journal of Legal Studies* 13:169–190.

Cook PJ, Molliconi S, Cole TB. 1995. Regulating gun markets. *Journal of Criminal Law and Criminology* 86(1):59–92.

Cummings P, Grossman DC, Rivara FP, Koepsell TD. 1997. State gun safe storage laws and child mortality due to firearms. *Journal of the American Medical Association* 278(13):1084–1086.

DeHaven H. 1942. Mechanical analysis of survival in falls from heights of fifty to one hundred fifty feet. *War Medicine* 2:586–596.

Evans L. 1991. *Traffic Safety and the Driver*. New York, NY: Van Nostrand Reinhold.

Farmer CM, Rettig RA, Lund AK. 1997. *Effect of 1996 Speed Limit Changes on Motor Vehicle Occupant Fatalities*. Arlington, VA: Insurance Institute for Highway Safety.

Fingerhut LA, Warner M. 1997. *Injury Chartbook. Health, United States, 1996–1997*. Hyattsville, MD: National Center for Health Statistics.

Fingerhut LA, Ingram DD, Felman JJ. 1992. Firearm homicide among black teenagers in metropolitan counties: Comparison of death rates in two periods, 1983 through 1985 and 1987 through 1989. *Journal of the American Medical Association* 267(22): 3054–3058.

GAO (General Accounting Office). 1987. *Drinking-Age Laws: An Evaluation Synthesis of Their Impact on Highway Safety*. Washington, DC: GAO. PEMD-87-10.

Greenfeld LA, Zawitz MW. 1995. *Weapons Offenses and Offenders*. Washington, DC: Bureau of Justice Statistics. Bureau of Justice Statistics Selected Findings. NCJ-155284.

Haddon W Jr. 1972. A logical framework for categorizing highway safety phenomena and activity. *Journal of Trauma* 12(3):193–207.

Haddon W Jr. 1980. Options for the prevention of motor vehicle crash injury. *Israel Journal of Medicine* 16:45–68.

Ikeda RM, Gorwitz R, James SP, Powell KE, Mercy JA. 1997. *Fatal Firearm Injuries in the United States, 1962–1994*. Atlanta, GA: National Center for Injury Prevention and Control. Violence Surveillance Summary Series, No. 3.

Jacobs JB. 1989. *Drunk Driving: An American Dilemma*. Chicago: University of Chicago Press.

Karlson TA, Hargarten SW. 1997. *Reducing Firearm Injury and Death: A Public Health Sourcebook on Guns*. New Brunswick, NJ: Rutgers University Press.

Kraus JF, Peek C. 1995. The impact of two related prevention strategies on head injury reduction among nonfatally injured motorcycle riders, California, 1991–1993. *Journal of Neurotrauma* 12(5):873–881.

Kraus JF, Peek C, McArthur DL, Williams A. 1994. The effect of the 1992 California motorcycle helmet use
law on motorcycle crash fatalities and injuries. *Journal of the American Medical Association* 272(19):1506–1511.

Lacey JH, Jones RK, Fell JC. 1997. The effectiveness of the Checkpoint Tennessee program. In: Mercier-Guyon C, ed. *Alcohol, Drugs, and Traffic Safety. Proceedings of the 14th International Conference on Alcohol, Drugs, and Traffic Safety*. Vol. 2. Pp. 969–975.

Lund AK, O'Neill B. 1986. Perceived risks and driving behavior. *Accident Analysis and Prevention* 18(5):367–370.

Mashaw JL, Harfst DL. 1990. *The Struggle for Auto Safety*. Cambridge, MA: Harvard University Press.

NAGHSR (National Association of Governors' Highway Safety Representatives). 1998. *National Association of Governors' Highway Safety Representatives*. [World Wide Web document]. URL http://www.naghsr.org/ (accessed May 1998).

National Committee (National Committee for Injury Prevention and Control). 1989. *Injury Prevention: Meeting the Challenge*. New York: Oxford University Press. Published as a supplement to the *American Journal of Preventive Medicine* 5(3).

NHTSA (National Highway Traffic Safety Administration). 1995. *The Case for Primary Enforcement of State Safety Belt Use Laws*. Washington, DC: NHTSA. DOT/HS 808 324.

NHTSA (National Highway Traffic Safety Administration). 1996. *Traffic Safety Facts, 1996. Alcohol*. Washington, DC: NHTSA.

NHTSA (National Highway Traffic Safety Administration). 1997. *Observed Safety Belt Use in 1996*. Research Note. Washington, DC: NHTSA.

NHTSA (National Highway Traffic Safety Administration). 1998. *The Effect of Increased Speed Limits in the Post-NMSL Era*. Report to Congress. Washington, DC: Department of Transportation.

NHTSA (National Highway Traffic Safety Administration) and FHWA (Federal Highway Administration). 1991. *Moving America More Safely. An Analysis of the Risks of Highway Travel and the Benefits of Federal Highway, Traffic, and Motor Vehicle Safety Programs*. Washington, DC: NHTSA and FHWA.

NSC (National Safety Council). 1997. *Accident Facts*. Itasca, IL: NSC.

OJJDP (Office of Juvenile Justice and Delinquency Prevention). 1996. *Reducing Youth Gun Violence: An Overview of Programs and Initiatives.* Washington, DC: U.S. Department of Justice. NCJ 154303.

Rand M. 1997. *Violence-Related Injuries Treated in Hospital Emergency Departments.* Bureau of Justice Statistics Special Report. Washington, DC: U.S. Department of Justice. NCJ-156921.

Reese JH. 1965. *The Legal Nature of a Driver's License.* Washington, DC: Automotive Safety Foundation.

Robinson KD, Teret SP, Vernick JS, Webster DW. 1996. *Personalized Guns: Reducing Gun Deaths Through Design Changes.* Baltimore, MD: Johns Hopkins Center for Gun Policy and Research.

Stapp JR. 1957. Human tolerance to deceleration. *American Journal of Surgery* 93(4):734–740.

Teret SP, Webster DW, Vernick JS, Smith TW, Leff D, Wintemute GJ, Cook PJ, Hawkins DF, Kellermann AL, Sorenson SB, DeFrancesco S. 1998. Support for new policies to regulate firearms: Results of two national surveys. *New England Journal of Medicine* 339(12):813–818.

Transport Canada. 1998. *Estimates of Seat Belt Use from Annual Surveys 1989–1997.* Ottawa, Ontario: Transport Canada.

TRB (Transportation Research Board, National Research Council). 1990. *Safety Research for a Changing Highway Environment.* Washington, DC: TRB.

Ulmer RG, Preusser CW, Preusser DF, Cosgrove LA. 1995. Evaluation of California's safety belt law change from secondary to primary enforcement. *Journal of Safety Research* 26(4):213–220.

Wagenaar AC. 1993. Research affects public policy: The case of legal drinking age in the United States. *Addiction* 88(Suppl.):758–818.

Waller JA. 1994. Reflections of a half century of injury control. *American Journal of Public Health* 84(4):664–670.

Weil DS, Knox RC. 1996. Effects of limiting handgun purchases on interstate transfer of firearms. *Journal of the American Medical Association* 275(22):1759–1761.

Wilkinson DL, Fagan J. 1996. Understanding the role of firearms in violence: The dynamics of gun events among adolescent males. *Law and Contemporary Problems* 59(1):55–90.

Williams AF, Preusser DF. 1997. Night driving restrictions for youthful drivers: A literature review and commentary. *Journal of Public Health Policy* 18(3):334–345.

Williams AF, Reinfurt D, Wells JK. 1996. Increasing seat belt use in North Carolina. *Journal of Safety Research* 27(1):33–41.

Zimring FE. 1996. Kids, guns, and homicide: Policy notes on an age-specific epidemic. *Law and Contemporary Problems* 59(1):25–38.

6

Trauma Care

The 1966 landmark report *Accidental Death and Disability: The Neglected Disease of Modern Society* was a clarion call to launch what it termed a "frontal attack" on the care of the injured. At the time, the problem of injury in the United States was met with public apathy, a dearth of 9-1-1 systems, and inadequate provision of care (NRC, 1966). Since then, much progress has been made in developing systems of care that strive to reduce injury-related morbidity and mortality. Trauma care systems deliver a continuum of prehospital, acute care, and rehabilitation services. Yet, despite their public health mission, only a handful of states have put into place comprehensive regional systems of trauma care, although some of the system elements are present in many states and communities (West et al., 1988; Bazzoli et al., 1995). Trauma care is integral to the injury field because it is critical to lessening the consequences of injury.

The purposes of this chapter are to describe trauma care systems, their organization, roles, and patient outcomes; to explore what is known about their costs and cost-effectiveness; to delve into the cardinal problem of financing the high cost of infrastructure and patient care, a problem that has been solved by some states through motor vehicle fees and other creative sources of financing; and to explore the impact of managed care on trauma care systems. The committee decided to focus on these issues rather than explore the fundamental issues related to trauma care and the rehabilitation sciences, since several other reports have discussed specific priorities for research in trauma care and rehabilitation (e.g., NCIPC [1993]; IOM [1991, 1997a]; NIH [1994]).

OVERVIEW OF TRAUMA CARE SYSTEMS

A trauma care system is an organized and coordinated effort in a defined geographic area to deliver the full spectrum of care to an injured patient, from the time of the injury through transport to an acute care facility and to rehabilitative care (Eastman et al., 1991; Mendeloff and Cayten, 1991). A trauma care system consists of three major providers—prehospital, acute care, and rehabilitation—that, when closely integrated, ensure a continuum of care. For general descriptions of prehospital, acute, and rehabilitative care, see Box 6.1. This chapter concentrates on prehospital and acute care rather than rehabilitation because the latter was the subject of two recent Institute of Medicine (IOM) reports (IOM, 1991, 1997a).

In a trauma system, the integration of prehospital, acute care, and rehabilitation providers is administered by a public agency whose cardinal roles are to provide leadership, coordinate service delivery, establish minimum standards of care, designate trauma centers (offering 24-hour specialized treatment for the most severely injured patients), and ensure system evaluation and refinement. Trauma care systems are best endowed with the following major clinical or operational components: medical direction, prevention, communication, training, triage, prehospital care, transportation, hospital care, public education, rehabilitation, and medical evaluation (ACEP, 1992; HRSA, 1992; ACS, 1993). How these components are configured, organized, and emphasized differs according to state, regional, and local circumstances, as there are many examples of trauma systems throughout the United States.

An overarching goal of a trauma care system is to match the severity of the injury to the most appropriate and cost-effective level of care in a geographic region (ACEP, 1992; HRSA, 1992; ACS, 1993). Patient matching is thought to be accomplished best by an inclusive trauma care system (i.e., one that harnesses the resources of all hospitals and trauma care providers in a community or region to meet the needs of all injured patients, the majority of whom [85–90 percent] are not severely injured; ACS [1993]). Most existing trauma systems are "exclusive" in orientation insofar as they focus mostly on the major trauma patient. Exclusive systems do not include all area hospitals, only prehospital providers and trauma centers to which the major trauma patient is triaged. Trauma centers are hospitals that are specially designed to care for the most critically injured patients. There are four levels of trauma center designation (Box 6.2), the pinnacle of which is the Level I center. Inclusive trauma care systems incorporate all hospitals and acute care facilities in a region to deliver quality care for all injured patients, regardless of severity. Inclusive trauma care systems marshal communitywide resources, broaden the number of stakeholders, enhance surveillance capacity, and seek to avert the overburdening of trauma centers with noncritically injured patients for whom expensive trauma center care is unnecessary. An inclusive philosophy of trauma care was espoused by federal legislation, the Trauma Care Systems Planning and Development Act of 1990 (P.L. 101-590), which until 1995 encouraged the development of, and provided funding for, inclusive systems (see later discussion of financing). The effectiveness of an inclusive system has yet to be empirically evaluated (NCIPC, 1993).

BOX 6.1
The Continuum of Care

Prehospital Emergency Medical Services (EMS) Prehospital care is the gateway to the trauma care system and a major determinant of patient outcome (Jacobs et al., 1984; Rutledge et al., 1993; Regel et al., 1997). The goals of prehospital care are prompt arrival at the scene, assessment of patients' needs through medically approved protocols for triage (the classification of injury severity and the selection of a hospital destination that matches patients with appropriate clinical resources); preliminary resuscitation and treatment; and rapid transport to the nearest, most appropriate acute care facility (ACS, 1993; Jacobs and Jacobs, 1993). Access to prehospital care is provided almost universally throughout the United States by a telephone call to 9-1-1 (NHTSA, 1997a). There are four levels of EMS providers: (1) first responder, (2) emergency medical technician (EMT)-Basic, (3) EMT-Intermediate, and (4) EMT-Paramedic. The paramedic has substantially more training than the others and is the provider of most advanced life support given outside the hospital.

Acute Care Hospitals and primary care providers diagnose and treat the majority of injured patients, but the cornerstone of the trauma care system is the trauma center. Trauma centers are highly sophisticated facilities geared to the most gravely injured. Four levels of trauma center, each with detailed qualifying criteria, have been established and revised by the American College of Surgeons (ACS, 1993). (See Box 6.2 for a description of Level I–IV trauma centers). Many states with the legal authority to designate trauma centers use the ACS's criteria for designation. Hospitals seeking designation in states where such formal authority is lacking often rely on verification by the ACS that they have met its criteria.

Rehabilitation Rehabilitation forms the final, and generally the longest, phase of treatment in a trauma care system. The goals of rehabilitation are to improve physical and mental health, reduce disability, and enhance personal autonomy and productivity. Rehabilitation is defined as the process by which physical, sensory, or mental capacities are restored or developed. It is a process that is accomplished through functional improvements in the patient, as well as through changes in the physical and social environment (IOM, 1997a). Rehabilitation is offered on an inpatient or outpatient basis in a designated hospital unit, a freestanding rehabilitation hospital, or in a clinic. In a model trauma care system, rehabilitation begins at the earliest stage possible after admission to an acute care hospital (HRSA, 1992; NCIPC, 1993).

BOX 6.2
Levels of Trauma Centers

Trauma centers are acute care facilities that are specially designed to care for the most critically injured patients. There are four types—or levels—of trauma centers, the qualifying criteria for which were established by the American College of Surgeons (ACS, 1993):

• *Level I*—A facility that meets criteria for a Level I trauma center has the highest degree of sophistication in treating the most severely injured patients. A Level I trauma center is a regional tertiary care facility required to have immediate availability of specialized surgeons, anesthesiologists, physician specialists, nurses, and resuscitation equipment. It also is required to conduct certain types of prevention and research activities.

• *Level II*—A facility that meets a Level II trauma center designation satisfies virtually all of the same clinical and facilities requirements as the Level I center, but is not required to conduct research and certain types of prevention activities. Most cities and suburban areas have Level I and/or II centers.

• *Level III*—A facility that meets a Level III trauma center designation is required to have emergency services and the availability of general surgeons, but it is not required to meet the extensive clinical and facilities criteria of a Level I or Level II center. A Level III center typically serves a rural area that does not have a Level I or Level II center.

• *Level IV*—A facility that meets a Level IV trauma center designation can be either a hospital or a clinic in a remote area where more sophisticated care is unavailable. It is a new classification added by the ACS in 1993 to accommodate patients in the most rural areas by linking them to higher levels of care. The key role of a Level IV center is to resuscitate and stabilize patients and arrange for their transfer to the closest, most appropriate level of trauma center.

The plight of rural areas has been a major factor propelling an inclusive philosophy of trauma care systems (Shackford, 1995). Rural emergency medical services have lagged behind their urban counterparts for a host of reasons, including greater transport times, insufficient volume of patients to maintain the skills of providers, and too sparse a population density to sustain local public financing (OTA, 1989; HRSA, 1990). In comparison with urban areas, rural areas experience higher mortality rates for motor vehicle crashes (Baker et al., 1987; Mueller et al., 1988; Flowe et al., 1995) and a higher proportion of deaths at the scene (Rogers et al., 1997b). To incorporate rural acute care facilities into an integrated system of care, the American College of Surgeons (ACS) created a new level of trauma center (Level IV) in 1993 and specified the organizational and clinical criteria needed for a facility to meet this level (Box 6.2). The facility may be a clinic or hospital, with or without a physician available. The purpose of this classification was to provide optimal care in remote areas with limited resources and, when necessary, to ensure linkage to higher levels of care.

Special Populations

Children and the elderly are among the special populations that merit emphasis by trauma care systems. Injury is the foremost cause of death among children above 1 year of age and the fifth leading cause of death for the elderly age 65 or over (Chapter 2). Congress authorized the Emergency Medical Services for Children (EMS-C) Program in 1984 to ensure state-of-the-art emergency medical care for injured children and adolescents and to ensure that pediatric services are integrated into trauma systems. The program funds demonstration, implementation, and targeted-issues grants to states and medical schools for the provision of emergency medical services geared to children (IOM, 1993; NIH, 1995). The program grew out of the awareness that children have unique physiological responses to illness and injury and that their treatment requires specific training, equipment, and approaches not ordinarily available in systems designed for adults. The program focuses on the entire continuum of pediatric emergency services, from injury prevention through prehospital, acute care, and rehabilitation services. The committee commends the collaborative efforts of the Maternal and Child Health Bureau (MCHB) and the National Highway Traffic Safety Administration (NHTSA) on the EMS-C Program and urges similar collaborative efforts between MCHB and the National Institute of Child Health and Human Development for investigator-initiated research in the areas of childhood injury epidemiology and prevention.

Research has demonstrated that specialized pediatric trauma care is associated with lower rates of pediatric morbidity and mortality compared with rates at adult trauma care centers (or national norms), although adult trauma centers with a pediatric component may be able to achieve outcomes comparable to those of pediatric trauma centers (Pollack et al., 1991; Fortune et al., 1992; Knudson et al., 1992; Nakayama et al., 1992; Cooper et al., 1993; Hall et al., 1993, 1996; Rhodes et al., 1993; Bensard et al., 1994; Hulka et al., 1997). As important, targeted pediatric injury prevention programs have been shown in population-based studies to result in substantial decreases in the incidence of serious childhood injuries (Davidson et al., 1994; Durkin et al., 1996). The National Pediatric Trauma Registry (NPTR), was established in 1985 to study the causes, circumstances, and consequences of injuries to children. Sponsored by the National Institute on Disability and Rehabilitation Research and by the American Pediatric Surgical Association, the NPTR has detailed information on over 50,000 cases of injuries to children. As of October 1996, there were 78 participating centers (pediatric trauma centers or children's hospitals with pediatric trauma units) located in 28 states, Puerto Rico, and Ontario, Canada (NPTR, 1998).

The elderly account for a disproportionate share of injury-related hospitalizations (see Chapter 2). Demographic projections suggest that their share of hospitalizations is likely to grow even more. The need for the full range of treatment efforts targeted to the elderly is especially critical, particularly the need for a seamless transition from prehospital to acute care to high-quality rehabilitation services tailored to their needs (IOM, 1997a). There is some evidence that the elderly with major trauma have an inferior quality of trauma care compared to other age groups. This problem may be the result of two factors: (1) inadequate triage criteria for dispatching an elderly patient to a trauma center, resulting in undertriage (Phillips et al., 1996; Ma, 1997), and (2) a higher risk of complications and death during hospitalization (DeMaria et al., 1987; Champion et al., 1989a; Finelli et al., 1989; Chen et al., 1995; Ma, 1997). More research is needed to identify causes, sequela, and interventions to ensure the highest quality of care for elderly patients.

System Management and State or Regional Agencies

It has long been recognized that trauma care systems are best managed on a regional basis by virtue of the opportunity to pool and centralize resources and the relative infrequency of major trauma (NRC, 1978; Eastman et al., 1987; Stewart et al., 1995). Major trauma generally accounts for a small percentage (10–12 percent) of overall injury admissions (MacKenzie et al., 1990; National Trauma Data Project, 1996). Injury admissions—of all types and levels of severity—ranged in 1993 from 6.19 to 9.02 admissions per thousand population (National Trauma Data Project, 1996). Consequently, state and regional agencies have come to play essential roles in establishing and coordinating regional and local trauma care systems, many of which receive assistance from the federal government.

Federal legislation since the 1970s, such as the Emergency Medical Services Systems Act of 1973 and the Trauma Care Systems Planning and Development Act of 1990, channeled funds to states and regions in order to cultivate the development of systems of care (Table 6.1 contains a chronology of federal trauma system legislation). The 1990 legislation not only authorized funding for development and planning activities (albeit unsustained funding; see later section on financing trauma systems), but also stipulated the creation of a Model Trauma Care System Plan (HRSA, 1992).

TABLE 6.1 Chronology of Trauma System Legislation

1966	*Highway Safety Act* authorizes funding for, and requires states to develop, regional EMS systems; also authorizes the Department of Transportation to develop standards for EMS provider training.
1973	*Emergency Medical Services Systems Act* (P.L. 93-154) authorizes additional federal guidelines and funding for the development of regional EMS systems.
1981	*Omnibus Budget Reconciliation Act* consolidates EMS funding into state preventive health and health services block grants under the Centers for Disease Control and Prevention (CDC).
1984	*Health Services, Preventive Health Services, and Home and Community-Based Services Act* (P.L. 98-555) authorizes the Emergency Medical Services for Children Program.
1990	*Trauma Care Systems Planning and Development Act* (P.L. 101-590) authorizes funding for state and regional trauma systems development.
1995	*Trauma Care Systems Planning and Development Act* is not reauthorized.

The Model Trauma Care System Plan offers a framework for states to build trauma care systems once they have procured legislative authority.[1] In broad terms, the plan calls for states to link prehospital, acute care, and rehabilitation providers through leadership, systems development, planning, and evaluation, and through securing financing for system administration and patient care (HRSA, 1992). More specifically, the plan exhorts states to designate trauma centers, establish trauma registries, and ensure, in concert with communities, that triage and transport protocols are in place for the timely assessment and movement of patients to the most suitable acute care facility. Bazzoli and coworkers (1995) found that the most common problem for states was to limit the number of designated trauma centers based on community need. The ACS (1993) underscored the importance of states' limiting the number of designated centers for two primary reasons: (1) trauma teams must treat sufficient numbers of major trauma patients to maintain their expertise, and (2) unnecessary duplication of centers yields excessively high societal health care costs (see also Goldfarb et al. [1996]). The importance of maintaining sufficient patient volume as a determi-

---

[1]By 1992, 41 state and regional agencies had legal authority to coordinate and regulate trauma care systems (Bazzoli et al., 1995). Regional agencies generally refer to counties or groups of counties (Bazzoli et al., 1995) or, occasionally to, private organizations. In the absence of legislation, states have little ability to require the routing of patients to trauma centers (Mendeloff and Cayten, 1991; Bazzoli et al., 1995).

nant of patient survival has been confirmed (Smith et al., 1990; Konvolinka et al., 1995). Still, there is no consensus on the amount of patient volume necessary for optimal performance of a trauma center (Moore, 1995).

Personnel and Training

More than 30 years ago, the National Research Council (NRC, 1966) spotlighted the paucity of trained emergency personnel at every level of care. The growth in the number of prehospital providers and the increase in their level of training are among the major achievements of the past three decades. The number of prehospital providers is estimated today at about 650,000 nationwide (W.E. Brown, National Registry of Emergency Medical Technicians, personal communication, 1998). Accompanying this growth has been the creation and standardization of the prehospital curriculum. Since the enactment of the 1966 Highway Safety Act, NHTSA has spearheaded the development of standardized curricula for multiple types of prehospital personnel (U.S. DOT, 1996b). In a series of evaluations conducted from 1988 to 1994, NHTSA found that 72.5 percent of 40 states used standardized curricula (primarily NHTSA's) in training courses for prehospital providers (U.S. DOT, 1995). NHTSA's FY 1997 budget for the EMS division responsible for curriculum development is $1.5 million. By virtue of its leadership and support for prehospital training and state highway grants, NHTSA is the federal agency with the most consistent and long-standing presence in trauma systems development (U.S. DOT, 1996b).

Certification of prehospital providers also has progressed, with all 50 states having some kind of certification procedure (BLS, 1997). However, there is much variability in requirements for certification (U.S. DOT, 1996b). Thirty-nine states certify prehospital providers who have passed written and practical examinations administered by the National Registry of Emergency Medical Technicians, a nonprofit certifying organization (NREMT, 1998). Yet, most states do not adhere to the registry's biennial reregistration requirement. Less than one quarter of the estimated 650,000 emergency medical technicians (EMTs) nationwide maintained their registration as of November 1997 (W.E. Brown, National Registry of Emergency Medical Technicians, personal communication, 1998).

There also has been considerable growth in the field of emergency medicine. The first emergency medicine residency program was formed in 1970. By 1998, the number of accredited residency programs had expanded to 120 (M. Schropp, Society for Academic Emergency Medicine, personal communication, 1998). The first certifying examination was given in 1980, one year after emergency medicine was recognized as a specialty by the American Medical Association Committee on Medical Education and the American Board of Medical Specialties. The number of board-certified emergency physicians catapulted to 15,202 by 1997 (American Board of Emergency Medicine, personal communication, 1998). The stature of the profession has also improved with the ascension of emergency medicine to full department status in many academic medical centers.

Finally, the profession of emergency nursing has grown and flourished. The field emerged as a nursing specialty around 1970, when the Emergency Nurses Association was formed. By 1997, membership in this organization rose to about 24,000, as did membership in related organizations such as the Society of Trauma Nurses. Emergency nurses practice mostly in the prehospital and acute care setting. They typically are responsible for assessing and initiating care to stabilize and resuscitate patients and for care during transport of critical care patients. The role of the emergency nurse in the prehospital arena is continuing to evolve (Adams and Trimble, 1994).

ROLE OF TRAUMA SYSTEMS IN PRIMARY PREVENTION, SURVEILLANCE, AND RESEARCH

Community-based primary prevention programs have been demonstrated to avert injury-related morbidity and mortality and to reduce health care costs. Trauma care systems have traditionally focused on secondary and tertiary prevention (i.e., efforts to reduce re-injury and to curtail the impact of an injury once it has occurred). Yet consensus has emerged that health professionals who manage trauma patients also should engage in primary prevention to keep an injury from occurring in the first place (U.S. DHHS, 1992; NCIPC, 1993; U.S. DOT, 1996a; Garrison et al., 1997). The rationale for broadening the role of trauma providers to include primary prevention is that these health professionals have unique and direct experience with, and knowledge of, the consequences of injury, as well as a professional obligation to improve health and safety and to control health care costs. After reviewing the biomedical literature on existing and recommended primary prevention activities for out-of-hospital providers (Kinnane et al., 1997), a consensus statement on prevention by the EMS community was prepared under the aegis of the National Association of EMS Physicians. The statement recommended leadership activities and knowledge areas that are either essential or desirable. Some of the leadership activities deemed to be essential were the provision of education to EMS providers on primary injury prevention, the protection of individual EMS providers from injury, and the collection and use of injury data (Garrison et al., 1997). Although a number of primary prevention programs by prehospital and acute care providers have been implemented in various states or regions, none has been evaluated as yet (Kinnane et al., 1997). The committee suggests that enhanced emphasis be placed on the development and evaluation of prevention programs by these providers, as well as by rehabilitation providers to prevent secondary complications of injuries. Further, the committee believes that primary injury prevention should be incorporated into training curricula and continuing medical education programs for prehospital and acute care providers. Finally, the committee believes that there are financial incentives for employers, insurers, and others who pay for health care to adopt injury prevention, a point discussed later in the section on health care financing.

Surveillance data from trauma systems are indispensable for monitoring outcomes, assessing system performance, determining the etiology and scope of the injury problem in a community, and influencing public policy. Yet no nationwide or nationally representative surveillance systems are operational for trauma systems as a whole nor for their separate elements (i.e., prehospital, acute care, and rehabilitation services). Most surveillance systems currently in place are kept by individual trauma centers as a condition of trauma center designation (Pollock and McClain, 1989).[2] In addition, although 48 percent of states have some type of hospital-based trauma registries, there is great variability in their nature, scope, purpose, and data elements (Shapiro et al., 1994). To instill greater uniformity, federal agencies and professional organizations have taken the initiative to develop and encourage the use of a variety of uniform data sets from prehospital, acute care, and rehabilitation providers. Working with the EMS community, NHTSA sponsored a conference in 1993, the final product of which was a proposed set of 81 uniform prehospital EMS data elements, either essential or desirable, for patient severity and treatment, cause of injury, response, and transfer times, but not for outcomes (under the rationale that these would have required linkages to the emergency department) (U.S. DOT, 1994). CDC's National Center for Injury Prevention and Control (NCIPC) supported the development of a uniform data set for 24-hour, hospital-based emergency departments, the Data Elements for Emergency Department Systems (DEEDS) (NCIPC, 1997a). The ACS developed, specifically for trauma centers, the National Trauma Data Bank to serve as a voluntary national repository of data from trauma centers. The Uniform Data System for Medical Rehabilitation was developed with support from the National Institute on Disability and Rehabilitation Research to capture the severity of patient disability and the outcomes of rehabilitation.

A number of states and regions have implemented laws that mandate inclusive trauma systems with comprehensive trauma registries. These registries include data retrieved from prehospital services, police and ambulance records, hospitals, rehabilitation centers, and medical examiners' files. These data systems are driven by E-codes (see Chapter 3) and have disease- and severity-specific information, as well as length of stay, morbidity and mortality, and charge information. Linkages between data sets covering prehospital, acute care, and rehabilitation providers are envisioned as a pivotal means of integrating information across trauma systems nationwide and of formulating public policy.

---

[2]ACS criteria require Levels I–III to collect minimal registry data, whereas Level IV is encouraged, but not required, to maintain a registry.

However, experience thus far points to the difficulty of performing such linkages for outcome studies (Copes et al., 1996). The committee supports the widespread adoption of uniform surveillance data sets, such as those recommended by NHTSA for prehospital care, by NCIPC for emergency department care, and by the ACS for trauma centers. Once adopted, demonstration projects should be developed to determine the most cost-effective means of establishing linkages between prehospital care, acute care, and rehabilitation data sets.

Research has been instrumental in the evolution of trauma systems. It has formed the underpinning for improved patient care and survival, reduced morbidity, and a national investment in trauma systems. In recognition of its vital role in advancing the trauma field, the ACS requires Level I trauma centers to conduct an active research program. Nevertheless, many prehospital, hospital, and rehabilitation providers do not participate in basic or clinical research, despite the existence of major gaps in knowledge across the entire spectrum, from basic research in tissue injury to health services research in trauma care systems.

There is a dearth of funding for research on trauma systems design, effectiveness, and cost-effectiveness. The existing research support is fragmentary at best, and there is no critical mass of support and leadership. The modest level of support comes mostly from NCIPC and the Agency for Health Care Policy and Research (AHCPR) (NCIPC, 1997b). NCIPC has sustained an investment in trauma systems research, even though its extramural research program is beset by funding limitations. The overall problem is that trauma systems research falls under health services research, an area that has not fared well in the research hierarchy and competition for resources. Health services research, despite a critical need, is a field whose recognition and importance have come only in the past decade, at a time of persistent pressures to reduce the federal budget deficit. Health services research has not grown to a level commensurate with its significance to society. As the major benefactor, AHCPR is among the newest and least-endowed agencies of the U.S. Department of Health and Human Services. The purview of AHCPR extends well beyond trauma systems to cover all areas of clinical practice. Expectations for a research center at the National Institutes of Health were temporarily aroused in 1994 with the publication of *A Report of the Task Force on Trauma Research*, a congressionally mandated report for research recommendations to launch a trauma research program, including research in trauma systems (NIH, 1994). However, the report went largely unnoticed; Congress did not appropriate funds for its implementation. A subsequent section of this chapter contains a recommendation to augment trauma systems evaluation and related research.

GROWTH IN TRAUMA CARE SYSTEMS

All indications point to a progressive increase in the development of trauma systems in the United States since the 1970s, yet documenting the growth is not easy. States vary in their ability to collect data, and there are no ongoing and systematic nationwide or nationally representative surveillance systems (U.S. DHHS, 1991).

The greatest growth appears to be in prehospital care. All but nonexistent in the 1960s, prehospital care has become ubiquitous today. In the early 1990s, the *Journal of Emergency Medical Services* (JEMS) began an annual survey of prehospital providers in the 200 most populous cities, the so-called JEMS 200 City Survey, which captures 25 percent of the U.S. population. Although the sample is not nationally representative and the methods and results are not peer reviewed, the survey is one of the only indicators of growth and trends. The 1995 survey found 9-1-1 access to be available in more than 99 percent of the cities surveyed, and 82 percent of surveyed cities have so-called enhanced 9-1-1 service, in which the caller's street address is automatically provided to the dispatcher (W. Stanton, National Emergency Number Association, personal communication, 1998).

The nationwide status of regional trauma system development has been evaluated about every five years since 1987 through voluntary surveys of state EMS directors or health departments. Before 1987, state efforts waxed and waned depending on the vicissitudes of federal, state, and local support (Bazzoli et al., 1995). By 1987, West and colleagues (1988) found only two states that had fulfilled eight components judged essential by the authors to constitute a regional trauma system (see Table 6.2); 19 states and the District of Columbia missed meeting one or more of the criteria; and 29 states had not yet started the process of trauma center designation. By 1992, when the survey was updated by Bazzoli and colleagues (1995), five states were judged to have met the eight criteria. More states would have qualified except that they had failed to limit the number of trauma centers, depending on community need. The survey also found that states lacked standardized policies for interhospital transfer and systemwide evaluation. The authors advocated that more research on useful and valid outcome measures be included in trauma systems registries in order to assess system effectiveness. Subsequent nationwide updates were conducted in 1996 by Goodspeed (1997) and in 1997 by Bass (1997). Both studies found 27 states reported an established trauma system (although the defining criteria for a system were left to state discretion by Goodspeed). Thus, there is evidence to suggest that the past decade has witnessed an increase in trauma systems. The increase is thought to be related to the availability of federal funding, especially through the catalytic role of the Federal Trauma Care Systems Planning and Development Act, which required state matching funds. However, the authorization for this legislation lapsed in 1995, and it remains to be seen whether states will continue to invest in trauma systems development and maintenance without federal assistance.

TABLE 6.2 Essential Criteria to Identify Regional Trauma Systems

Legal authority to designate trauma centers
Formal process to designate trauma centers
Use of ACS criteria for classifying trauma centers
Out-of-area survey team for trauma center designation
Number of trauma systems limited by need (i.e., volume of patients or population of
    the area)
Written triage criteria
Ongoing monitoring system
Statewide trauma center coverage

SOURCE: West et al. (1988).

Although the surveys cited above provide insight into trauma systems development, they do not identify the actual growth in the number of trauma centers, as opposed to systems, nationwide. In an effort to identify hospitals either formally designated or self-designated as trauma centers between 1980 and 1991, Bazzoli and MacKenzie (1995) found 471 trauma centers. More recent figures from the ACS Committee on Trauma, which began a program to verify centers in 1987, reveal that, from 1987 to 1997, 285 hospitals were verified by the ACS as trauma centers (G. Strauch, American College of Surgeons, personal communication, 1998).

Rehabilitation is among the fastest-growing provinces of health care, with the number of freestanding rehabilitation hospitals and inpatient units increasing by more than 100 percent between 1985 and 1994 (IOM, 1997a). Even though injury patients account for a minority of all rehabilitation patients, their use of rehabilitation services is likely to increase for two key reasons: (1) the increased survival of more injured patients (HRSA, 1992) and (2) reduced lengths of stay in acute care services or hospitals, instituted in response to cost containment policies (IOM, 1997a). Nevertheless, there is anecdotal information about the lack of coordination between rehabilitation and acute care providers. The committee endorses full-fledged coordination between rehabilitation and acute care providers in an inclusive trauma system (for a complete discussion of rehabilitation research and the effectiveness of acute care interventions, see IOM [1997a]).

OUTCOMES OF TRAUMA CARE SYSTEMS

Does the establishment of trauma systems increase trauma patients' survival? This is a seminal question governing trauma systems research since the 1970s. Many outcome studies have focused on "preventable mortality" (i.e., the percentage of deaths retrospectively judged to have been preventable had optimal care been available from a trauma system). Although estimates vary, some studies have found preventable deaths to range as high as 20–40 percent of deaths due to injury (Trunkey and Lewis, 1991). These figures translate into nationwide annual estimates of approximately 20,000 to 25,000 lives saved (Champion and Teter, 1988). Nonetheless, studies of preventable deaths are beset by methodological limitations (Cales and Trunkey, 1985; Roy, 1987; Mendeloff and Cayten, 1991; MacKenzie et al., 1992). The purpose of this section is not to review comprehensively the peer-reviewed, published literature on patient outcomes with trauma systems, but rather to point to some illustrative studies, including more recent studies employing refined methodologies.

One noteworthy study of preventable mortality assessed the implementation of a regional trauma system in San Diego County, California (Shackford et al., 1986). The study found that after the implementation of a regional trauma system, the proportion of preventable fatalities fell from 13.6 to 2.7 percent. Such studies have been instrumental in stimulating the wider adoption of trauma systems.

Other approaches that are more objective than studies of preventable mortality have been developed to assess the benefits of trauma systems implementation. The Trauma and Injury Severity Score (TRISS) offers a means of predicting patient mortality based on injury severity, age, and revised trauma score (blood pressure, respiratory rate, and Glasgow Coma Scale for brain injury) (Boyd et al., 1987). With TRISS, the actual death rate in a hospital or trauma center can be compared to the predicted death rate from a large national data set of seriously injured trauma center patients voluntarily submitted to the Major Trauma Outcome Study (Champion et al., 1990). Champion and colleagues (1992) employed TRISS to assess longitudinally a reduction in trauma deaths in a center undergoing improvements from 1977 to 1982. They found an average of 13.4 more survivors per 100 seriously injured patients treated per year over the course of the improvements. Similarly, Stewart and colleagues (1995) found with TRISS that designation of a Canadian hospital as a trauma center led to a reduction in unexpected deaths from motor vehicle crashes from 8.8 percent before its designation to 3.6 percent after designation.

A newer method of evaluating outcomes related to trauma system implementation relies on population-based registries. The first study to capitalize on a comprehensive statewide population-based registry was performed by Mullins and coworkers (1994). They analyzed mortality outcomes among 70,350 patients who were hospitalized with injuries before and after institution of a trauma system in the Portland, Oregon metropolitan area. They found that the adjusted rate of mortality at Level I trauma centers was lowered by one-third compared to the pre-trauma system rate (the adjusted odds ratio for death declined from 1.00 before system establishment to 0.65 afterward). The impact was significant enough to be detected as an overall decline in the regional injury death rates, according to their analyses of two vital statistics databases. They also determined that the Portland metropolitan trauma system, through its prehospital triage criteria, was successful at shifting more seriously injured patients to trauma centers. Similar results were found when the authors broadened their analysis to cover five categories of injury across the entire state of Oregon before and after the implementation of a statewide trauma system (Mullins et al., 1996). A more recent publication reinforced earlier findings, demonstrating that mortality improvements were attributable to the introduction of the trauma system rather than to concurrent improvements in new technologies and treatments (Mullins et al., 1998).

The studies cited above focus on the hospital phase of care. There is scanty knowledge of outcomes in the prehospital (Spaite et al., 1993) and rehabilitation phases of care (IOM, 1997a). For example, there is incomplete understanding of the effectiveness of many widely used prehospital interventions, such as fluid repletion, its nature and timing, as a means of patient resuscitation (NIH, 1994). There is another critical gap in research on outcomes relating to morbidity, in both the short and the long term (NIH, 1994). Measures of morbidity have to transcend the traditional medical model to encompass measures of productivity, disability, and quality of life. Morbidity outcomes also need to be tracked post-discharge from acute and rehabilitative care. Additionally, research on the design and effectiveness of trauma systems must take into account the differences between trauma systems that are related to the mechanism of injury (e.g., blunt versus penetrating trauma) in each system.

In summary, studies demonstrate that acute trauma care reduces patient mortality. However, very few studies have addressed improved long-term morbidity with trauma systems (Rhodes et al., 1988) and improved quality of care (Shackford et al., 1986). Much work remains in order to demonstrate the benefits of trauma care in relation to morbidity. Additional work also is necessary to identify which elements of a trauma system are most responsible for reductions in morbidity and mortality. Research that identifies the most effective elements is difficult to perform for the following reasons: the elements have to be carefully defined and measured for comparative analysis, major trauma itself requires better definition, and an appropriate comparison group has to be identified as a control population.

RESEARCH ON TREATMENT OUTCOMES AND CLINICAL EFFECTIVENESS

Evaluating outcomes of trauma systems often depends on the availability of research measures for evaluating patient outcomes and clinical effectiveness. Research is needed to develop more reliable and valid measures of (1) injury severity and case mix and (2) short- and long-term outcomes that are sensitive to changes over time and to differences in treatment. These two areas are discussed below.

Injury Severity and Case Mix

Indicators used as a basis for assessing the severity of an injury include anatomical descriptors for assessing the extent of tissue damage; the mechanism of the injury; the physiological response of the body to the injury; and a priori or host factors such as age, gender, and coexisting disease that mediate the response of the body to the injury. There is general consensus that all four indicators or parameters are important for characterizing the impact of an injury or a constellation of injuries on outcome. More research is needed to improve the measurement of each parameter and to develop better models that establish the relationship between these parameters and outcomes, as discussed below.

The Abbreviated Injury Scale (AIS) has become a standard for measuring the extent of tissue damage (AAAM, 1990), yet its usefulness in detailed clinical studies of trauma involving specific organ systems is limited. Other classifications have been developed, such as to classify solid organ injuries (Moore et al., 1995) and long-bone fractures (Muller et al., 1990). The harmonization of these classifications should be encouraged. The AIS rates the severity of single injuries only. The Injury Severity Score (ISS) (Baker and O'Neill, 1976), defined as the sum of the squares of the maximum AIS obtained in each of the three most severely injured body regions, is currently the most widely used method for assessing the combined effect of multiple injuries. However, recent work has pointed to inadequacies of the ISS (Copes et al., 1988; Cayten et al., 1991). Alternatives such as the Anatomic Profile (Copes et al., 1990) and the New Injury Severity Score (Osler et al., 1997) have been proposed in order to account more adequately for the severity of multiple injuries to a single body system and for the important contribution of head injury in predicting outcome. These newer methods must be evaluated more broadly before their widespread use.

For large, population-based studies, use of the AIS (and its derivatives for scaling multiple injuries) is often not practical, since it takes, on average, between 10 and 20 minutes to score a single patient. Alternative scoring systems based on the International Classification of Diseases (ICD) have been proposed (MacKenzie et al., 1989; Rutledge et al., 1997) Although not as detailed a classification as the AIS, the clinical modification of the Ninth Revision of the ICD (ICD-9CM) does provide an alternative set of anatomic descriptors that is useful for characterizing the nature of traumatic injuries. Given the widespread use of the ICD, the further development and evaluation of ICD-based scoring systems should receive high priority .

The Revised Trauma Score (RTS)—based on the Glasgow Coma Score, systolic blood pressure, and respiratory rate—is the most widely used measure of injury severity based on physiologic parameters (Champion et al., 1989b). Although it has been shown to be a good predictor of mortality when combined with age and mechanism of injury, the RTS is inaccurate when the patient either is under the influence of drugs or alcohol or is intubated, paralyzed, or both (Offner et al., 1992). In addition, RTS values fluctuate over time and are sensitive to prehospital treatment. Further work is needed to better understand how these factors affect RTS values and how this information can be used to identify which values obtained over the course of time and treatment should be used retrospectively as fixed-point indicators of severity. In addition, further research is necessary to better characterize the physiologic response to injury at the extremes of age.

Statistical modeling techniques have been used to combine information on the anatomic descriptors of tissue damage, the physiologic response of the body to the injury, age, preexisting chronic conditions, and mechanism of injury in order to produce estimates of the probability of survival. The two most widely used models are the TRISS and ASCOT (A Severity Characterization of Trauma), both of which are based on the AIS, elements of the RTS, age, and mechanism of the injury (Champion et al., 1994, 1996). Refinements of TRISS and ASCOT have been proposed (Cayten et al., 1991). In addition, models using ICD-based versus AIS-based measures of severity have been introduced (Rutledge et al., 1997). Research is needed to validate existing models and to develop new models where necessary. Common databases and standard measures of scale performance should be employed.

Finally, and perhaps most importantly, research is needed to extend existing approaches or to develop new approaches for modeling outcomes other than death, including resource utilization and functional outcomes. Existing measures of severity and case mix have been developed principally for use in studies of mortality and are inadequate for assessing severity in terms of hospital length of stay, treatment costs, or disability (Bull, 1985; MacKenzie et al., 1986; Rutledge et al., 1998). With increasing attention to the determinants and consequences of nonfatal injuries, several efforts have been undertaken to develop a companion to the AIS that maps AIS injury descriptors into scores that better reflect probable degree of impairment or disability when the patient survives the injury (AAAM, 1994; MacKenzie et al., 1996; McClure and Douglas, 1996). Additional work is under way to develop approaches for predicting hospital length of stay and charges (Rutledge et al., 1998). High priority should be given to the evaluation of these approaches across the wide range of injury types and severities.

Outcome Measures

Evaluation of the effectiveness of trauma care has traditionally focused on survival. However, as more lives are saved, attention also is shifting to nonfatal outcomes. However, in measuring nonfatal outcomes following trauma, it is important to move beyond the use of narrowly defined measures of morbidity, impairment, and performance in basic activities of daily living to include more global measures of health status and health-related quality of life (HRQOL). Ultimately, the goal of good trauma care is the restoration of function that will allow the patient to resume his or her normal everyday activities. Although numerous measures of health status and HRQOL have been proposed in the literature, few have been applied to the study of trauma care and rehabilitation. There is an urgent need for broader use of these measures and for the development of standard approaches to assess trauma outcomes. The challenges are summarized below.

The Functional Independence Measure (FIM) (Keith et al., 1987) has gained wide acceptance in the field of medical rehabilitation as a measure of the "burden of care" associated with an illness or injury. The FIM score is generally assigned by a caregiver on the basis of direct observations of performance, although more recently developed telephone versions of the FIM rely on the individual's own assessment of his or her performance. Although further testing of the FIM is warranted, it holds promise as an effective tool for assessing the impact of inpatient rehabilitation on outcomes following serious trauma. However, the FIM does not encompass broader issues of outcome related to role activity, psychological well-being, and general health perceptions. It has also been criticized for its lack of sensitivity to the range of disabilities associated with traumatic brain injury.

Less frequently applied in the evaluation of trauma care and rehabilitation have been the wide array of health status and HRQOL measures. Although these measures vary widely in form and content, they share two important characteristics. First, they all measure function across multiple domains, including not only physical health, but also mental and cognitive health, social function, role function, and general health perceptions. Second, and even more important, health status and HRQOL measures assess outcomes from the patient's or consumer's perspective through the use of well-constructed questionnaires. One of the more important developments in health care over the past several years has been the recognition that the patient's point of view is important in evaluating the success of alternative therapies (Ware, 1995). Increasingly, patient-oriented measures of health status are playing a central role in health care evaluations (Relman, 1988). Examples of health status measures that have been used in measuring outcomes following trauma include the Sickness Impact Profile (Bergner et al., 1985), the General Health Status Measure Short Form-36 (Ware and Sherbourne, 1992), the Quality of Well-Being Scale (Kaplan et al., 1989; Holbrook et al., 1998), and the Rand Health Insurance Study Measures for Child Health Status (Eisen et al., 1980). However, their application has not been widespread, and important questions remain regarding their discriminate validity and their responsiveness to different treatments and to changes over time. Few studies have compared and contrasted available measures across the wide range of types and severities of injuries. Methodological research is critical in identifying and promoting the use of appropriate measures. An important issue is the extent to which available measures are sensitive to the cognitive deficits and behavioral changes that often accompany head injury.

Broad application of appropriate health status and HRQOL measures using standard protocols is essential for developing benchmarks for trauma outcomes. Substantial progress has been made over the past decade in establishing hospital-based trauma registries and defining the minimal data set needed for quality improvement activities. Typically, however, registries are not designed to collect information on outcomes beyond hospital mortality and morbidity. Efforts are needed to extend the current concept of a trauma registry to include information on longer-term and nonfatal outcomes to develop norms for outcomes other than mortality. Clearly, significant challenges exist in developing and maintaining such registries. First, there is a need for practical tools that can be applied routinely at low cost. Considerable effort has been focused over the past several years in developing shortened versions of some of the longer, time-consuming instruments. It will be important to evaluate these instruments for their sensitivity and responsiveness to the broad range of trauma patients. Second, effective and efficient systems for tracking patients are needed to facilitate assessment of outcomes at uniform time periods postinjury for patients who do and do not receive postacute care. Guidelines for developing and maintaining these registries are critical to ensure that information on long-term outcomes is collected with attention to data quality.

In assessing outcomes using health status and HRQOL measures, it will be important to simultaneously collect information on patient risk factors. Even with high-quality measures of outcome, determining the influence of trauma care and rehabilitation on these outcomes is difficult without an understanding of patient risk factors (MacKenzie et al., 1987; Wilson and Cleary, 1995). In part, this is because some of the greatest observed differentials in health outcomes are related more to patient risk factors than to the receipt of medical care. Thus, the analysis of clinical outcomes must take into account the complex interactions between the health care system and patient factors in order to effectively identify the potential for intervention and how this potential might vary for different subgroups of the population.

COSTS OF TRAUMA CARE SYSTEMS

There has been scanty systematic study of the overall cost of trauma systems (Mendeloff and Cayten, 1991). The reasons are essentially twofold: (1) Costs are incurred by multiple organizations (i.e., public agencies, and prehospital, acute care, and rehabilitation providers); and (2) costs fall under multiple categories, such as administration and planning, infrastructure and equipment, communications, additional staffing, and patient care. For simplicity, these costs reduce to either patient care or system infrastructure. Infrastructure costs, which are generally shouldered by public agencies, vary greatly depending on whether the trauma system is built de novo or whether elements of the system (e.g., prehospital care) are already in place. A state or region already equipped with an array of prehospital, acute care, and rehabilitation services geared for all types of trauma incurs modest additional costs to establish a trauma system, primarily for public administration, trauma center designation, and coordination; whereas a region without a continuum of care and with no public commitment to systemwide integration may incur substantial start-up and maintenance expenditures. The degree of public costs, for both start-up and maintenance, varies depending on how sophisticated a system is desired. However, there is no formal study of nationwide public and private costs for trauma systems.

Hospital charges, at 55 percent of the total costs of injury, represented the largest single type of direct cost (Rice et al., 1989). Using data from the 1984, 1985, and 1986 National Hospital Discharge Surveys, MacKenzie and coworkers (1990) determined that hospital, including trauma center, expenditures for all types of trauma in 1985 totaled $11.4 billion (inclusive of professional fees). This study also estimated that 25 percent of the total charges (or $2.8 billion) would be incurred by trauma centers treating the severely injured if such centers were available throughout the United States. Even though only 12 percent of trauma patients are severely injured, they disproportionately incur 26 percent of the charges (MacKenzie et al., 1990). Goldfarb and colleagues (1996) used a large national hospital discharge database to find that the average charge per hospital stay for severely injured patients in 1987 ranged from $12,891 to $28,464. The highest charges were incurred at Level I trauma centers that were part of a formal system. The lowest average charges for the severely injured were incurred at hospitals that were neither publicly designated nor self-designated as trauma centers. The study controlled for patient severity and hospital and community characteristics. A separate study of 12,088 trauma center admissions over a five-year period (1989–1993) by O'Keefe and colleagues (1997) found per-patient costs at a single regional trauma center to average $15,032 for victims of all ages with blunt and penetrating injuries. Several categories of complications greatly enhanced costs, such as pneumonia, adult respiratory distress syndrome, and acute kidney failure. According to 1995 data from the Health Services Cost Review Commission in Maryland, the mean hospital charge for a trauma admission is about 40 percent higher than that for a non-trauma admission (H. Champion, University of Maryland, Baltimore, personal communication, 1998).

There appear to be few studies of prehospital or rehabilitation costs for patients with injuries. The IOM (1997a) noted some studies that combine acute care and rehabilitation charges for a subset of the most severely injured, those with spinal cord and traumatic brain injuries. It also noted studies of total medical expenditures for people with disabling conditions, yet only a fraction of these people were disabled as a result of injury. Consequently, there is a noticeable lack of studies strictly of rehabilitation charges for injured patients of varying levels of severity. Since there is increasing recognition that a significant portion of an injured patient's clinical and financial experience occurs in the rehabilitation setting, a major challenge yet to be addressed is to measure objectively patients' outcomes and costs, including unreimbursed costs, of prehospital through rehabilitative care.

Cost-Effectiveness of Trauma Care Systems

The cost-effectiveness of trauma care systems only recently has begun to be explored. Miller and Levy (1995) were among the first to study the cost-effectiveness of these systems. Using 217,000 randomly sampled workers' compensation claims from 17 states (1979–1988), these investigators examined the cost-effectiveness in terms of lowered direct medical costs and increased worker productivity. They determined that, in states with trauma care systems, hospital and nonhospital medical care payments for acute care and rehabilitation for four types of injuries were, on average, 5–18 percent less costly per episode than those in states without such systems. Likewise, productivity (in terms of days at work) was enhanced. Extrapolating their figures to the nation as a whole, the authors estimated that if trauma systems were implemented nationwide, savings of $10.3 billion (in 1988 dollars) would be realized in increased productivity and lower medical payments. The largest portion of savings would be from productivity gains ($7.1 billion). The authors were careful to point out the limitations of their data set, namely, that results may not generalize to nonworker populations and to certain types of injury (e.g., head injuries). With enhanced productivity accounting for such a large proportion of savings, it may be difficult to establish the cost-effectiveness of trauma systems for older patients. The authors also acknowledged that their analysis fails to include potential indirect effects of trauma care systems on cost.

Targeted studies have addressed the cost-effectiveness of select elements of prehospital and rehabilitation care. For example, a recently published analysis of 13 previously published data sets found that helicopter medical transport is cost-effective in terms of cost per year of life saved, and is more cost-effective than other emergency medical interventions (Gearhart et al., 1997). Helicopter and ground transport directly from the scene of injury to a trauma center led to significantly shorter lengths of stay and charges than did matched interhospital transfers (i.e., patients transferred to a trauma center from a local hospital; Schwartz et al. [1989]). A study in a rural area found substantial delays, averaging about 70 minutes, between the time of arrival of the patient at a referring emergency department (ED) and the time a request is made by that ED for emergency helicopter transport to a trauma center (Garrison et al., 1989). Despite these findings, the use of helicopters is not systematized. Maryland and Connecticut are among the few states with centralized dispatch of helicopters.

Paramedic EMS in the treatment of prehospital cardiopulmonary arrest were found to be more cost-effective than heart, liver, and bone marrow transplantation and chemotherapy for acute leukemia (Valenzuela et al., 1990). Likewise, early, aggressive, and expert application of rehabilitation in brain injury and spinal cord injury patients is associated with economic savings (Cope and O'Lear, 1993). Much research remains to be performed on the cost-effectiveness of rehabilitation services for many other types of injuries (U.S. DHHS, 1992; IOM, 1997a).

Research undertaken thus far indicates that trauma systems and select elements of systems are cost-effective for some groups. Yet far more research must be conducted on the cost-effectiveness of trauma care systems and system characteristics such as organization, configuration, and elements of care (Spaite et al., 1993; NIH, 1994). For example, research is critically needed to determine which elements of prehospital, acute, and rehabilitative care are the most cost-effective in reducing patient morbidity and mortality. Better methods are needed for arriving at true costs, rather than charges, and better methods are needed for capturing outcomes in terms of later productivity (NIH, 1994). There may be some populations, such as the elderly, for whom cost-effectiveness is difficult to establish. For such vulnerable populations, continued public support is likely to be necessary. The key is to devise adequate sources of financing for trauma systems and patient care.

FINANCING OF TRAUMA SYSTEMS

This section covers public and private financing of trauma systems. The first part discusses federal and state funding for system infrastructure, and later sections cover the financing of patient care and the advent of managed care. The availability of financing is a prime determinant of trauma systems development, proliferation, and endurance.

History of Federal and State Support for Trauma Systems

For the past three decades, federal and state governments have assumed much of the responsibility for trauma systems development. A major impetus came from the publication of *Accidental Death and Disability: The Neglected Disease of Modern Society* (NRC, 1966). Another major factor was awareness of the military's prowess at triage, transport, and field hospital care in Korea and Vietnam. Federal and state support, however, has not been consistent. The record of support has been erratic, shifting over time, depending on the vicissitudes of legislative and public support, competing budget priorities, and health care costs. The history of federal and state support is captured in more detail elsewhere (Boyd, 1983; IOM, 1993; Mustalish and Post, 1994). Nevertheless, a few general observations and legal milestones are worth chronicling (Table 6.1).

Since the passage of the 1966 Highway Safety Act, the federal role traditionally has been to provide leadership, technical assistance, and systemwide models and guidelines for states and regions; to establish curricula for EMS providers; and to offer financial support to states for planning and infrastructure. States have assumed responsibility for dispersing federal and state funds; developing, coordinating, and administering systems; designating trauma centers; and ensuring quality. Yet both federal and state activities historically have concen-

trated upon the development of prehospital EMS care. It was not until 1990, with the passage of the Federal Trauma Care Systems Planning and Development Act (P.L. 101-590), that a broader approach to trauma systems, one that systematically organizes prehospital care, acute care, and rehabilitation,
was promulgated. This legislation, which called for an inclusive approach to trauma systems development, authorized grants to states and regions for planning, implementing, and monitoring statewide trauma care systems. The Division of Trauma and EMS (DTEMS) was established by the Health Resources and Services Administration (HRSA) to serve as a focal point, implement the legislation, and offer technical assistance to states.

The five-year history of P.L. 101-590 was marked by unfulfilled expectations because appropriations fell substantially short of the $60 million authorization, and states had difficulty during and after the second year in procuring matching funds (Hackey, 1995). Federal appropriations ranged from $4.4 million to 4.9 million from 1992 to 1995 (U.S. Executive Office of the President, 1992–1995). DTEMS was dissolved in 1995 when the legislation was not reauthorized, apparently the result of indiscriminate congressional efforts to reduce the federal deficit rather than to rebuke the program (ACS, 1995). There is some evidence that during its years of implementation, the legislation began to achieve its purpose, insofar as many more states began to launch or fully develop trauma care systems. Still, by 1997, only half of the states reported having trauma systems (Bass, 1997; Goodspeed, 1997).

Current Federal and State Funding for Trauma Care Systems

In a recent survey, 49 states and the District of Columbia reported the receipt of $14.5 million in FY 1996 for EMS and trauma systems funding (Goodspeed, 1997). The funds emanated mostly from block and categorical grants to states and regions and were not necessarily targeted to trauma systems development. Funds are distributed by three federal agencies: CDC, NHTSA, and HRSA.[3] Actual federal funding appears to be higher than that reported by states, but cannot be known with precision. Under block or formula grant funding, states are not required to report on the amounts that they allocate specifically to trauma system development. Block and formula grants are designed to give wide discretion to states, in contrast to categorical grant programs, such as that jointly administered by HRSA and NHTSA for the EMS-C Program.

---

[3]In FY 1997, the estimated funding for state and regional trauma systems was $11.9 million from the CDC Preventive Health and Health Services Block Grant and $12.5 million from the Emergency Medical Services for Children (EMS-C) Program sponsored by HRSA and NHTSA. An estimate of trauma system funding from the NHTSA Section 402 State and Community Formula Grants was not available.

States expend significant resources for trauma care systems, well in excess of the federal resources they receive, but there is no ongoing monitoring of annual amounts nationwide. A recent survey found that, in 1996, states spent more than $161.6 million on EMS and trauma care combined. The states' average annual per capita expenditure was $0.57 (Goodspeed, 1997). The methods by which states finance EMS and trauma care systems vary markedly. Methods include direct legislative appropriations (from general revenues or earmarked funds), fees for vehicle or driver licenses and motor vehicle violations, and other tax revenues (Swor, 1994; Goodspeed, 1997). Some states and localities finance EMS via subscriptions (e.g., residents voluntarily can pre-pay for ambulance services through an annual fixed fee, whereas those who do not subscribe are charged the full cost if they use the service). Local tax subsidies and fee-for-service billings (some of which are paid by third-party insurers) are the two most important sources of revenues for prehospital care (Stout, 1994).

In summary, trauma systems development is a shared responsibility of federal, state, and local agencies. The federal role has diminished substantially with the lapse in authorization of the 1990 Federal Trauma Care Systems Planning and Development Act. Consequently, there is no longer a focal point at the federal level to cultivate trauma systems development.

The committee supports a greater national commitment to, and support of, trauma care systems at the federal, state, and local levels, and recommends the reauthorization of trauma care systems planning, development, and outcomes research at the Health Resources and Services Administration.

To ensure the success of this recommendation, resources should be provided to stimulate the development and evaluation of trauma systems in states and regions with the greatest need for systems development. Further, states and regions should adhere to the Model Trauma System Care Plan for guidance about trauma systems design (HRSA, 1992); ensure that their trauma systems collect surveillance and outcome information related to all system elements, including rehabilitation (systems should perform periodic evaluations, especially of outcomes); and finance trauma systems development, coordination, and implementation with funds from dedicated revenue streams, such as surcharges on motor vehicle registration, motor vehicle violations, and other mechanisms.

Financing of Patient Care

The financing of patient care is the Achilles' heel of trauma systems. A well-cited publication has referred to the financing problem as a "crisis in trauma care reimbursement" (Champion and Mabee, 1990). One survey of 313 trauma centers in 1992 found that 58 percent reported serious financial problems and another 36 percent reported minor financial problems (Eastman et al., 1994). From 1983 to 1990, 66 trauma centers closed, with economic strains ranked as four of the five most important reasons for closure (Dailey et al., 1992). Although the pace of closures appears to have abated more recently (Bazzoli et al., 1995), the current changes wrought by managed care may imperil trauma systems once again (see below).

Several interrelated factors explain the economic strains on trauma centers (GAO, 1991; Dailey et al., 1992; Hackey, 1995). The first is the high cost of care and overhead relative to other types of care. The second factor is the growth in uncompensated care. From 1984 to 1994, the percentage of uninsured Americans grew from 15.4 to 17.8 percent (HRSA, 1995). The problem of uncompensated care is compounded in urban and public hospitals, especially due to increases in violent injury during the 1980s and early 1990s (Mendeloff and Cayten, 1991; Bazzoli et al., 1996). The third factor is inadequate patient care financing by Medicare and Medicaid (MacKenzie et al., 1991; Mendeloff and Cayten, 1991; Hackey, 1995). For example, Medicare's prospective reimbursement system, which has been adopted by some state Medicaid programs, did not adequately adjust reimbursement rates to account for the greater severity of patients' injuries seen in trauma centers, although Medicare did make an adjustment for this problem in 1991 (Dailey et al., 1992; Bazzoli et al., 1996). Medicare and Medicaid are among the mix of major payers of patient care in trauma centers, and the recovery rates to hospitals are among the lowest (Figure 6.1).

The most important sources of patient care financing for trauma center care are, in decreasing order of recovery rate,[4] private insurance and workers' compensation, Medicare, Medicaid, and self-pay (Eastman et al., 1991, 1994). In terms of the percentage of total trauma care charges, the leaders are workers' compensation and private insurance (i.e., health insurance and auto insurance) at 42.8 percent of charges, followed by Medicaid at 19.1 percent and Medicare at 13.5 percent (Figure 6.1). With this mix of payers and recovery rates, Eastman and coworkers (1994) found that trauma centers experienced an overall loss of 8.4 percent of costs. Yet when they proceeded to stratify the data by service location (urban, suburban, and rural), a more complex picture emerged: trauma centers in urban and suburban areas reported losses at 11.7 and 5.7 percent, respectively, whereas trauma centers in rural areas had the most favorable financial performance—the only area of the three to show a small aggregate surplus of 3.7 percent (although only 11 rural centers were studied). A more recent study at a rural trauma center in Vermont attributes its financial profitability to lower injury severity among patients and a more favorable payer mix, with about 50 percent of injury patients being covered by private insurance (Rogers et al., 1997a).

---

[4]Recovery rate is the percentage of costs recovered by total revenues received (Eastman et al., 1991, 1994).

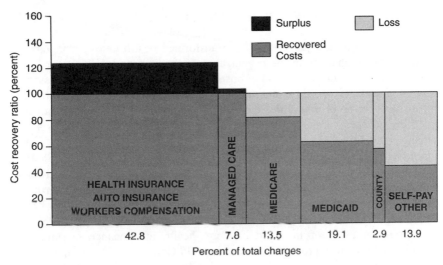

FIGURE 6.1 Reimbursement profile for all service areas. SOURCE: Eastman et al. (1994). Reprinted with permission from Lippincott, Williams and Wilkins.

The cost-recovery profile presented in Figure 6.1, although limited to a sample of trauma centers surveyed in 1992, illustrates the general principle that the most generous rates of recovery for patient care costs are from fee-for-service health insurance, auto insurance, and workers' compensation. This profile, however, fails to capture the great degree of expansion of managed care into the private and public sectors (see following section). As managed care continues to infiltrate the health care market, the ability of trauma centers and hospitals to shift costs from publicly to privately insured patients is jeopardized. This trend is likely to present new challenges in trauma care financing, the viability of trauma centers, and the quality of patient care in the future.

The increasing cost of patient care provides financial incentives for payers such as employers and health insurers to embrace injury prevention, both in occupational and in nonoccupational settings. Prevention programs have the potential to reduce health care costs. With an effective prevention program, reductions in health care costs may even be experienced in the short term (i.e., while the enrollee is still covered), compared to prevention programs for chronic conditions, such as heart disease, where cost reductions are more likely to be experienced in the long term (i.e., after enrollment has lapsed). The immediacy of prevention payoffs for injuries is likely an important consideration for payers. Payers should be eager to support injury prevention programs with their potential for short-term results because enrollee turnover tends to be high.

ADVENT OF MANAGED CARE

The managed care juggernaut has transformed health care. Managed care entails dramatic changes in the organization, financing, and delivery of health services, all in pursuit of containing costs, increasing access to health insurance through greater affordability, and maintaining quality (IOM, 1989, 1997b). The impact has been so profound that the diminishing numbers of providers not governed by managed care are compelled to respond with cost-cutting measures to remain competitive. Enrollment in managed care has burgeoned from virtual obscurity a decade ago to more than 70 percent of working Americans in 1995 (Foster Higgins, 1995). Millions more are covered through Medicaid and Medicare (Retchin, 1997), where the greatest growth in managed care is occurring. In 1996, 13.3 million Medicaid beneficiaries were enrolled in some form of managed care, a fourfold increase since 1991 (Kaiser Family Foundation, 1998). The most common types of managed care are health maintenance organizations (HMOs) and preferred provider organizations (PPOs), in which a group of hospitals or physicians provides services to plan members at discounted rates, or mixes of the two (Gold et al., 1995). In most PPOs and some HMOs, emergency care is provided through contracts with select EDs and trauma centers, whereas other HMOs provide emergency services directly.

Although the configurations of plans vary widely, managed care generally employs a common set of methods to attain the goal of cost containment, including selective contracting, special financing structures through capitation or discounted fees, benefit structures, and mechanisms for monitoring or managing services (IOM, 1996). From the point of view of the trauma patient, the latter is among the most significant because of the "gatekeeping" functions of managed care organizations (MCOs). Gatekeeping typically requires the patient or the provider to seek pre-authorization to receive payment for emergency care. The intent of preauthorization is to discourage ED use for patients who do not require such care. Although it is strictly for payment purposes, preauthorization is often misunderstood as preauthorization for treatment. However, federal law (the Emergency Medical Treatment and Active Labor Act of 1985) requires that all emergency patients be evaluated or screened and, if necessary, stabilized in the emergency room before release or transfer (GAO, 1991).[5]

What is the impact of managed care on trauma systems? The simple answer is that the full verdict is not yet in, and may never be, because of the dynamic nature of managed care and the difficulty of securing funding for research on its impact. Most of the accusations against managed care surround gatekeeping functions in relation to ED use—accusations that have prompted several states to

---

[5]Nevertheless, there is evidence that the denial of payment authorization serves as a powerful incentive for patients to choose to leave the emergency room (Derlet, 1997; Young and Lowe, 1997).

pass, and Congress to consider, proposed legislation to protect consumers (Derlet and Young, 1997; ACEP, 1998). Specifically, managed care has been charged with the delay of emergency care through preauthorization requirements; denial or undercoverage at EDs that are not part of a managed care network of providers; inadequate information about the use of 9-1-1; and premature discharge from acute care or rehabilitation (ACEP, 1993, 1998; Kilborn, 1997). The net effect may be an interruption in the continuity of care and poorer patient outcomes (Derlet, 1997). Counterbalancing these charges are the purported benefits of managed care. Among them is the possibility of promoting a better match between available resources and patient needs; reducing unnecessary costs; and emphasizing prevention, cost-effectiveness, data acquisition, and the use of treatment guidelines (IOM, 1996). What may be lost amidst the entry of managed care into trauma systems is the fact that some underlying goals of managed care and trauma care are similar, particularly the emphasis on prevention and on a match between available resources and patient needs. Congress is currently considering the passage of proposed federal legislation requiring public and private health insurance coverage for ED visits that any "prudent layperson" considers to be medically necessary.

The remainder of this section describes the modest body of peer-reviewed literature on the impact of managed care on trauma systems utilization, costs, and outcome. To place this literature in the context of managed care across all types of health care, a comprehensive literature analysis of studies since 1980 found HMOs, in comparison with fee-for-service plans, to have lower hospital admission rates, shorter lengths of stay (LOS), the same or more physician office visits per enrollee, less use of expensive procedures and tests, greater use of preventive services, mixed results on outcomes, and somewhat lower enrollee satisfaction with services (Miller and Luft, 1994).

With respect to managed care and trauma systems, the main measures of utilization have been 9-1-1 access, emergency room visits, and LOS. In terms of 9-1-1 access, one study found that virtually all Chicago-based HMOs surveyed in the late 1980s advised enrollees in case of emergency to contact the HMO office, primary physician, or a toll-free number, whereas only one HMO advised enrollees to go to the nearest hospital, yet made no mention of calling 9-1-1 (Hossfeld and Ryan, 1989). This study may be limited in applicability or dated, but it was among the first and only study of its kind. In another study, ED visits were reduced by at least 15 percent during one hospital's transition to managed care that was mandated by the State of Connecticut for all Medicaid recipients (Powers, 1997). Since access to emergency services is crucial, it is important for research to monitor the impact of managed care on trauma system access and related outcomes.

Under managed care, LOS would be expected to be lower for trauma patients. Yet two published studies that bear either directly or indirectly on LOS offer conflicting results. In the first study, Campbell and coworkers (1995) found that the mean LOS for 89 HMO trauma center patients in San Francisco from 1989 to 1993 were actually higher than those for non-HMO controls matched for age, injury severity, and other characteristics. In fact, one subset of HMO patients, those transferred from the trauma center to the HMO hospital, had the longest LOS. The authors speculate that the possible reasons for the increased LOS among transferred patients are the disruption in continuity of care, problems in discharge planning, and medical complications that occur after transfer. On the other hand, a study of 3,141 admissions from 1990 to 1992 to a Seattle trauma center found LOS to be similar among motor vehicle crash patients with and without commercial insurance (Rhee et al., 1997). (Those without commercial insurance were either Medicaid or self-pay.) Although this study did not specifically compare managed care and fee-for-service patients, it found no effect of payer status on utilization. Part of the difficulty of monitoring LOS among managed care and fee-for-service patients is that LOS has declined in general in response to nationwide trends in cost containment.

Outcomes under managed care have been studied with respect to mortality and morbidity, but studies are sparse and not necessarily comparable. In the study by Campbell and coworkers cited above, HMO patients experienced lower mortality rates (4.1 percent) relative to non-HMO patients (9.9 percent), after adjustment for severity of injury and other factors, but HMO patients were younger, more often male, and more likely to have blunt injuries. The study by Rhee and colleagues (1997) found no differences in mortality between patients with commercial insurance and those without, but as pointed out above, the study was not of managed care per se. On the other hand, Young and Lowe (1997) found gatekeeping by managed care to be associated with adverse outcomes. After reviewing solicited case reports of 29 patients denied authorization by MCOs for ED payment, they determined that 14 percent had adverse outcomes (mortality and morbidity), 14 percent were at increased risk, and 72 percent were near misses (i.e. cases in which adverse outcomes were averted by ED care despite denial of authorization). Their findings confirmed earlier published reports about adults and children being denied authorization for ED payment (Derlet and Young, 1997). These findings are disturbing and warrant examination in a larger, random sample in which there is no selection bias.

The quest for cost containment also is significantly felt in EMS. There are several important and interrelated trends transforming EMS: (1) the consolidation of small, independent public and private EMS providers into large, publicly traded corporations that can realize economies of scale; (2) increased contracting between MCOs and EMS agencies in capitated or risk-sharing agreements; and (3) the development of new triage guidelines for EMS dispatchers designed to steer non-emergency calls away from the EMS system to more appropriate community resources (Neely, 1997; Neely et al., 1997; NHTSA, 1997b). It is important to monitor these trends with respect to their impact on EMS access, utilization, cost, and patient outcomes. The development of new triage guidelines is a special concern because of the potential for undertriage, which occurs when patients are not administered the emergency services they need. Public health professionals are concerned that the development of new triage guidelines is being driven more by cost containment pressures than by empirical evaluation to ensure their effectiveness in matching patient needs with available resources. With one exception (Neely, 1998), very few such evaluations have been published thus far.

Managed care has extensively penetrated rehabilitation services in some major cities and is growing rapidly elsewhere (DeJong et al., 1996). There is a paucity of research on the impact of managed care on rehabilitation services. So many questions remain unanswered that a blueprint for research on managed care and people with disabilities has been developed (U.S. DHHS, 1995; IOM, 1997a). Although 70 percent of working Americans are enrolled in managed care, the need to demonstrate the relationship between quality of trauma care and rehabilitation and costs and outcomes is important for all Americans. This information is needed for defining best practices and for shaping treatment guidelines. It is also essential to the development of innovative service delivery models that benefit the patient while attending to the escalating costs of health care.

The committee recommends intensified trauma outcomes research, including research on the delivery and financing of acute care services and rehabilitation. The committee envisions that HRSA and other appropriate federal agencies (e.g., NCIPC, AHCPR) will collaborate on this research.

Specific areas of research that should be addressed include the following:

• the cost-effectiveness of specific clinical and service interventions to establish best practices in trauma care;
• the most efficient and effective strategies for organizing and financing the delivery of both acute care services and rehabilitation, including the impact of managed care arrangements on access to services, quality of care, and outcomes; and
• the development of improved methods for measuring the severity of injury, particularly for those at high risk of adverse outcomes.

Finally, managed care accrediting organizations should support the development, coordination, and implementation of trauma care systems. They should mandate, as a condition of facility accreditation, participation in an inclusive trauma care system in states and regions with such systems and should promote the development of trauma care systems in states and regions without them.

SUMMARY

Great strides have been made over the past decades in developing trauma systems covering a continuum of prehospital, acute care, and rehabilitation services. Public health organizations and providers have embraced the need for a broader, more inclusive philosophy that shifts the focus from the trauma center to a system of trauma care that attends to the needs of all trauma patients over the full course of treatment.

Trauma care is lifesaving, yet expensive. The costs of trauma systems development should be shared by federal, state, and local governments. About half of the states report having some kind of trauma systems, although their nature and extent are not well documented. Some of the most successful statewide trauma systems have flourished with dedicated sources of funding through motor vehicle fees and other creative approaches. Research has begun to demonstrate that the investment in systems of care can be cost-effective in terms of long-term health care costs and productivity. However, there always may be vulnerable populations, such as the elderly, for whom cost-effectiveness may be difficult to demonstrate. More research is needed on vulnerable populations, patient outcomes, system configuration, and cost-effectiveness. A focal point at the federal level has to be reinstated to support research and to cultivate the growth of state and regional trauma systems. A federal program had been in place until 1995, when budget pressures led to the program's demise.

The financing of patient care continues to constrain trauma systems. The growth of managed care has placed further financial burdens on hospitals and trauma centers. The impact of managed care on trauma patient access, utilization, quality, and financing is essential to monitor but has been largely unexamined in the peer-reviewed biomedical literature. Financing constraints reinforce the public health imperative of primary injury prevention.

REFERENCES

AAAM (Association for the Advancement of Automotive Medicine). 1990. *The Abbreviated Injury Scale.* Des Plaines, IL: AAAM

AAAM (Association for the Advancement of Automotive Medicine). 1994. *The Injury Impairment Scale, 1994.* Des Plaines, IL: AAAM.

ACEP (American College of Emergency Physicians). 1992. Guidelines for trauma care systems. *Annals of Emergency Medicine* 22:1079–1100.

ACEP (American College of Emergency Physicians). 1993. *America's Health Care Safety Net, Emergency Medicine: 1968–1993 and Beyond.* Dallas, TX: ACEP.

ACEP (American College of Emergency Physicians). 1998. *ACEP* [World Wide Web document]. URL http://www.acep.org (accessed January 1998).

ACS (American College of Surgeons). 1993. *Resources for Optimal Care of the Injured Patient.* Chicago: ACS.

ACS (American College of Surgeons). 1995. Trauma funding is threatened. *Bulletin of the American College of Surgeons* 80:7.

Adams BL, Trimble MP. 1994. Nurses. In: Kuehl AE, ed. *Prehospital Systems and Medical Oversight,* 2d edition. St. Louis: Mosby-Year Book. Pp. 76–80.

Baker SP, O'Neill B. 1976. The injury severity score: An update. *Journal of Trauma* 16(11):882–885.

Baker SP, Whitfield MA, O'Neill B. 1987. Geographic variation in mortality from motor vehicle crashes. *New England Journal of Medicine* 316:1384–1387.

Bass R. 1997. *Data Obtained from a Survey by the National Association of State EMS Directors.* Presented to the National Association of EMS Physicians, EMS Research Meeting, July 10. Lake Tahoe, NV.

Bazzoli GJ, MacKenzie EJ. 1995. Trauma centers in the United States: Identification and examination of key characteristics. *Journal of Trauma* 38(1):103–110.

Bazzoli GJ, Madura KJ, Cooper GF, MacKenzie EJ, Maier RV. 1995. Progress in the development of trauma systems in the United States: Results of a national survey. *Journal of the American Medical Association* 273(5):395–401.

Bazzoli GJ, Meersman PJ, Can C. 1996. Factors that enhance continued trauma center participation in trauma systems. *Journal of Trauma* 41(5):876–885.

Bensard DD, McIntyre RC, Moore EE, Moore FA. 1994. A critical analysis of acutely injured children managed in an adult level I trauma center. *Journal of Trauma* 35:384–393.

Bergner M, Bobitt RA, Carter WB, Gilson BS. 1985. The SIP: Development and final revision of a health status measure. *Medical Care* 19:787–805.

BLS (Bureau of Labor Statistics). 1997. *Occupational Outlook Handbook* [World Wide Web document]. URL http://stats.bls.gov/oco/ocos101.htm (accessed July 1998).

Boyd CR, Tolson MS, Copes WS. 1987. Evaluating trauma care: The TRISS method. *Journal of Trauma* 27:370–378.

Boyd DR. 1983. The history of emergency medical systems in the United States of America. In: Boyd DR, Edlich RF, Mioik SH, eds. *Systems Approach to Emergency Medical Care.* Norwalk, CT: Appleton-Century-Crofts.

Bull JP. 1985. Disabilities caused by road traffic accidents and their relation to severity scores. *Accident Analysis and Prevention* 17:355–366.

Cales RH, Trunkey DD. 1985. Preventable trauma deaths: A review of trauma care systems development. *Journal of the American Medical Association* 254(8):1059–1063.

Campbell AR, Vittinghoff E, Morabito D, Paine M, Shagoury C, Praetz P, Grey D, McAninch JW, Schecter WP. 1995. Trauma centers in a managed care environment. *Journal of Trauma* 39(2):246–251.

Cayten CG, Stahl WM, Murphy JG, Agarwal N, Byrne DW. 1991. Limitations of the TRISS Method for interhospital comparisons: A multihospital study. *Journal of Trauma* 31(4):471–482.

Champion HR, Mabee MS. 1990. *An American Crisis in Trauma Care Reimbursement.* Washington, DC: Washington Hospital Center.

Champion HR, Teter H. 1988. Trauma care systems: The federal role. *Journal of Trauma* 28(6):877–879.

Champion HR, Copes WS, Buyer D, Flanagan ME, Bain L, Sacco WJ. 1989a. Major trauma in geriatric patients. *American Journal of Public Health* 79(9):1278–1282.

Champion HR, Sacco WJ, Copes WS, Gann DS, Gennarelli TA, Flanagan, ME. 1989b. A revision of the trauma score. *Journal of Trauma* 29(5):623–629.

Champion HR, Copes WS, Sacco WJ, Lawnick MM, Keast SL, Bain LW, Flanagan ME, Frey CF. 1990. The major trauma outcome study: Establishing national norms for trauma care. *Journal of Trauma* 30:1356–1365.

Champion HR, Sacco WJ, Copes WS. 1992. Improvement in outcome from trauma center care. *Archives of Surgery* 127:333–338.

Champion HR, Copes WS, Sacco WJ. 1994. The major trauma outcome study: Establishing norms for trauma care. *Journal of Trauma* 36:499–503.

Champion HR, Copes WS, Sacco WJ, Frey CF, Folcroft JW, Hoyt DB, Weigelt JA. 1996. Improved predictions from A Severity Characterization of Trauma (ASCOT) over Trauma and Injury Severity Score (TRISS): Results of an independent evaluation. *Journal of Trauma* 40:40–49.

Chen B, Maio RF, Green PE, Burney RE. 1995. Geographic variation in preventable deaths from motor vehicle crashes. *Journal of Trauma* 38(2):228–232.

Cooper A, Barlow B, DiScalla C, String D, Ray K, Mottley L. 1993. Efficacy of pediatric trauma care: Results of a population-based study. *Journal of Pediatric Surgery* 31:72–77.

Cope DN, O'Lear J. 1993. A clinical and economic perspective on head injury rehabilitation. *Journal of Head Trauma Rehabilitation* 8:1–14.

Copes WS, Champion HR, Sacco WJ, Lawnick MM, Keast SL, Bain LW. 1988. The injury severity score revisited. *Journal of Trauma* 28(1):69–77.

Copes WS, Champion HR, Sacco WJ, Lawnick MM, Gann DS, Gennarelli T, MacKenzie E, Schwaitzberg S. 1990. Progress in characterizing anatomic injury. *Journal of Trauma* 30(10):1200–1207.

Copes WS, Stark MM, Lawnick MM, Tepper S, Wilderson D, DeJong G, Brannon R, Hamilton BB. 1996. Linking data from national trauma and rehabilitation registries. *Journal of Trauma* 40(3):428–436.

Dailey JT, Teter H, Cowley RA. 1992. Trauma center closures: A national assessment. *Journal of Trauma* 33:539–547.

Davidson LL, Durkin MS, Kuhn L, O'Connor P, Barlow B, Heagarty MC. 1994. The impact of the Safe Kids/Healthy Neighborhoods Injury Prevention Program in Harlem, 1988 through 1991. *American Journal of Public Health* 84:580–586.

DeJong G, Wheatley B, Sutton J. 1996. Perspective and analysis: Medical rehabilitation undergoing major shakeout in advanced managed care markets. *Bureau of National Affairs' Managed Care Reporter* 2:138–141.

DeMaria E, Kenney PR, Merriam MA, Casanova LA, Gann DS. 1987. Survival after trauma in geriatric patients. *Annals of Surgery* 206(6):738–743.

Derlet RW. 1997. Locked gates: Profit and pain. *Academic Emergency Medicine* 4:1099–1100.

Derlet RW, Young GP. 1997. Managed care and emergency medicine: Conflicts, federal law, and California legislation. *Annals of Emergency Medicine* 30:292–300.

Durkin MS, Kuhn L, Davidson LL, Laraque D, Barlow B. 1996. Epidemiology and prevention of severe assault and gun injuries to children in an urban community. *Journal of Trauma* 41:667–673.

Eastman AB, Lewis FR, Champion HR, Mottox KL. 1987. Regional trauma system design: Critical concepts. *American Journal of Surgery* 154:79–87.

Eastman AB, Rice CL, Bishop GS, Richardson JD. 1991. An analysis of the critical problem of trauma center reimbursement. *Journal of Trauma* 31:920–960.

Eastman AB, Bishop GS, Walsh JC, Richardson JD, Rice CL. 1994. The economic status of trauma centers on the eve of health care reform. *Journal of Trauma* 36(6):835–844.

Eisen M, Donald CA, Ware JE, Brook RH. 1980. *Conceptualization and Measurement of Health for Children in the Health Insurance Study.* Santa Monica, CA: RAND Corporation. Publication No. R–2313.HEW.

Finelli FC, Jonsson J, Champion HR, Morelli S, Fouty WJ. 1989. A case control study for major trauma in geriatric patients. *Journal of Trauma* 29(5):541–548.

Flowe KM, Cunningham PR, Foil B. 1995. Rural trauma systems in evolution. *Surgery Annual* 27:29–39.

Fortune JB, Sanchez J, Graca L, Haselbarth J, Kuehler DH, Wallace JR, Edge W, Feustel PJ. 1992. A pediatric trauma center without a pediatric surgeon: A four-year outcome analysis. *Journal of Trauma* 33(1):130–137.

Foster Higgins. 1995. *National Survey of Employer Sponsored Health Plans, 1995*. New York: Foster Higgins.

GAO (General Accounting Office). 1991. *Trauma Care: Lifesaving System Threatened by Unreimbursed Costs and Other Factors*. Washington, DC: GAO. HRD-91-57.

Garrison HG, Benson NH, Whitley TW. 1989. Helicopter use by rural emergency departments to transfer trauma victims: A study of time-to-requests intervals. *American Journal of Emergency Medicine* 7:384–386.

Garrison HG, Foltin GL, Becker LR, Chew JL, Johnson M, Madsen GM, Miller DR, Ozmar BH. 1997. The role of emergency medical services in primary injury prevention. *Annals of Emergency Medicine* 30(1):84–91.

Gearhart PA, Wuerz R, Localio AR. 1997. Cost-effectiveness analysis of helicopter EMS for trauma patients. *Annals of Emergency Medicine* 30:500–506.

Gold MR, Hurley R, Lake T, Ensor T, Berenson R. 1995. A national survey of the arrangements managed-care plans make with physicians. *New England Journal of Medicine* 333(25):1678–1683.

Goldfarb MG, Bazzoli GJ, Coffey RM. 1996. Trauma systems and the costs of trauma care. *Health Services Research* 31(1):71–95.

Goodspeed DG. 1997. Benchmarking emergency medical services: Trauma systems funding in the United States. *Best Practices and Benchmarking in Healthcare* 2(2):45–51.

Hackey RB. 1995. Politics of trauma system development. *Journal of Trauma* 39(6):1045–1053.

Hall JR, Reyes HM, Meller JL, Stein RJ. 1993. Traumatic death in urban children, revisited. *American Journal of Diseases of Children* 147:102–107.

Hall JR, Reyes HM, Meller JL, Loeff D3, Dembek R 1996. The outcome for children with blunt trauma is best at a pediatric trauma center. *Journal of Pediatric Surgery* 31(1):72–76.

Holbrook TL, Anderson JP, Sieber WJ, Browner D, Hoyt DB. 1998. Outcome after major trauma: Discharge and 6-month follow-up results from the Trauma Recovery Project. *Journal of Trauma* 45(2):315–324.

Hossfeld G, Ryan M. 1989. HMOs and utilization of emergency medical services: A metropolitan survey. *Annals of Emergency Medicine* 18(4):374–377.

HRSA (Health Resources and Services Administration). 1990. *Success and Failure: A Study of Rural Emergency Medical Services*. Prepared by the National Rural Health Association. Rockville, MD: HRSA.

HRSA (Health Resources and Services Administration). 1992. *Model Trauma Care System Plan*. Rockville, MD: HRSA Division of Trauma and Emergency Medical Systems.

HRSA (Health Resources and Services Administration). 1995. *Five-Year Plan: Emergency Medical Services for Children, 1995–2000*. Washington, DC: Emergency Medical Services for Children National Resource Center.

Hulka F, Mullins RJ, Mann NC, Hedges JR, Rowland D, Worrall WH, Sandoval RD, Zechnich A, Trunkey DD. 1997. Influence of a statewide trauma system on pediatric hospitalization and outcome. *Journal of Trauma* 42:514–519.

IOM (Institute of Medicine). 1989. *Controlling Costs and Changing Patient Care? The Role of Utilization Management.* Washington, DC: National Academy Press.

IOM (Institute of Medicine). 1991. *Disability in America: Toward a National Agenda for Prevention.* Washington, DC: National Academy Press.

IOM (Institute of Medicine). 1993. *Emergency Medical Services for Children.* Washington, DC: National Academy Press.

IOM (Institute of Medicine). 1996. *Pathways of Addiction: Opportunities in Drug Abuse Research.* Washington DC: National Academy Press.

IOM (Institute of Medicine). 1997a. *Enabling America: Assessing the Role of Rehabilitation Science and Engineering.* Washington, DC: National Academy Press.

IOM (Institute of Medicine). 1997b. *Managing Managed Care: Quality Improvement in Behavioral Health.* Washington, DC: National Academy Press.

Jacobs BB, Jacobs L. 1993. Prehospital emergency medical services. In: Kravis TC, Warner CG, Jacobs LM, eds. *Emergency Medicine*, 3d edition. New York: Raven Press. Pp. 1–29.

Jacobs LM, Sinclair A, Beiser A, D'Agostino RB. 1984. Prehospital advance life support: Benefits in trauma. *Journal of Trauma* 24(1):8–13.

Kaiser Family Foundation. 1998. Fact sheet: Medicaid and Managed-Care. [World Wide Web document]. URL http://www.kff.org:80/archive/health_policy/kcfm/mmcare/mmcare.html (accessed May 1998).

Kaplan RM, Anderson JB, Wu AW, Mathers WC, Kozin F, Orenstein D. 1989. The quality of well-being scale: Applications in AIDS, cystic fibrosis and arthritis. *Medical Care* 27(3):S27–S43.

Keith RA, Granger CV, Hamilton BB, Sherwin FS. 1987. The functional independence measure: A new tool for rehabilitation. In: Eisenberg MG, ed. *Advances in Clinical Rehabilitation.* Vol. 1. New York: Springer. Pp. 6–18.

Kilborn PT. 1997. Fitting managed care into emergency rooms. *New York Times*, December 28, p. 10.

Kinnane JM, Garrison HG, Coben JH, Alonso-Serra HM. 1997. Injury prevention: Is there a role for out-of-hospital emergency medical services? *Academic Emergency Medicine* 4(4):306–312.

Knudson MM, Shagoury C, Lewis FR. 1992. Can adult trauma surgeons care for injured children? *Journal of Trauma* 32(6):729–737.

Konvolinka CW, Copes WS, Sacco WJ. 1995. Institution and per surgeon volume vs. survivor outcome in Pennsylvania's trauma centers. *American Surgeon* 170:333–340.

Ma MH-M. 1997. *System Performance and Appropriateness of Care for Elderly Trauma Patients.* Doctoral dissertation. Johns Hopkins University, Baltimore, MD.

MacKenzie EJ, Shapiro S, Moody M, Siegel JH, Smith RT. 1986. Predicting posttrauma functional disability for individuals without severe brain injury. *Medical Care* 24(5):377–387.

MacKenzie EJ, Shapiro S, Smith RT, Siegel JH, Moody M, Pitt A. 1987. Influencing return to work following hospitalization for traumatic injury. *American Journal of Public Health* 77(3):329–334.

MacKenzie EJ, Morris JA, Edelstein SL. 1989. Effect of pre-existing disease on length of stay in trauma patients. *Journal of Trauma* 29(6):757–765.

MacKenzie EJ, Morris JA, Smith GS, Fahey M. 1990. Acute hospital costs of trauma in the U.S.: Implications for regionalized systems of care. *Journal of Trauma* 30(9):1096–1103.

MacKenzie EJ, Steinwachs DM, Ramzy AI, Ashworth JW, Shankar B. 1991. Trauma case mix and hospital payment: The potential for refining DRGs. *Health Services Research* 26(1):5–26.

MacKenzie EJ, Steinwachs DM, Bone LR, Floccare DJ, Ramzy AI. 1992. Inter-rater reliability of preventable death judgments. The Preventable Death Study Group. *Journal of Trauma* 33(2):292–302.

MacKenzie EJ, Damiano A, Miller T, Luchter S. 1996. The development of the functional capacity index. *Journal of Trauma* 41(5):799–807.

McClure RJ, Douglas RM. 1996. The public health impact of minor injury. *Accident Analysis and Prevention* 28:443–451.

Mendeloff JM, Cayten CG. 1991. Trauma systems and public policy. *Annual Review of Public Health* 12:401–424.

Miller RH, Luft HS. 1994. Managed care plan performance since 1980: A literature analysis. *Journal of the American Medical Association* 271:1512–1519.

Miller TR, Levy DT. 1995. The effect of regional trauma care systems on costs. *Archives of Surgery* 130:188–193.

Moore EE. 1995. Trauma systems, trauma centers, and trauma surgeons: Opportunities in managed competition. *Journal of Trauma* 39(1):1–11.

Moore EE, Cogbill TH, Jurkovich GJ, Malangoni MA, Shackford SR, Champion HR. 1995. Organ injury scaling: Spleen and liver (1994 Revision). *Journal of Trauma* 38(3):323–324.

Mueller BA, Rivara, FB, Bergman A. 1988. Urban-rural location and a risk of dying in a pedestrian-vehicle collision. *Journal of Trauma* 28:91–94.

Muller ME, Nazarian S, Koch P, Schatzker J. 1990. *Classification of Long Bone Fractures*. Berlin: Springer-Verlag.

Mullins RJ, Veum-Stone J, Helfand M, Zimmer-Gembeck M, Hedges JR, Southard PA, Trunkey DD. 1994. Outcome of hospitalized injured patients after institution of a trauma system in an urban area. *Journal of the American Medical Association* 271(24):1919–1924.

Mullins RJ, Veum-Stone J, Hedges JR, Zimmer-Gembeck MJ, Mann NC, Southard PA, Helfand M, Galnes JA, Trunkey DD. 1996. Influence of a statewide trauma system on location of hospitalization and outcome of injured patients. *Journal of Trauma* 40(4):536–545.

Mullins RJ, Mann NC, Hedges JR, Worrall W, Jurkovich GJ. 1998. Preferential benefit of implementation of a statewide trauma system in one of two adjacent states. *Journal of Trauma* 44(4):609–616.

Mustalish AC, Post C. 1994. History. In: Kuehl AE, ed. *Prehospital Systems and Medical Oversight*. 2d edition. St. Louis: Mosby-Year Book. Pp. 3–23.

Nakayama DK, Copes WS, Sacco W. 1992. Difference in trauma care among pediatric and nonpediatric trauma centers. *Journal of Pediatric Surgery* 27(4):427–431.

National Trauma Data Project. 1996. *A Report to the Division of Trauma and Emergency Medical Systems, Health Resources and Services Administration*. Conducted by John V. Udell, Augusta, ME.

NCIPC (National Center for Injury Prevention and Control). 1993. *Injury Control in the 1990s: A National Plan for Action. A Report to the Second World Conference on Injury Control*. Atlanta, GA: Centers for Disease Control and Prevention.

NCIPC (National Center for Injury Prevention and Control). 1997a. *Data Elements for Emergency Department Systems (DEEDS)* [World Wide Web document]. URL http:www.cdc.gov/ncipc/pub-res/deedspage.htm (accessed December 1997).

NCIPC (National Center for Injury Prevention and Control). 1997b. *Inventory of Federally Funded Research in Injury Prevention and Control.* Atlanta, GA: NCIPC.

Neely K. 1997. Demand management: The new view of EMS? *Prehospital Emergency Care* 1(2):114–118.

Neely K. 1998. *Can Emergency Medical Service Dispatchers Identify Callers Suitable For Non-Emergency Medical Service Resources?* Presentation at the 1998 Society for Academic Emergency Medicine Research Forum, Steamboat Springs, CO. January 1998.

Neely K, Drake ME, Moorhead JC. 1997. Multiple options and unique pathways: A new direction for EMS? *Annals of Emergency Medicine* 30:797–799.

NHTSA (National Highway Traffic Safety Administration). 1997a. *Emergency Access: Extending the Nation's Emergency Medical Safety Net.* Washington, DC: NHTSA.

NHTSA (National Highway Traffic Safety Administration). 1997b. Working with managed care organizations. *EMS and Managed Care Bulletin.* [World Wide Web document]. URL http://www.nhtsa.dot.gov:80/people.injury/ems/bulletin/bullet97. htm (accessed July 1998).

NIH (National Institutes of Health). 1994. *A Report of the Task Force on Trauma Research.* Bethesda, MD: NIH.

NIH (National Institutes of Health). 1995. *Disease-Specific Estimates of Direct and Indirect Costs of Illness and NIH Support.* Bethesda, MD: NIH.

NPTR (National Pediatric Trauma Registry). 1998. *The National Pediatric Trauma Registry.* [World Wide Web document]. URL http://www.nemc.org/rehab/ nptrhome.htm (accessed September 1998).

NRC (National Research Council). 1966. *Accidental Death and Disability: The Neglected Disease of Modern Society.* Washington, DC: National Academy Press.

NRC (National Research Council). 1978. *Emergency Medical Services at Midpassage.* Washington, DC: National Academy Press.

NREMT (National Registry of Emergency Medical Technicians). 1998. *NREMT* [World Wide Web document]. URL http://www.nremt.org (accessed January 1998).

Offner PJ, Jurkovich GJ, Gurney J, Rivara FP. 1992. Revision of TRISS for intubated patients. *Journal of Trauma* 32(1):32–35.

O'Keefe GE, Maier RV, Diehr P, Grooseman D, Jurkovich GJ, Conrad D. 1997. The complications of trauma and their associated costs in a level I trauma center. *Archives of Surgery* 132(8):920–924.

Osler T, Baker S, Long W. 1997. A modification of the Injury Severity Scale that both improves accuracy and simplifies scoring. *Journal of Trauma* 43:922–926.

OTA (Office of Technology Assessment). 1989. *Rural Emergency Medical Services— Special Report.* Washington, DC: OTA. OTA-H-445.

Phillips S, Rond PC, Kelly SM, Swartz PD. 1996. The failure of triage criteria to identify geriatric patients with trauma: Results from the Florida Trauma Triage Study. *Journal of Trauma* 40(2):278–283.

Pollack MM, Alexander SR, Clarke N, Ruttimann UE, Tesselaar HM, Bachulis AC. 1991. Improved outcomes from tertiary center pediatric intensive care: A statewide comparison of tertiary and nontertiary facilities. *Critical Care Medicine* 19(2):150–159.

Pollock DA, McClain PW. 1989. Trauma registries: Current status and future prospects. *Journal of the American Medical Association* 226:2280–2283.

Powers RD. 1997. Medicaid managed care and the emergency department: The first 100 days. *Journal of Emergency Medicine* 15(3):393–396.

Regel G, Stalp M, Lehmann U, Seekamp A. 1997. Prehospital care, importance of early intervention on outcome. *Acta Anaesthesiologica Scandinavica Supplementum* 110:71–76.

Relman AS. 1988. Assessment and accountability: The third revolution in medical care. *New England Journal of Medicine* 319:1220–1222.

Retchin SM. 1997. Heterogeneity of health maintenance organizations and quality of care. *Journal of the National Cancer Institute* 89(22):1654–1655.

Rhee PM, Grossman D, Rivara F, Mock C, Jurkovich G, Maier RV. 1997. The effect of payer status on utilization of hospital resources in trauma care. *Archives of Surgery* 132(4):399–404.

Rhodes M, Aronson J, Moerkirk G, Petrash E. 1988. Quality of life after the trauma center. *Journal of Trauma* 28(7):931–938.

Rhodes M, Smith S, Boorse D. 1993. Pediatric patients in an "adult" trauma center. *Journal of Trauma* 35:384–393.

Rice DP, MacKenzie EJ, Jones AS, Kaufman SR, deLissovoy GV, Max W, McLoughlin E, Miller TR, Robertson LS, Salkever DS, Smith GS. 1989. *Cost of Injury in the United States.* San Francisco, CA: Institute for Health and Aging, University of California and Injury Prevention Center, The Johns Hopkins University.

Rogers FB, Osler TM, Shackford SR, Cohen M, Camp L. 1997a. Financial outcome of treating trauma in a rural environment. *Journal of Trauma* 43(1):65–72.

Rogers FB, Shackford SR, Hoyt DB, Camp L, Osler TM, MacKersie RC, Davis JW. 1997b. Trauma deaths in a mature urban vs. rural trauma system. *Archives of Surgery* 132(4):376–381.

Roy PD. 1987. The value of trauma centers: A methodological review. *Canadian Journal of Surgery* 30:17–22.

Rutledge R, Fakhry SM, Meyer A, Sheldon GF, Baker CC. 1993. An analysis of the association of trauma centers with per capita hospitalization and death rates from injury. *Annals of Surgery* 218(4):512–524.

Rutledge R, Hoyt D, Eastman AB, Sise MJ, Velky T, Canty T, Wachtel T, Osler TM. 1997. Comparison of the ISS and ICD-9 diagnoses codes as predictors of outcome in injury. *Journal of Trauma* 42(3):477–489.

Rutledge R, Osler T, Emery S, Kromhout-Schiro S. 1998. The end of ISS and the TRISS: ICISS outperforms both ISS and TRISS as predictors of trauma patient survival, hospital charges and hospital length of stay. *Journal of Trauma* 44:41–49.

Schwartz RJ, Jacobs LM, Yaezel D. 1989. Impact of pre-trauma center care on length of stay and hospital charges. *Journal of Trauma* 29:1611–1615.

Shackford SR. 1995. The evolution of modern trauma care. *Surgical Clinics of North America* 75(2):147–156.

Shackford SR, Hollingworth-Fridlund P, Cooper GF, Eastman AB. 1986. The effect of regionalization upon quality of trauma care as assessed by concurrent audit before and after institution of a trauma system: A preliminary report. *Journal of Trauma* 26(9):812–820.

Shapiro MJ, Cole KE, Keegan M, Prasad CN, Thompson RJ. 1994. National survey of state trauma registries—1992. *Journal of Trauma* 37(5):835–840.

Smith JS, Martin LF, Young WW, Macioce DP. 1990. Do trauma centers improve outcome over non-trauma centers? The evaluation of regional trauma care using discharge abstract data and patient management categories. *Journal of Trauma* 30(12):1533–1538.

Spaite DW, Valenzuela TD, Meislin HW. 1993. Barriers to EMS system evaluation: Problems associated with field data collection. *Prehospital and Disaster Medicine* 8:S35–S40.

Stewart TC, Lane PL, Stefanits T. 1995. An evaluation of patient outcomes before and after trauma center designation using trauma and injury severity score analysis. *Journal of Trauma* 39:1036–1040.

Stout JL. 1994. System financing. In: Roush WR, ed. *Principles of EMS Systems*. Dallas: American College of Emergency Physicians. Pp. 451–473.

Swor R. 1994. Funding strategies. In: Kuehl AE, ed. *Prehospital Systems and Medical Oversight*, 2d edition. St. Louis: Mosby-Year Book. Pp. 76–80.

Trunkey D, Lewis FR. 1991. Preventable mortality. In: Trunkey D, Lewis FR, eds. *Current Therapy of Trauma*, 3d edition. Philadelphia, PA: Decker. Pp. 3–4.

U.S. DHHS (Department of Health and Human Services). 1991. *Healthy People 2000: National Health Promotion and Disease Prevention Objectives*. Washington, DC: U.S. Government Printing Office. (PHS) 91–50212.

U.S. DHHS (U.S. Department of Health and Human Services). 1992. *Position Papers from the Third National Injury Conference, Setting the National Agenda for Injury Control in the 1990s, April 22–25, 1991, Denver, CO*. Washington, DC: DHHS.

U.S. DHHS (Department of Health and Human Services). 1995. *Managed Care for People with Disabilities: Developing a Research Agenda*. Washington, DC: U.S. DHHS.

U.S. DOT (Department of Transportation). 1994. *Uniform Pre-Hospital EMS Data Conference Final Report, 1994*. Washington, DC: U.S. DOT. DOT-3P0061.

U.S. DOT (Department of Transportation). 1995. *EMS Systems Development: Results of the Statewide EMS Assessment Program*. Washington, DC: U.S. DOT. DOT-3P0067.

U.S. DOT (Department of Transportation). 1996a. *Consensus Statement on the EMS Role in Primary Injury Prevention*. Washington, DC: U.S. DOT. DOT-3P0081.

U.S. DOT (Department of Transportation). 1996b. *Emergency Medical Services: Agenda for the Future*. Washington, DC: U.S. DOT. DOT HS 808 441; NTS-42.

U.S. Executive Office of the President, Office of Management and Budget. 1992–1995. *Budget of the United States Government Fiscal Years 1992–1995*. Washington, DC: U.S. Government Printing Office.

Valenzuela TD, Criss EA, Spaite D, Meislin HW, Wright AL, Clark L. 1990. Cost effectiveness analysis of paramedic emergency medical services in the treatment of prehospital cardiopulmonary arrest. *Annals of Emergency Medicine* 19(12):1407–1411.

Ware JE. 1995. The status of health assessment 1994. *Annual Review of Public Health* 16:327–354.

Ware JE, Sherbourne CD. 1992. The MOS 36-Item Short-Form Health Survey (SF-36). *Medical Care* 30:473–483.

West JG, Williams MJ, Trunkey DD, Wolferth CC. 1988. Trauma systems: Current status—future challenges. *Journal of the American Medical Association* 259(24):3597–3600.

Wilson IB, Cleary PD. 1995. Linking clinical variables with health-related quality of life: A conceptual model of patient outcomes. *Journal of the American Medical Association* 273(1):59–65.

Young GP, Lowe RA. 1997. Adverse outcomes of managed care gate keeping. *Academic Emergency Medicine* 4(12):1129–1135.

7

State and Community Response

Further progress in reducing the burden of injuries not only depends on concerted research and treatment efforts but also requires a strengthened focus on prevention implementation. Great strides have been made in developing injury prevention strategies that have been shown to be successful in promoting safety and reducing injury morbidity and mortality (Chapter 4). In most cases, injury prevention is best achieved through a multifaceted approach that utilizes the range of available prevention strategies (Box 7.1). However, widespread implementation of proven injury prevention strategies is often impeded by political, social, and economic barriers.

In large measure, prevention is a local effort. Because the implementation of prevention measures frequently involves interacting with individuals and families (e.g., providing education, distributing safety measures such as bike helmets), it is at the state and community levels that most prevention programs are implemented. As problems and needs are identified, public support is garnered at the local level, and a number of organizations (including hospitals, schools, civic groups, athletic leagues, businesses, and fire and police departments) frequently work together to address injury hazards and concerns. Therefore, local capacity to develop, implement, and evaluate prevention interventions must be supported.

This chapter first provides a brief overview of the broad landscape of state, local, and nonprofit efforts that are involved in addressing different facets of the injury problem. The remainder of the chapter discusses several steps that need to be taken to move toward more systematic and widespread implementation of injury prevention programs.

BOX 7.1
Child Passenger Safety Seats: An Example of the Lessons Learned and the Challenges Faced in Implementing an Efficacious Injury Prevention Strategy

Child passenger safety seats were developed to protect children and are known to be efficacious in reducing the risk of death and injury in car crashes. From 1988 to 1995, the motor vehicle occupant death rate declined 18 percent for children less than 1 year of age. (SAFE KIDS, 1998b).

The efforts contributing to the increase in the use of safety seats are indicative of the multiple approaches needed to implement injury prevention measures and include:

- legislatively mandated child seat use in all states and the District of Columbia;
- education of police regarding enforcement of child passenger safety laws;
- development of a national certification program to train child passenger safety specialists;
- development and dissemination of educational and technical material for health care practitioners, safety professionals, car dealers, and the general public;
- advances in crash testing technology and biomechanics that led to specific safety requirements;
- establishment of low-cost safety-seat loaner programs;
- increases in hospital policies requiring discharge of newborns in child safety seats;
- investment by corporate entities (e.g., Johnson & Johnson, General Motors, Allstate, State Farm) in national campaigns such as SAFE KIDS;
- provision of technical assistance, seed funds, and mini grants to local agencies by state governor highway safety offices and state health departments; and
- policy statements on the use of child occupant restraints by professional organizations such as the American Academy of Pediatrics, the American Public Health Association, and the American School Health Association.

Given the success of this intervention, there are still problems in implementation. It is estimated that 35 percent of children 4 years old and under are riding unrestrained and that nearly 80 percent of children riding in child safety seats are improperly restrained (SAFE KIDS, 1998b). In short, even proven injury prevention interventions require a multifaceted approach. A reduction in injuries is achieved only after a long period of intervention and sustained attention to the issue.

Because of their number and diversity, it is difficult to quantify the total extent of government, community, and private-sector endeavors in the injury field. At the state and local levels of government, many agencies are charged with protecting the public's well-being, including health and safety (Table 7.1). Although all of these agencies may not consider themselves part of the injury field per se, each is an integral component of broader safety efforts to prevent or reduce injuries.

Private-sector organizations, ranging from corporations to foundations and other nonprofit organizations, provide substantive support for injury prevention through injury-related advocacy, sponsorship of research, and implementation of prevention programs. A number of individuals and groups have started grassroots organizations on injury prevention, often turning personal tragedies into dedicated injury prevention efforts. All of these endeavors have an impact on increasing public awareness about injury, providing funding for injury prevention programs, and galvanizing support for the implementation of injury prevention goals. Nonprofit organizations garner financial support (and often volunteer support) from concerned citizens, small businesses and corporate sponsorship, philanthropic foundations, and through state and federal government agencies. For-profit corporations and businesses also contribute to safety efforts by implementing employee safety programs (often providing information about both on-the-job and off-the-job safety issues), focusing on product safety, and providing consumer education. The examples provided in Box 7.2 reflect only a snapshot of the numerous nonprofit, foundation, and grassroots efforts dedicated to injury prevention. The examples were chosen to reflect the diversity of ongoing injury efforts. Additionally, a number of professional organizations focus their attention on injury issues (Box 7.3). These organizations often develop educational materials, sponsor continuing education classes and workshops, hold conferences to discuss ongoing research, and support injury prevention programs.

Although the current response is impressive, it is also fragmented. Many of the organizations and agencies focus on a specific cause of injury (e.g., sports, vehicles, fires), type of injury (e.g., spinal cord injury, burns), or target population (children, teenagers, elderly). As depicted throughout this report, one of the prime opportunities for the injury field is to leverage the resources and expertise of the numerous agencies, organizations, and individuals interested in reducing injuries. Additionally, it is important for the injury field to focus educational efforts on legislators, administrators, manufacturers, and the media, to continue to inform them about the effectiveness and cost-effectiveness of injury prevention and to keep them updated on new developments.

BOX 7.2
Examples of Nonprofit Organizations

Brain Injury Association (BIA): Founded in 1980, the BIA works to increase awareness and promote prevention of brain injury. Additionally, it works through state associations and in conjunction with health care facilities to develop a network of community services and support groups for individuals with brain injury and their families. Administered by the BIA, the American Academy for the Certification of Brain Injury Specialists has developed a three-level certification program for individuals working in brain injury rehabilitation (BIA, 1998).

The California Wellness Foundation: Targeting youth violence prevention as one of its five key strategic initiatives, the foundation funds grants on policy change, funds research grants, encourages grassroots leadership through community leadership awards, strengthens postgraduate programs through academic fellowship grants, and supports community action by providing resources and technical assistance for pilot programs.

Insurance Institute for Highway Safety (IIHS): Sponsored by more than 80 automobile insurance companies, IIHS is a nonprofit research organization that focuses on the primary factors involved in automobile collisions: human factors, vehicle crashworthiness and safety features, the physical environment, and legal measures. The Highway Loss Data Institute, one of the two major components of IIHS, gathers, analyzes, and publishes data on vehicles and their insurance losses. In 1992, IIHS opened the Vehicle Research Center, which utilizes full-scale crash testing and investigation of on-the-road crashes to collect and analyze information on vehicle crashworthiness and the implications of safety measures on occupant protection.

Mothers Against Drunk Driving (MADD): MADD has worked for the past 17 years to raise awareness about the often fatal consequences of drunk driving, to look for effective solutions to drunk driving and underage drinking problems, and to provide support to victims of drunk driving crashes. Started by a small group of California women after the death of a teenager, the nonprofit association now has over 600 local chapters throughout the United States and receives both individual and corporate support (MADD, 1998).

Continued

BOX 7.2 *Continued*

National Fire Protection Association (NFPA): NFPA has worked since 1896, to educate the public and develop codes and standards for fire safety. The membership of the nonprofit organization has over 68,000 individuals and 100 organizations (NFPA, 1998). Through technical committees, the NFPA has developed more than 300 codes and standards, known collectively as the National Fire Code. Additionally, the NFPA is active in developing and disseminating educational materials and its safety programs include the Fire Prevention Week activities and the Learn Not to Burn curriculum.

National SAFE KIDS Campaign: Founded in 1987, SAFE KIDS promotes childhood safety through the implementation of community-based strategies and is an example of a nationwide collaborative effort between the private and public sectors. SAFE KIDS is sponsored by the Children's National Medical Center, Johnson & Johnson, General Motors Corporation, Bell, First Alert, Toy Manufacturers of America, Gas Appliance Manufacturers Association, National Fire Protection Association, the Health Resources and Services Administration (HRSA), the National Highway Traffic Safety Administration (NHTSA), the Maternal and Child Health Bureau (MCHB), and the U.S. Fire Administration (SAFE KIDS, 1998a). SAFE KIDS supports over 240 state and local injury prevention coalitions, each of which draws on a diversity of local resources, including school systems, fire departments, local hospitals, civic organizations, and parks and recreation departments.

National Safety Council: Although federally chartered in 1913, the Council is a not-for-profit, nongovernmental organization with over 18,500 members representing business, labor, industry, and government. The Council works both through topic-oriented divisions (e.g., agriculture, construction, labor, motor transportation, utilities, youth activities) and state and local chapters. The Council provides training, education programs, consulting, and advocacy leadership with the goal of improving safety and environmental health.

Snell Memorial Foundation: Founded in 1957, the Foundation is dedicated to improving sport helmet safety and develops standards for helmets including those used in bicycling, equestrian events, motorcycle riding, skiing, and auto racing. Additionally, prior to Snell certification, the Foundation conducts extensive testing to evaluate the extent of the helmet's protection.

BOX 7.3
Examples of Professional Organizations

American Academy of Pediatrics, Section on Injury and Poison Prevention
American Association for the Surgery of Trauma
American College of Emergency Physicians, Trauma Care and Injury Control Committee
American College of Surgeons, Committee on Trauma
American Pediatric Surgical Association, Committee on Trauma
American Public Health Association, Injury Control and Emergency Health Services Section
American School Health Association, National Task Force for Injury Prevention
American Society of Safety Engineers
American Trauma Society
Association for the Advancement of Automotive Medicine
Emergency Nurses Association
Human Factors Society
Institute of Transportation Engineers
Intelligent Transportation Society of America
International Association of Chiefs of Police
International Association of Fire Chiefs
International Association of Fire Fighters
International Council on Alcohol, Drugs, and Traffic Safety
International Society for Child and Adolescent Injury Prevention
International Trauma Anesthesia and Critical Care Society
National Association of Governors' Highway Safety Representatives
National Association of State Fire Marshalls
Society of Automotive Engineers
Society of Trauma Nurses
State and Territorial Injury Prevention Directors' Association

---

As illustrated above, many agencies, organizations, and individuals work on some facet of injury prevention. However, the state and community response is often hampered by federal and state funding constraints and a lack of awareness of injury prevention measures. The committee has identified five areas that, if successfully addressed, could optimize proven strategies for prevention: (1) strengthening the public health infrastructure; (2) building and encouraging collaboration and coalitions of state and local safety agencies and organizations; (3) improving training and technical assistance; (4) improving the translation of research findings into practice; and (5) increasing public awareness and advocacy.

TABLE 7.1 State and Local Government Agencies and Organizations

Agency or Organization	Infrastructure	Injury Focus	Examples of Funding Sources for Injury Activities
Child Death Review Teams (CDRTs)	All states have state and/or local CDRTs; some state teams are legislatively mandated	• Gather and analyze data on the circumstances surrounding child deaths • Make recommendations on measures to prevent future childhood deaths	• Funding sources vary widely
Child Protective Services	State agencies	• Screen and investigate cases of child abuse and neglect; assist families in finding solutions	• State appropriations
Emergency Medical Services (EMS) Agencies	Transport services in every state; more than 600,000 regional or local EMS providers	• Care of the injured person at the scene and transportation to hospitals	• Preventative Health and Human Services block grants • State appropriations • EMS for Children grants
Fire Service Agencies	More than 31,500 county, city, local, or district fire departments	• Fire fighting and rescue operations • Fire prevention programs, and broader fire and life safety education programs	• State and local taxes
Labor and Occupational Offices	25 states operate their own occupational safety and health agencies; the Occupational Safety and Health Administration (OSHA) runs the programs in other states	• Investigate injuries in the workplace • Develop and implement prevention programs • Provide input on regulations	• Multiple sources: OSHA, state appropriations

Law Enforcement Agencies	State, county, municipal, and other local juris-dictional police or law enforcement agencies	• Enforce laws (e.g., driving under the influence, safety belt and child safety seat laws) • Provide prevention measures (e.g., sobriety checkpoints, bicycle and motorcycle safety programs)	• State and local taxes
Poison Control Centers	85 centers nationwide	• Provide information about poisonings and appropriate treatment protocols • Involved in poisoning prevention	• State appropriations • Municipal funding • Hospital or university funding
Public Health Departments	• Each state has a state health department • Over 3,000 local health departments	• Use surveillance data to identify injury problems • Implement and evaluate injury prevention programs	• Federal block grants: Maternal and Child Health (MCH) and PHHS • State appropriations

SOURCES: NRC (1993); Garrison et al. (1997); NACCHO (1998); NFPA (1998).

STRENGTHENING THE PUBLIC HEALTH INFRASTRUCTURE

The strengthening of a well-developed injury prevention program in the state health department is the foundation for state and local injury prevention efforts. In many states, however, this key element is only a fledgling effort. There is wide disparity between states in the extent to which injury prevention is a priority program at the health department level. A 1988 survey of state and territorial health departments found that 10 states had a separate injury program or unit devoted solely to injury prevention (Harrington et al., 1988). Forty percent of the states or territories allocated one full-time equivalent (FTE) or less to injury prevention, and the major sources of funding for state injury prevention efforts were MCH block grants, and PHHS block grants (Harrington et al., 1988).

This picture seems to have changed little in the intervening 10 years. The committee and staff interviewed state personnel from 30 state departments of health and found that there is still wide disparity in the size and funding of injury prevention programs independent of state size and population: 3 of the 30 states have extensive injury programs with 14–23 FTEs and more than $1.5 million in funding, whereas 8 of the 30 states have 1.5 FTEs or less devoted to injury prevention. The primary sources of funding continue to be MCH and PHHS block grants, and the majority of states have only limited direct state funding. Little funding for state capacity building is available from the National Center for Injury Prevention and Control (NCIPC) and the funding that is made available is often earmarked for specific programs of NCIPC interest. Consequently, locally prioritized prevention programs often lack needed resources. Injury prevention programs are administratively placed in a variety of different divisions of the state health department (e.g., epidemiology, health promotion, maternal and child health, chronic disease prevention, EMS, environmental health). Program placement is important in that it may influence not only the division's priorities for the injury prevention program but also the specific injuries that the program may target (e.g., maternal and child health may target only childhood injuries).

The State and Territorial Injury Prevention Directors' Association (STIPDA)[1] Safe States initiative outlines five core elements necessary for a well-developed injury prevention program: (1) statewide and local data collection and analysis; (2) program design, implementation, and evaluation; (3) coordination and collaboration; (4) technical support and training; and (5) policy development (STIPDA, 1997). In some cases, components (e.g., surveillance) may be administratively located in separate divisions of the health department, and close collaboration between divisions is crucial.

---

[1]STIPDA is a national organization made up of designated members from every state health department. STIPDA's mission is to sustain, enhance, and promote the ability of state, territorial, and local health departments to reduce death and disability from injury.

Data and Surveillance

To set priorities for injury prevention programs, state and local practitioners need morbidity and mortality injury data (see Chapter 3). However, data collected at the local and community levels have not always been available. In the past 10 years a number of specialized, topic-specific state and local surveillance systems (e.g., traumatic brain injury surveillance, firearm injury surveillance) have been funded as demonstration projects by federal agencies. Unfortunately, funding for such programs has generally been intermittent or time limited, preventing long-term implementation, analysis, evaluation, or dissemination (see Chapter 3).

Local hospital discharge data that are accompanied by an external cause-of-injury code (E-codes) are also useful for developing injury prevention interventions (see Chapter 3). These data provide a perspective on the more serious injuries that require hospitalization, allow comparisons to be made with other medical conditions and diseases, and pinpoint localities with higher than normal injury incidence, which then may be targeted for specific programs and resources. Almost half of the states now require E-coding, which allows this information to be routinely analyzed and available on a statewide basis (Chapter 3). However, practitioners cannot access community data directly from the local hospital because such data are available only from a central collecting agency. Other untapped sources of injury data include records of emergency departments, EMS and police investigations. However, those records often are not computerized or not linked to hospital data or other data sets, and unresolved issues of confidentiality make it difficult—if not impossible—to trace the injuries in a useful way for targeted prevention interventions. Technical assistance by state personnel trained in injury surveillance methods can help communities and local professionals access, analyze, and transform locally collected data into useful information

Strategic Planning

As states embrace injury prevention efforts and work toward strengthening their injury prevention programs, it is important to incorporate injury prevention into many diverse strategic planning processes and documents. For example, the *State of Utah Annual Plan for Maternal and Child Health* devotes sections to injury control and youth suicide prevention (Utah Department of Health, 1997); New York's Highway Safety Strategic Plan contains a section on injury (Klein et al., 1997); and the Emergency Preparedness and Injury Control Program of the California Department of Health Services has produced a five-year strategic plan dedicated to injury prevention. The California Department of Health Services' strategic plan for 1993–1997 contains specific objectives for reducing injury morbidity and mortality and suggests mechanisms for incorporating injury prevention efforts into other health department and state agency programs (California Department of Health Services, 1992). California's plan is noteworthy because it was developed with the input of local practitioners and researchers and used annual injury conferences to facilitate this consensus-building process (Kelter, 1997).

Annual state health plans should establish injury prevention goals, specific performance indicators, and outcome measures for monitoring unintentional injury, suicide, and violence. The plans should include specific actions for the integration of injury prevention within existing service delivery mechanisms in relevant state agencies. Similar efforts should be made for planning documents related to transportation, social services, criminal justice, and other state functions. An important component of all state programs should be the inclusion of careful evaluation of all implemented injury programs.

Technical Assistance

Strengthening, and in some cases, building the public health infrastructure could be greatly facilitated by direct technical assistance to state and local injury programs. As discussed in Chapter 8, the committee supports an increased role for NCIPC in providing technical assistance. This could be accomplished in a number of ways. One approach would be to team states having extensive and long-standing injury programs with states that have new, inexperienced, or fledgling programs. Sharing expertise and lessons learned would hasten the maturation of new injury programs and could be linked to incentives for both members of the state teams. Another model would be to use regional offices to provide technical assistance directly to states within the region. A third approach would utilize technical assistance teams composed of multidisciplinary staff (e.g., state health commissioner, injury program manager, epidemiologist, health educator) with field experience in injury prevention at the state and local levels. Such a team could conduct site visits and assist state health injury prevention staff in developing specific action plans, identifying means to overcome state and local barriers, and providing follow-up technical assistance at regularly scheduled intervals. A potential resource for assembling such teams is STIPDA, which through its membership from every state can access the needed expertise of personnel who have developed similar injury prevention programs in other states and localities. The site visit team approach was utilized by NHTSA to assist state EMS agencies in the development and implementation of state level EMS plans.

Funding

Funding for injury prevention programs by the public and private sectors has been inadequate when compared to the magnitude of the injury problem (see

Chapter 2) and what is already known about prevention. Available funding for state and local public health departments has frequently been too restrictive, has placed an emphasis on the development of separate and categorical programs, and generally has received limited state appropriations. A federal commitment is needed to provide the funding to sustain state injury prevention programs, similar to the Section 402 formula grant funding from NHTSA that is used to support state highway safety offices and the Governors' Highway Safety Program. Further, it is critical that program funding include monies for a strong evaluation component. Evaluation is integral to improving program effectiveness, but too often receives limited or no specific funding.

Federal Funding

Federal funding for injury prevention programs in state and local health departments comes from multiple funding streams including MCH and PHHS block grants.[2] Little funding, however, is made available for state and local capacity building (i.e., instituting and maintaining an ongoing injury prevention program).

From FY1989 to 1993, the NCIPC funded 15 state and community-based injury prevention capacity-building grants (totaling $3.9 million per year) with the goal of developing, expanding, or improving injury programs. An evaluation of these grants (Hersey et al., 1995) found that they had been used successfully to support and strengthen injury prevention infrastructures in the 15 locations and recommended expansion of the program to support core injury programs in all 50 states. However, because of funding constraints, by the mid-1990s, NCIPC began to transform these grants into more focused cooperative agreements that targeted specific proven interventions, such as smoke detectors and bicycle helmets, or specific surveillance efforts, such as head and spinal cord injuries, burns, or firearm injuries. States without established injury programs, however, found it difficult to compete for these cooperative agreements, thus, in FY 1997, NCIPC introduced new cooperative agreements for Basic Injury Program Development similar to, but smaller in scale than, the former capacity-building grants. The awards, made to only four states at $75,000 per year for three years, are for the development of a state plan to establish or strengthen injury prevention activities. It is difficult to build a state infrastructure for injury prevention with such limited and short-term funding. Increased federal funding is needed to provide capacity-building funds while allowing practitioners to set local priorities for implementing injury prevention interventions (see Chapter 8).

---

[2]MCH block grants are administered by MCHB of the HRSA. PHHS block grants are administered by the Centers for Disease Control and Prevention's National Center for Chronic Disease Prevention and Health Promotion.

State and Local Funding

State-funded support for injury prevention generally has not been forthcoming. Some states have initiated creative funding mechanisms for injury programs; examples include special "Kids Plate" vehicle license tags (e.g., SAFE KIDS license plate in Connecticut, Kids Plates in California), court-imposed fines for car seat and bike helmet violations, and fines for driving under the influence of alcohol.

The majority of states have been unable to garner support for a line item in their budgets specifically for injury prevention. Injury prevention is usually combined with large, multimillion dollar "family and community health" or "preventive health services" budgets, which makes it difficult for state-level injury staff to claim any of these dollars for injury prevention. It is important for advocacy organizations and injury practitioners (through organizations such as STIPDA) to educate state legislators, health commissioners, and their staffs about the scope of the injury problem and the effectiveness of prevention interventions so that they will be willing to support increased state funding.

At the community level, injury prevention is frequently implemented through coalitions of nonprofit organizations, local businesses, and community agencies (e.g., schools, fire departments, day-care centers). As a result, funding comes from a variety of sources, including foundations, federal and state programs, and community organizations, and is used to implement specifically targeted programs (e.g., conflict resolution, bike helmet giveaways) but not to support core functions.

Thus, it is crucial that state-level injury prevention programs be able to supply the financial and technical assistance needed at the local level to conduct core elements of injury programs: needs assessment, program evaluations, staff training, local data surveillance, and other technical assistance. The committee supports the development of a core injury program in each state's department of health. In the committee's view the program must have state and federal support to provide adequate staffing and resources for statewide injury prevention services (see recommendation in Chapter 8).

The committee recommends strengthening the state infrastructure in injury prevention by development of core injury prevention programs in each state's department of health. To accomplish this goal, funding, resources, and technical assistance should be provided to the states. Support for such programs should be provided by the National Center for Injury Prevention and Control in collaboration with state and local governments.

Integrating Injury Prevention Efforts into Health Care Delivery

One of the goals of injury prevention efforts should be the integration of injury prevention strategies, policies, and messages into existing programs of service delivery, routine activities of health professionals, and priority initiatives of professional associations. Such integration expands the population that can be reached and increases the likelihood of the institutionalization of injury prevention. For example, childhood injury prevention education can be incorporated into a variety of settings where families receive health and social services, including prenatal care clinics; primary health care settings; Women, Infants, and Children clinics; and parenting classes.

Inasmuch as the costs of providing treatment for injuries are often borne by the injured person's health insurance provider, there is the potential for considerable cost savings through the prevention or amelioration of injuries. Thus, injury prevention should be integrated into the clinical care and prevention programs of managed care organizations. Opportunities include collecting and analyzing their own data on injuries using E-codes; using hospital community benefits programs (mandated in 12 states) to implement domestic violence programs; conducting screening and anticipatory guidance activities; providing patients with incentives for safe behaviors; and training providers on injury prevention issues.

There are many additional opportunities for integrating injury prevention into health care. These include the incorporation of developmentally appropriate injury prevention counseling into visits to pediatric and prenatal clinics, as well as home visits. Relevant professional organizations can embrace injury prevention as an integral component of practice and can issue guidelines and policy statements. Injury practitioners should provide their expertise to managed care organizations in order to facilitate the integration of injury prevention into managed care plans and practices. Federal agencies can foster integration by including injury prevention within existing service delivery, planning, and policy documents (e.g., block and training grant applications). For example, the MCHB has recently included youth suicide and motor vehicle crashes as 2 of 18 national maternal and child health performance measures that states must report annually (HRSA, 1997).

COLLABORATION AND COALITION BUILDING

One of the strengths of the injury prevention field is the broad base of stakeholders concerned about reducing injury morbidity and mortality. As discussed above, injury prevention is part of broader public safety efforts at the state and local levels, and numerous federal, state, and local agencies and organizations have a mandate to ensure public safety. Additionally, there are nonprofit organizations, for-profit corporations and businesses, and foundations that have the resources, energy, and expertise to contribute to injury prevention efforts. To increase the impact and reach of injury prevention programs and to maximize the expertise and resources available, injury prevention and safety professionals have to expand collaborative activities and work together to develop and support state and community coalitions.

Collaboration

Partnerships are needed within the different divisions of the state health department as well as with other state and local agencies (e.g., highway safety, criminal justice, fire services, education, law enforcement, emergency medical services). The advantages of multiagency collaboration include gaining access to a wider population, combining different approaches and expertise, sharing data relevant to injury, and better use of resources.

Currently formalized linkages across agencies are often discouraged because of grant restrictions and competition for state dollars, and it has been easier to develop and implement separate categorical funding programs. However, efforts are being made to enhance collaborative efforts. Several states have injury prevention task forces or interagency coalitions; for example, the Illinois Injury Control Work Group brings together more than 40 members representing every office in the state health agency, as well as other state agencies and nonprofit organizations; Vermont has a multidisciplinary team working on unintentional injury and occupational health as part of its Healthy Vermonters 2000 program; and Virginia has a statewide coalition on children's safety.

To foster multidisciplinary collaboration between state highway safety and public health professionals around traffic safety issues, NHTSA funded an assessment of the traffic safety activities of state highway safety offices and public health departments and of their perceptions of one another's activities (EDC, 1994). As a result, NHTSA's 10 regional offices are currently sponsoring collaborative programs and training, including regional workshops for state health and highway safety staff.

To encourage intra- and interagency collaboration at the state and local levels, federal agencies can mandate collaborative activities in federal requests for proposals and require joint activities and/or advisory board representation. Data-sharing efforts can be supported by federal and state agencies, especially among hospitals and public health, law enforcement, EMS, criminal justice, and education agencies. Interagency collaboration can be modeled at the federal level by holding joint conferences, creating joint funding streams, and maintaining interagency communication. An example is the Lifesavers Conference, a highway safety conference with participants from many fields including traffic safety, transportation, public health, injury prevention, and law enforcement. The conference has multiple funders (including corporations, nonprofit organizations, and state and federal agencies) with the common goal of reducing injury morbidity and mortality and promoting highway safety.

Local, state, and federal leadership and collaboration is also needed to support poison control centers. Poison control centers coordinate care for poison victims from the point of exposure to information sources and therapies, as well as serving as a locus for prevention, training, and research on poisoning. The number of poison control centers in the United States has declined steadily over the past two decades and is currently precariously low (Litovitz et al., 1994). Currently, many poison control centers face serious funding constraints while others face closure, and no one federal agency is responsible for sponsorship (Poison Control Center Advisory Work Group, 1996). Yet, it has been estimated that poison control centers prevent an estimated 50,000 hospitalizations and 400,000 doctors' visits annually (Poison Control Center Advisory Work Group, 1996). The committee urges federal leadership in supporting and sustaining poison control centers in the United States.

Coalition Building

At the community level, injury prevention becomes the responsibility of numerous organizations and agencies. Day-care facilities, nursing homes, schools, police and fire departments, civic organizations, athletic leagues, families, and numerous other groups all implement measures to prevent or minimize injuries. As a result of this diverse group of stakeholders, coalitions have been found to be particularly useful as a means of pooling resources, targeting specific injury problems, and educating the interested parties on effective injury prevention interventions (National Committee, 1989).

Injury prevention coalitions range in the degree of formality and the breadth of their mission and activities. Grassroots coalitions have been started by concerned parents, health professionals, and other individuals. For example, the San Francisco Bay Area Coalition on Drowning Prevention advocated for a change in county ordinances to require safety measures for backyard pools (National Committee, 1989). Other coalitions are nationwide efforts and include the National SAFE KIDS Campaign which works through more than 240 state and local coalitions to promote children's safety efforts (SAFE KIDS, 1998a). Safe Communities, a program initiated by NHTSA, strives to reduce traffic safety injuries by working at the community level through broad coalitions of public safety officials, medical services providers, civic and industry leaders, and citizens (NHTSA, 1998; see Chapter 8).

Since injury prevention is often most successful at the local level, where specific injury problems can be addressed, coalition building is crucial to strengthening the nation's response to the injury problem. Financial and technical assistance is needed from federal and state government agencies and from the private for-profit and nonprofit sectors.

TRAINING AND TECHNICAL ASSISTANCE

In 1985, *Injury in America* identified the shortage of trained injury prevention professionals and scientists as a major impediment to the development of the field (NRC, 1985); this continues to be a significant barrier. Additionally, further education on injury prevention has to be incorporated into the education of health care professionals so that nurses, physicians, physician assistants, and nurse practitioners can integrate injury prevention into their clinical practice.

Training Injury Prevention Practitioners

The need to train practitioners is confirmed by surveys of the staffs of state health departments, traffic safety agencies, and schools of public health (Harrington et al., 1988; Dana et al., 1990; Miara et al., 1990). A 1990 survey found that only 25 percent of health department personnel and 20 percent of traffic safety professionals had graduate-level coursework in injury epidemiology or prevention. Additionally, 92 percent of health department personnel and 47 percent of traffic safety staff requested additional training (Miara et al., 1990).

Most states do not currently have the resources to conduct training and continuing education for local agencies, nor do they have the capacity to keep current on the latest research and its application. Moreover, career paths are not well defined for injury prevention practitioners, and training opportunities are not readily available or accessible (in fact, state and local practitioners often have difficulty in obtaining travel approval to attend out-of-state conferences or training programs). Training and continuing education most often occur through state and national conferences and via sessions on injury prevention at the annual meetings of national professional organizations (e.g., the American Public Health Association). A one-week training course has been restarted recently by the Johns Hopkins Center for Injury Research and Policy. Although these developments are positive signs, they are of no value to those who cannot attend because of funding constraints.

Federal agencies provide training that is most often focused on specific injury topics. MCHB provides technical assistance to state maternal and child health agency staff through the Children's Safety Network (CSN) National Injury and Violence Prevention Resource Center. This information is targeted to maternal and child health practitioners and is focused on child and adolescent injury prevention. NHTSA offers regional workshops on traffic safety topics. The National Institute for Occupational Safety and Health (NIOSH) funds 15 Education and Research Centers (ERCs), primarily at universities, that offer continuing education courses in occupational health and safety. The Indian Health Service (IHS) offers an Injury Prevention Specialist Fellowship program that allows 10 to 20 IHS field staff to receive training in the use of data collection systems and the development of intervention strategies. These efforts are critical to the continued education of injury professionals; however, additional opportunities are needed.

An interesting interdisciplinary model currently under development is a national satellite training program on violence prevention for education, public health, justice, and community-based professionals. Each of the six parts of the curriculum will involve a three-hour national broadcast supplemented by two hours of facilitated training on site and a website for follow-up. The primary sponsors are the Office of Safe and Drug Free Schools in the U.S. Department of Education, MCHB, the Office of Juvenile Justice and Delinquency Prevention, NCIPC, and IHS. This unique collaboration recognizes that practitioners with a different perspective need a common language and approach. A teleconference offered in June 1997 through the University of North Carolina Injury Prevention Research Center shows promise as a method for providing education.

Federal leadership is needed to prepare a cadre of trained injury prevention practitioners and to continue to keep them informed of best practices. The 1993 agenda-setting report *Injury Control in the 1990s: A National Plan for Action* identified the training of injury professionals as one of its 22 recommendations (NCIPC, 1993). Specific elements of the proposed approach included the following:

- the development of a national injury control training plan;
- collaboration among federal agencies that fund training of professionals (e.g., engineers and police) to incorporate an injury prevention component;
- funding for Injury Control Research Centers (ICRCs) to enable them to provide training to state and local safety professionals, as well as to faculties of health professional schools;
- designation and funding of a resource center to collect and disseminate curricula and learning materials; and
- support for the inclusion of injury in the core curricula of medical schools.

These recommendations have not been fully implemented and appear stalled because several federal agencies bear the responsibility for coordination, funding, and implementation. The committee believes that the 1993 NCIPC training recommendations should be implemented and that training should be a key mission of NCIPC (see Chapter 8), in collaboration with other federal agencies.

In addition to focusing on specific injury topics, training should emphasize program development, implementation, and evaluation processes. Further, practitioners should be integrally involved in research on the practice of prevention. While this may be considered the primary function of researchers, practitioners are ideally positioned to provide feedback about the effectiveness and utility of prevention interventions through the evaluation process. This role may require expanded training and would necessitate greater two-way communication between practitioners and researchers. The committee believes that this more integrative process will result in more effective prevention interventions.

Core curricula for injury practitioners have to be developed through a consensus and peer review process. One model is the EMS curriculum development process conducted by NHTSA. Training curricula should include information on working with culturally diverse populations. Professionals working in the field, whether focused on childhood injury, teen violence, driver safety, domestic violence, or injury problems of the elderly, must be able to address these concerns in the context of varied socioeconomic levels and cultures.

The ICRCs and ERCs, located throughout the United States, are excellent resources and potential sites for training programs. However, current funding for such centers is limited and would have to be increased in order to expand their mandate. Consideration should be given by multiple federal agencies to the expansion of training opportunities for state and local injury prevention professionals.

The committee recommends the expansion of training opportunities for injury prevention practitioners by the relevant state and federal agencies (e.g., NCIPC, NHTSA, MCHB, and NIOSH) in partnership with key stakeholders such as STIPDA. Training should emphasize program development, implementation, and evaluation as well as participation in program research.

Training Health Care Professionals in Injury Prevention

Comprehensive curricula materials should be developed to allow the subject of injury prevention and treatment to be integrated into the curricula of medical and nursing schools and schools of public health. The Educating Professionals in Injury Control series funded by the Pew Charitable Trust may serve as a model; however, it requires updating and expansion for the multiple causes of injury (EDC, 1990). With its modular format, the series has a flexible design that allows different disciplines to adapt the materials (including lectures, slides, and case studies) for their own use. Despite a positive evaluation by faculty users on the modules relating to firearms, fire and burns, falls in the elderly, and general injury prevention principles, modules for other causes of injury have not yet been developed.

Materials have been developed to assist pediatricians and others in injury prevention counseling. The American Academy of Pediatrics (AAP) provides a set of standard, developmentally appropriate protocols in its Injury Prevention Program (TIPP) for pediatricians who are counseling patients up to age 12 on injury and violence prevention. The AAP has also developed the Steps to Prevent Firearm Injury (STOP) program which provides a training tape for pediatricians on how to counsel about firearms issues.[3] Similar protocols are needed for other types of injuries, settings, ages, and providers.

Technical Assistance

Training must be accompanied by technical assistance to support states and communities in developing and implementing practical injury prevention plans, building and sustaining an injury prevention infrastructure, evaluating prevention programs, and making the transition from research to practice. Technical assistance must be conducted by experienced professionals who know how to overcome state and local barriers to program implementation and are knowledgeable about conducting evaluation studies. For example, the CSN's National Injury and Violence Prevention Resource Center provides technical assistance by developing publications and resources that synthesize best practice from different disciplines; conduct needs assessments and site visits; assisting states in overcoming institutional barriers in implementing prevention programs; developing or facilitating the development of continuing education programs for state and local practitioners; operating a national resource library and website; and representing the interests of practitioners in national forums and committees. Additional examples include the National Children's Center for Rural and Agricultural Health and Safety recently funded by NIOSH and the National Program for Playground Safety funded by the Centers for Disease Control and Prevention.

Many of the federal agencies discussed in Chapter 8 are involved in technical assistance to states and communities, and the committee supports continuation of these efforts. Further, the committee supports an increased technical assistance role for NCIPC, particularly in providing assistance (including the site-visit teams discussed earlier in this chapter) to state health departments.

In addition to implementing technical assistance mechanisms, there should be a periodic assessment to determine the status of injury prevention programming and capacity, the specific barriers that must be overcome to enhance implementation, and the needs for technical assistance and training. A survey, such as the 1988 survey of state health departments (Harrington et al., 1988), should be updated and the results used to develop a technical assistance plan for states.

INTEGRATING RESEARCH AND PRACTICE

As described in Chapter 4, emphasis is needed on evaluating prevention interventions in real-world settings so that effective interventions can move from research and demonstration projects to wide-scale dissemination. A recent NCIPC

---

[3]STOP 2, an educational program developed for all health care providers, by the Center to Prevent Handgun Violence with funding from the Metropolitan Life Foundation, is now available.

publication, *Demonstrating Your Program's Worth*, provides a guide to assist injury practitioners and researchers in evaluating injury prevention programs (Thompson and McClintock, 1998). Local injury prevention practitioners need applied information on best practices based on current research. Likewise, practitioners can provide valuable input to researchers on areas requiring future research. Best practices should be informed by an overall assessment of evidence-based research and current practices in the field. Resource libraries, such as the Trauma Foundation's Injury and Violence Prevention Library, facilitate the flow of information from research to practice (Craig et al., 1998). This function is crucial to the success of state and local injury prevention efforts and consideration should be given to expanding the library and information networking efforts at NCIPC.

The 1989 report *Injury Prevention: Meeting the Challenge* provided information on then-current prevention interventions from a multidisciplinary perspective (National Committee, 1989). The report was designed to serve as a tool to adapt and combine research findings in light of local data and available resources. It reviewed interventions in terms of those proven effective (e.g., bicycle helmets), those that were promising (e.g., raising alcohol taxes to reduce availability), those ineffective or counterproductive (e.g., painted crosswalks), and creative ideas whose efficacy was unknown and should be studied (e.g., designated driver and safe ride programs). There is a need for additional and updated resources that provide information on effective prevention interventions.

Such an effort could be linked to reviews of evidence-based research on injury interventions, such as those conducted through the Cochrane Collaboration,[4] and should be disseminated widely through technical assistance efforts. Cochrane Collaboration reviews relevant to the injury field have been completed on childhood injury prevention (Rivara et al., 1998) and falls in the elderly (Gillespie et al., 1998), and are in progress on a number of other injury topics.

One of the difficulties in facilitating the translation of research into policy and practice is the limited communication between practitioners and researchers. Vehicles that may be utilized for synthesizing and disseminating research findings include publication of newsletters (e.g., NHTSA's *Traffic Tech Transfer Series*), publication of bulletins on topics of recent research (e.g., NIOSH's *Alert* series), and an annual conference to foster bi-directional communication between practitioners and researchers.

PUBLIC AWARENESS AND ADVOCACY

A crucial challenge faced by injury prevention professionals is the lack of public and legislative awareness of the scope of injury morbidity and mortality

---

[4]Cochrane Collaboration reviews are systematic reviews of controlled trials of health care interventions conducted by international panels of experts (Cochrane Collaboration, 1998).

and the utility of potential interventions. Many members of the general public as well as many policy makers still believe that injuries are "accidents" that just happen. This perception often precludes policy makers from identifying injury prevention as a discrete public health issue and limits the earmarking of federal and state dollars for injury research and for the development of prevention programs.

Raising Public Awareness

The breadth of the injury field has resulted in a number of advocacy and nonprofit organizations that generally focus on one type or cause of injury (e.g., BIA, MADD) or one population of concern (e.g., National SAFE KIDS Campaign). These organizations have a significant contribution to make to their issues of concern and to the broader field of injury prevention; together they can raise the visibility of injury prevention, build a broad base of support, and provide a recognizable constituency for the field of injury prevention and treatment. Policy makers' attitudes and interest in this field will not change easily without a change in society's attitudes and perception of the field. The field has to engage existing social marketing techniques to determine the messages that should be employed to raise the profile of injury prevention research and focus the public's and policy makers' attention on the preventability of injuries.

Advocacy

Public education, advocacy, and constituency building are key elements of modern public health practice at the state and community levels. Proactive "marketing" of public health is needed to arouse public awareness and concern, to counteract complacency or sluggishness, and to prod policy makers into action. The need for injury officials and program directors to embrace advocacy as a core professional role is a recurrent theme in the field (Rivara, 1997). According to the Institute of Medicine (IOM) report *The Future of Public Health*, educating legislators and political leaders "on public health issues and on the rationale for strategies advocated and pursued by the health department" is a key element of public health leadership (IOM, 1988). Eight years later, another IOM (1996, p. 39) committee noted:

> Even when promising solutions exist, public health agencies too often have difficulty generating support for intervention among elected officials and the general public. A key struggle for [public health leaders] is making the benefits of community-based, population-wide public health activities and initiatives more recognizable, and finding allies who will speak on behalf of those initiatives and the unique role for government public health agencies in carrying [them] out. . . .

These important activities—public education, constituency building, and advocacy—must be carried on with due regard for long-standing legal constraints on "lobbying," which are designed to limit contact with legislators, directly or through grassroots efforts concerning specific legislative proposals. Federal grantees may not use federal funds for lobbying, and nonprofit organizations lose their tax-exempt status if they devote too much of their activities to lobbying. However, these restrictions on lobbying still leave the organizations free to engage in a wide range of educational activities. Unfortunately, many organizations in the injury field appear to be unsure about the boundaries between advocacy and lobbying and thus are uncertain about the legitimate scope of educational and constituency-building efforts. Nonprofit organizations in the injury field should understand the federal and state rules that govern lobbying. By better understanding these rules, nonprofit organizations can maximize their effectiveness as advocates for the public's health, while minimizing the likelihood that they will jeopardize their nonprofit legal status.

The federal government itself has recognized that changes in state and local policy are often necessary to help effectuate national public health policy goals. Many Healthy People 2000 goals focus on state legislative action (U.S. DHHS, 1990). Congress often makes state eligibility for federal program support conditional upon state legislative action (e.g., the 21-year-old minimum drinking age). In many situations, however, Congress is not so directive, relying instead on public education and local constituency building to arouse public support and eventually achieve state and local legislative action. It is well understood that nonprofit organizations interested in public health issues devote substantial resources to public education and issue advocacy, even though their lobbying for a specific piece of legislation is restricted.

Thus, advocacy for national public health objectives by federal grantees and nonprofit organizations is often encouraged by federal policy. Against this background, the committee believes that recent proposals to curtail advocacy by federal grantees and nonprofit organizations are troubling. For example, proposals have been made to preclude federal grants to organizations that spend more than a specified amount on "political advocacy," thereby broadening the constraints and compelling the use of nonfederal funds by these organizations (Moody, 1996). In the committee's view, the achievement of national public health priorities, including injury prevention objectives, would be significantly impeded if Congress were to broaden traditional constraints on lobbying by federal grantees and nonprofit organizations beyond their long-accepted meanings and boundaries to include advocacy. Traditional restrictions adequately carry out the federal government's legitimate interest in avoiding taxpayer-subsidized political activity and the distortion of the political process to which subsidized political activity might lead. More sweeping restrictions on the advocacy of ideas or positions not only would have a chilling effect on constitutionally protected activities by federal grantees and tax-exempt organizations, but would also undermine the U.S. government's strong interest in promoting public understanding of and support for national public health objectives. The committee urges Congress to preserve its customary support for public health advocacy.

SUMMARY

Although it is difficult to quantify the total extent of government, community, and private-sector endeavors in the injury field, there is a wide range of ongoing efforts, many of which have begun or expanded within the past 20 years. Although the current response is impressive, it is also fragmented. A core injury prevention program is needed in each state that can implement (and assist other agencies and organizations in implementing) injury prevention interventions. State injury prevention programs require a sustained federal commitment to funding and to providing technical assistance to the states. Further, training opportunities for state and local injury prevention practitioners should be expanded. Beyond the public health arena, numerous safety organizations and agencies have an important role to play in injury prevention efforts. Collaboration between state agencies and coalition building, particularly at the local level, are crucial for addressing injury prevention.

As new prevention interventions are developed and evaluated, ongoing information exchange between researchers and practitioners is needed that will facilitate the implementation of new interventions and the refinement of these interventions to meet real-world demands. A final component of strengthening the state and local response is raising public awareness and increasing advocacy efforts. Both the general public and policy makers need information on the effectiveness of injury prevention measures in order to make informed decisions and choices.

REFERENCES

BIA (Brain Injury Association). 1998. *1996–1997 Annual Report.* Washington, DC: BIA.

California Department of Health Services. State Injury Control Advisory Task Force. 1992. *Strategic Plan for Injury Prevention and Control in California, 1993–1997.* Sacramento, CA: California Department of Health Services.

Cochrane Collaboration. 1998. *The Cochrane Collaboration.* [World Wide Web document]. URL http://hiru.hirunet.mcmaster.ca/cochrane/ (accessed June 1998).

Craig A, Tremblay-McGaw R, McLoughlin E. 1998. Injury prevention in the information age: The Injury and Violence Prevention Library. *Injury Prevention* 4(2):150–154.

Dana AJ, Gallagher SS, Vince CJ. 1990. *Survey of Injury Prevention Curricula in Schools of Public Health.* Paper presented at the annual meeting of the American Public Health Association, October 2, 1990, New York City. Newton, MA: Education Development Center.

EDC (Education Development Center, Inc.), Johns Hopkins Injury Prevention Center. 1990. *Educating Professionals in Injury Control (EPIC)*. Newton MA: EDC.

EDC (Education Development Center, Inc.). 1994. *Motor Vehicle Injury Prevention: An Assessment of Highway Safety and Public Health Activities in Selected States*. Washington, DC: National Highway Traffic Safety Administration.

Garrison HG, Foltin GL, Becker LR, Chew JL, Johnson M, Madsen GM, Miller DR, Ozmar BH. 1997. The role of emergency medical services in injury prevention. *Annals of Emergency Medicine* 30(1):84–91.

Gillespie LD, Gillespie WJ, Cumming R, Lamb SE, Rowe BH. 1998. *Interventions to Reduce the Incidence of Falling in the Elderly* [World Wide Web document]. URL http://som.flinders.edu.au/fusa/cochrane/cochrane/revabstr/ab000340.htm (accessed April 1998).

Harrington C, Gallagher SS, Burgess LL, Guyer B. 1988. *Injury Prevention Programs in State Health Departments: A National Survey*. Boston, MA: Harvard School of Public Health, Massachusetts Department of Maternal and Child Health.

Hersey JC, Abed J, Butler MO, Diver AR, Mitchell K. 1995. *Reducing the Burden of Injury: An Evaluation of CDC Injury Grant Programs. Final Report*. Arlington, VA: Battelle. Report to the Centers for Disease Control and Prevention, National Center for Injury Prevention and Control and the Office of Program Planning and Evaluation.

HRSA (Health Resources and Services Administration). 1997. *Title V Block Grant Program Guidelines*. Rockville, MD: HRSA, Maternal and Child Health Bureau.

HRSA (Health Resources and Services Administration). 1998. *Emergency Medical Services for Children. FY 1997 Report*. Rockville, MD: HRSA.

IOM (Institute of Medicine). 1988. *The Future of Public Health*. Washington, DC: National Academy Press.

IOM (Institute of Medicine). 1996. *Healthy Communities: New Partnerships for the Future of Public Health*. Washington, DC: National Academy Press.

Kelter A. 1997. Reinventing injury prevention in California: A model for reinventing local public health programs. *Journal of Public Health Management and Practice* 3(6):30–34.

Klein SH, O'Connor P, Fuhrman JM. 1997. Injury prevention capacity building in New York State: Federal support played a significant role. *Journal of Public Health Management and Practice* 3(6):17–24.

Litovitz T, Kearney TE, Holm K, Soloway RA, Weisman R, Oderda G. 1994. Poison control centers: Is there an antidote for budget cuts? *American Journal of Emergency Medicine* 12(5):585–599.

MADD (Mothers Against Drunk Driving). 1998. *About MADD*. [World Wide Web document]. URL http://www.madd.org/ (accessed May 1998).

Miara C, Gallagher SS, Malloy P. 1990. *National Survey of the Training Needs of Health Department & Traffic Safety Injury Control Professionals*. Paper presented at the annual meeting of the American Public Health Association, October 2, 1990, New York. Newton, MA: EDC and Harvard Injury Control Center.

Moody AE. 1996. Conditional federal grants: Can the government undercut lobbying by non-profits through conditions placed on federal grants? *Boston College Environmental Affairs Law Review* 24:113–158.

NACCHO (National Association of County and City Health Officials). 1998. *NACCHO Overview*. [World Wide Web document]. URL http://www.naccho.org/overview/index.html (accessed May 1998).

National Committee (National Committee for Injury Prevention and Control). 1989. *Injury Prevention: Meeting the Challenge.* New York: Oxford University Press. Published as a supplement to the *American Journal of Preventive Medicine* 5(3).

NCIPC (National Center for Injury Prevention and Control). 1993. *Injury Control in the 1990s: A National Plan for Action. A Report to the Second World Conference on Injury Control.* Atlanta, GA: Centers for Disease Control and Prevention.

NFPA (National Fire Protection Association). 1998. *National Fire Protection Association: A Century of Service.* [World Wide Web document]. URL http://www.nfpa.org (accessed July 1998).

NHTSA (National Highway Traffic Safety Administration). 1998. Safe Communities. [World Wide Web document]. URL http://www.nhtsa.dot.gov/safecommunities/ (accessed June 1998).

NRC (National Research Council). 1985. *Injury in America: A Continuing Public Health Problem.* Washington, DC: National Academy Press.

NRC (National Research Council). 1993. *Understanding Child Abuse and Neglect.* Washington, DC: National Academy Press.

Poison Control Center Advisory Work Group. 1996. *Final Report of the Poison Control Center Advisory Work Group.* Report to the National Center for Injury Prevention and Control and the Maternal and Child Health Bureau.

Rivara FP. 1997. Should we be advocates for injury prevention? *Injury Prevention* 3(3): 158–159.

Rivara FP, Beahler C, Patterson MQ, Thompson DC, Zavitkovsky A. 1998. *Systematic Reviews of Childhood Injury Prevention Interventions.* [World Wide Web document]. URL http://weber.u.washington.edu/~hiprc/childinjury/ (accessed April 1998).

SAFE KIDS (National SAFE KIDS Campaign). 1998a. National SAFE KIDS Campaign. [World Wide Web document]. URL http://www.safekids.org (accessed July 1998).

SAFE KIDS (National SAFE KIDS Campaign). 1998b. *Safe Kids at Home, at Play, and on the Way: A Report to the Nation on Unintentional Childhood Injury.* Washington, DC: National SAFE KIDS Campaign.

STIPDA (State and Territorial Injury Prevention Directors' Association). 1997. *Safe States: Five Components of a Model State Injury Prevention Program and Three Phases of Program Development.* Oklahoma City, OK: STIPDA.

Thompson NJ, McClintock HO. 1998. *Demonstrating Your Program's Worth: A Primer on Evaluation for Program to Prevent Unintentional Injury.* Atlanta, GA: National Center for Injury Prevention and Control.

U.S. DHHS (Department of Health and Human Services). 1990. *Healthy People 2000: National Health Promotion and Disease Prevention Objectives.* Washington, DC: U.S. DHHS.

Utah Department of Health. 1997. *State of Utah Annual Plan for Maternal and Child Health.* Salt Lake City: Utah Department of Health.

8

Federal Response

The purpose of this chapter is to evaluate the current federal response to the problem of injury and to make recommendations to strengthen that response for the future. The federal government's collective response spans the work of numerous agencies in nearly all cabinet-level departments (Table 8.1). These agencies have far-ranging missions, varying approaches, and differing levels of commitment to preventing injuries. Since the federal effort is so multifaceted and diverse, the committee chose to focus on eight agencies for which it felt that its recommendations would significantly advance the injury field. For each agency, this chapter contains a description of the agency's mission, resources, and injury-related programs, followed by the committee's assessment and recommendations. However, the committee did not restrict itself to an agency-by-agency assessment. An effective federal response relates to more than just the sum of its parts, especially when the "parts" are dispersed across dozens of agencies. Consequently, the final portion of this chapter emphasizes the need to avert fragmentation through cooperation, coordination, and leadership, so as to reduce the toll of injuries. The eight federal agencies covered in this chapter are (1) the National Highway Traffic Safety Administration (NHTSA) of the Department of Transportation; (2) the Consumer Product Safety Commission (CPSC); (3) the Occupational Safety and Health Administration (OSHA) of the Department of Labor; (4) the National Institute for Occupational Safety and Health (NIOSH); (5) the National Institutes of Health (NIH); (6) the Maternal and Child Health Bureau (MCHB) of the Health Resources and Services Administration (HRSA);

(7) the Office of Justice Programs (OJP) of the Department of Justice; and (8) the National Center for Injury Prevention and Control (NCIPC).[1]

The committee's evaluations and recommendations are based on insights gained from an array of activities it sponsored over the course of 18 months. The activities included workshops, public meetings, site visits, surveys, written testimony, and extensive interviews of, and discussions with, federal and state leaders in injury prevention and treatment. The committee identified the following overarching themes: the need to strengthen research at some agencies; the need to encourage more emphasis on research planning and priority setting; and the need to enhance funding for research, training, and programs in select areas.

NATIONAL HIGHWAY TRAFFIC SAFETY ADMINISTRATION

The National Highway Traffic Safety Administration was created by the Highway Safety Act of 1970 as the successor to the National Highway Safety Bureau, itself the product of highway safety legislation passed in 1966. NHTSA's mission is "to save lives, prevent injuries and reduce traffic-related health care and other economic costs. The agency develops, promotes, and implements effective educational, engineering, and enforcement programs toward ending preventable tragedies and reducing economic costs associated with vehicle use and highway travel" (NHTSA, 1994). NHTSA's traffic safety activities span research, surveillance, programs, public education, and regulation. The focus is primarily on prevention and acute care, rather than on rehabilitation.

Regulation

NHTSA's regulatory activities are authorized separately under the National Traffic and Motor Vehicle Safety Act of 1966. This legislation mandates the establishment and enforcement of safety standards for new motor vehicles and motor vehicle equipment. These standards relate to windshields, headlights, occupant protection systems, brakes, and side impact protection, among other items. NHTSA's safety standards are developed through a formal rule-making process, after which NHTSA enforces the standards through compliance investigations. Compliance investigations are often triggered by the approximately 1,500 reports received from the public per month about alleged safety problems. NHTSA also develops standards for collision bumpers, odometers, fuel economy, and theft prevention under the Motor Vehicle Information and Cost Savings Act. Since the 1970s, NHTSA has shifted its regulatory strategy away from

---

[1]NCIPC and NIOSH are part of the Centers for Disease Control and Prevention (CDC), which is within the Department of Health and Human Services, as are the NIH and HRSA.

TABLE 8.1 Federal Agencies Involved in Injury Prevention and Treatment

Agency	Injury Focus
Consumer Product Safety Commission	Consumer products
Department of Agriculture	Farm safety
Department of Commerce National Institute of Standards and Technology	Safety materials
Department of Defense	Safety of military personnel
Department of Education National Institute on Disability and Rehabilitation Research	Rehabilitation
Department of Energy	Worker safety
Department of Health and Human Services Administration for Children and Families Children's Bureau	Child abuse
Administration on Aging	Safety of older Americans
Agency for Health Care Policy and Research	Injury outcomes, managed care

Centers for Disease Control and Prevention
    National Institute for Occupational Safety and
      Health
	Occupational safety

National Center for Injury Prevention and
      Control
	Intentional and unintentional
	    injuries

National Center for Chronic Disease Prevention and Health Promotion	Injury prevention
National Center for Environmental Health	Disabilities
Health Resources and Services Administration Maternal and Child Health Bureau	Children's safety
Indian Health Service	Native American populations
National Institutes of Health National Institute on Aging	Elderly populations
National Institute on Alcohol Abuse and Alco- holism	Alcohol

National Institute of Arthritis and Musculoskele-
      tal and Skin Diseases
	Fractures, musculoskeletal
	    injury

National Institute of Child Health and Human
      Development
        National Center for Medical Rehabilitation
        Research
	Rehabilitation

National Institute on Drug Abuse	Drugs, violence
National Institute of General Medical Sciences	Wounds, shock, burns
National Institute of Mental Health	Suicide, abuse
National Institute of Neurological Disorders and Stroke	Spinal cord injury, CNS injury
Substance Abuse and Mental Health Services Administration	Violence and suicide prevention

TABLE 8.1 *Continued*

Agency	Injury Focus
Department of Housing and Urban Development	Youth violence
Department of Justice	
Office of Justice Programs	Crime, violence, and justice
Bureau of Justice Statistics	Statistics
National Institute of Justice	Violence
Office of Juvenile Justice and Delinquency Prevention	Juvenile crime and justice
Department of Labor	
Bureau of Labor Statistics	Occupational safety statistics
Occupational Safety and Health Administration	Occupational safety
Department of Transportation	
Federal Aviation Administration	Aviation safety
Federal Highway Administration	Highway safety
Federal Railroad Administration	Railroad safety
Federal Transit Administration	Public transportation safety
National Highway Traffic Safety Administration	Highway and traffic safety
U.S. Coast Guard	Boating safety
Department of the Treasury	
Bureau of Alcohol, Tobacco, and Firearms	Alcohol and firearms
Department of Veterans Affairs	Rehabilitation, treatment of injury
Federal Emergency Management Agency	
U.S. Fire Administration	Fire safety
National Science Foundation	Biomechanics, violence, biomedical engineering
National Transportation Safety Board	Investigation

standard setting to greater reliance on mandatory recalls, a shift paralleled by the Consumer Product Safety Commission (CPSC). The impetus for this transformation has been judicial review, among other factors (Mashaw and Harfst, 1990; Dewees et al., 1996).

Resources and Structure

In FY 1997, NHTSA was appropriated $300 million. Its 632 FTEs (full-time equivalents) were divided among seven branches and five offices serving the administrator. A significant portion of NHTSA's budget, about 55 percent in

FY 1997, was devoted to financing state programs authorized under Section 402 of the Highway Safety Act. The largest single program is the "Section 402 State and Community Formula Grants," which support performance-based highway safety programs planned and managed by states in order to reduce highway crashes, deaths, and injuries. Formula grants for state programs under Section 402 are similar to block grants in that they are awarded on the basis of a state's population and public road mileage in relation to national figures. In FY 1997, the Federal Highway Administration (FHWA) merged its Section 402 highway-related safety grant program with NHTSA's Section 402 traffic safety grant program and the resulting State and Community Formula Grants Program is now administered by NHTSA. From 1992 to 1998, a total of $887 million was allocated to the states.

NHTSA also funds incentive grants to states, including Alcohol Incentive Grants, which enable states to reduce safety problems related to driving while impaired by alcohol.[2] In comparison to formula grants, states are eligible for alcohol grants only if they have met specific criteria, such as administrative driver license actions, graduated licensing systems, and sanctions for repeat offenders. These funds are used to encourage states to enact strong, effective anti-drunk driving legislation; improve enforcement of drunk driving laws; and promote the development and implementation of innovative programs to combat impaired driving. In 1997, 38 states received a total of $25.5 million for this program.

Research

NHTSA conducts a research program on vehicle and traffic safety. Its traffic safety research—funded at approximately $6 million annually—focuses on behavioral research and emphasizes alcohol and drugs, occupant protection, and driver fatigue and inattention. Vehicle safety research, the larger of the two research programs—funded at about $30 million annually—stresses crashworthiness (biomechanics, air-bag and occupant safety); crash avoidance (directional control, braking, rollover stability, and intelligent transportation systems); high fuel efficiency vehicles; and crash testing in an in-house facility.

NHTSA supports its research largely through contracts, although some research is performed internally (TRB, 1990). Contracts are awarded competitively after publication of a request for proposals (RFP) and a structured internal review process according to published criteria (unless contracts are sole source). Contract recipients are typically either private firms or universities. NHTSA does not sponsor investigator-initiated research through an extramural grant program, with the exception of one program on intelligent transportation systems. NHTSA also does not sponsor a formal research training program.

---

[2]In FY 1998, alcohol grants were consolidated under the Section 402 program.

Surveillance

NHTSA conducts surveillance activities through its National Center for Statistics and Analysis, which received about $20 million in FY 1997. This center houses two major data systems, the Fatality Analysis Reporting System (FARS) and the National Automotive Sampling System (NASS). FARS tracks all motor vehicle crashes on public roads that result in a fatality. Begun in 1975, it is used to monitor trends in traffic safety and evaluate the impact of motor vehicle safety standards. FARS relies on a designated person within each state who, under contract to NHTSA, extracts and codes 100 data elements on the crash, the vehicles, and the people involved. These elements are obtained from the analysis of multiple state information systems, including police accident reports, vital and death certificates, coroner or medical examiner reports, hospital records, and emergency medical service reports.

Surveillance of all types of traffic crashes, which involve both deaths and injuries, is the focus of the NASS. This system is made up of two separate surveillance systems, both of which are representative samples of traffic crashes. The oldest, the Crashworthiness Data System, formed in 1979, depends on thorough crash investigations conducted by 24 field research teams studying about 5,000 crashes annually. The research teams measure crash damage, interview crash victims, and review medical records to ascertain the nature and severity of injuries. Among the uses of this system are detailed data on the crash performance of passenger cars, the evaluation of safety systems and designs, and improved understanding of the relationship between the injuries and severity of the crash.

The second system, created in 1988, is the General Estimates System (GES). This system is a nationally representative probability sample of police-reported crashes. Eligibility for sampling depends on a police accident report having been filed; the crash having involved at least one motor vehicle; and the result being either property damage, injury, or death. GES samples about 50,000 police reports each year covering 400 police jurisdictions in 60 selected areas in the United States. NHTSA publishes an annual compilation of data on traffic-related injuries and deaths, including trend data, from FARS and GES (NHTSA, 1996).

Assessment and Recommendation

Substantial improvements in motor vehicle safety have been achieved over the past 25 years (see Chapter 5). Although many factors have contributed to this success, including increased urbanization and improved highway design, NHTSA's activities have undoubtedly played a major contributing role (Graham, 1993). NHTSA has effectively led the motor vehicle safety field by promulgating science-based vehicle safety standards; supporting, evaluating and disseminating safety programs at the state and local levels; and forging research partnerships with universities.

State and Local Programs

NHTSA has developed an outstanding program of assisting state and local governments to combat motor vehicle injuries. NHTSA's grant programs authorized under Section 402 of the Highway Safety Act have been instrumental in the development of a national infrastructure. NHTSA studies have found some state programs to be not only highly effective but also cost-effective in terms of lives saved relative to costs incurred (NHTSA, 1991, 1995). In addition to its grant programs, NHTSA plays a leadership role through the conduct of national evaluations that guide states and communities in moving interventions into practice. For example, its research has examined the impact of state laws relating to blood alcohol levels, seat belt use, and motorcycle helmets. Research results, in turn, are widely distributed to states. They have been pivotal in the passage of state laws to curtail drunk driving and promote helmet usage, among other areas.

NHTSA also is to be applauded for recruiting new types of stakeholders who are concerned about injury prevention at the local level. NHTSA wisely recognized that the traditional stakeholders (e.g., health care professionals, emergency medical technicians, safety advocates) must be expanded to include law enforcement, business, local government, and schools. NHTSA has fostered the development of the Network of Employers for Traffic Safety, a public and private partnership that encourages employers to integrate traffic into their safety management systems. With coordinators in approximately 30 states, the network's major activities include training in traffic safety management practices and an emphasis on safety awareness programs such as BeltAmerica 2000, the employer component of Buckle Up America! and National Drive Safely@Work Week. At the community level, NHTSA has forged the Safe Communities program designed to integrate injury control at the community level (NHTSA, 1997). Guided by the philosophy that communities are in the best position to design innovative solutions to all of their injury problems, NHTSA launched Safe Communities in 1995 with assistance from federal, state, and local partners. NHTSA provides leadership, resources (through Section 402 grants), and technical assistance. To qualify as a Safe Community, a community must meet four criteria: (1) it uses injury data analysis and linkage to define its injury problem; (2) it expands partnerships, especially with health care providers and businesses; (3) it involves citizens and seeks their input in program design and implementation; and (4) it creates an integrated and comprehensive injury control system.

Research and Training

In order to fulfill its regulatory role, NHTSA has a strong applied research portfolio that is conducted through contract and internal research. Contract research is most appropriate when the purpose is not to answer fundamental questions but to identify and evaluate different methods of achieving agreed-upon goals. However, it is less likely than grant research to produce innovation because it is driven by agency need and is not subject to independent peer review.

The committee urges NHTSA to expand its investigator-initiated research program and to implement greater reliance on external peer review for both its contract and grant programs. It is crucial to encourage the publication of results from all types of NHTSA-funded research in peer-reviewed scientific journals, and NHTSA may consider accepting publication of journal articles in the peer-reviewed literature in lieu of final reports. NHTSA currently cosponsors one small investigator-initiated research program, the IDEA program (Ideas Deserving of Exploratory Analysis) which funds innovative research in intelligent transportation systems. The program is jointly sponsored by NHTSA, FHWA, and the Federal Railroad Administration with the peer-review process administrated by the NRC's Transportation Research Board (TRB).

To promote greater scientific innovation and quality the committee believes that NHTSA needs to establish formal procedures for independent review of its research plans. One NHTSA research office recently published a five-year draft strategic plan for its research program in the *Federal Register.* [3] In addition to seeking comments, the office plans to follow up with meetings involving outside experts. This is an important step, especially because NHTSA controls much of the country's agenda on highway safety research. The approach taken by the Federal Highway Administration (FHWA) may serve as a model for NHTSA. FHWA asked the National Research Council's Transportation Research Board (TRB) to review its research plans covering a large amount of research through many different programs. [4] Since 1991, a TRB committee, [5] consisting of a wide-ranging group of experts in transportation and related fields, has reviewed research plans and made recommendations to the FHWA. A similar strategy could be adopted by NHTSA to improve the quality of its contract research portfolio.

Following the creation of the federal highway safety program in 1966, there was an expansion of extramural research capacity that endured through the early 1970s. When funding leveled off and actually decreased somewhat in constant dollars, many researchers left the field. More recently, funding has expanded somewhat, primarily in engineering disciplines, but there is a "missing generation" in between. Over the next decade, most of the leadership developed during the early years is destined to retire, without seasoned replacements. If a field of study is to remain vibrant, there must be a commitment to continuity of training and research support, both to attract and train new researchers and to sustain and nourish the growth of those already in the field. Unlike programs for other major health problems and other programs in DOT, funding in highway safety does not include support for graduate study. In order to attract young investigators to the field, support could be provided for graduate education in biomechanics, biosta-

[3]The Office of Research and Traffic Records, Research and Evaluation Division.

[4]Research spending amounted to $201 million in FY 1993 (TRB, 1994).

[5]The Research and Technology Coordinating Committee.

tistics, engineering, epidemiology, health education, psychology, or any of a number of other disciplines that are relevant to highway safety research. Longer-term research support also is needed if serious researchers are to commit to careers in the field.

The committee recommends that NHTSA expand its investigator-initiated research program, conduct periodic and independent peer review of its research and surveillance programs, and provide training and research support to sustain careers in the highway traffic safety field.

CONSUMER PRODUCT SAFETY COMMISSION

The Consumer Product Safety Commission is an independent regulatory, research, and educational agency established in 1972 by the Consumer Product Safety Act. This legislation mandated CPSC to "protect the public against unreasonable risks of injuries and deaths associated with consumer products." CPSC has jurisdiction over approximately 15,000 types of consumer products that collectively are associated with about 21,400 deaths and 29 million injuries annually (CPSC, 1996a). CPSC's purview does not extend to motor vehicles; food and drugs; or alcohol, tobacco, and firearms. The mission of the CPSC is "simple and nonpartisan: saving lives and keeping families safe in their homes" (CPSC, 1996a). The breadth of this mission is reflected by the fact that CPSC enforces five separate statutes, the earliest of which was the 1953 Flammable Fabrics Act.[6]

CPSC's major activities are to develop product safety standards, most of which are voluntary; to ban products for which safety standards cannot effectively eliminate a hazard and to recall and/or require repair or replacement of defective products; to collect data and conduct research on potential product hazards; and to educate consumers. CPSC also operates a toll-free hotline for consumers to report unsafe products or product-related injuries. The number of calls has gradually escalated in recent years, with 288,000 such calls in FY 1998.

Resources and Structure

In FY 1998, CPSC had a budget of $45 million and 480 FTEs. For the past five years CPSC's budget has remained stable; however, from 1974 to 1996 its inflation-adjusted budget decreased by about 60 percent (GAO, 1997). CPSC

---

[6]The statutes administered by CPSC are the Consumer Product Safety Act, the Federal Hazardous Substances Act, the Flammable Fabrics Act, the Poison Prevention Packaging Act, and the Refrigerator Safety Act.

houses three operational offices: compliance, field operations, and hazard identification and reduction. The latter office is the site of CPSC's internal research and surveillance activities. CPSC does not provide grant funds to states or universities for injury research or programs.

Regulation

CPSC, as indicated above, has at its disposal several approaches to regulation through its standard-setting and recall authorities. With respect to the former, CPSC relies far more heavily on voluntary, rather than mandatory, standards for product performance or labeling. Its declining use of formal rulemaking is partially attributable to the Consumer Product Safety Act Amendments of 1981, which made rulemaking requirements more stringent; they require CPSC to employ a voluntary, rather than a mandatory standard when it finds that the voluntary standard can adequately address the hazard and that substantial compliance is likely (GAO, 1997). By its own account, CPSC has worked with industry for the past two decades to develop more than 300 voluntary standards, while issuing less than 50 mandatory standards (CPSC, 1996b). CPSC also has shifted its emphasis from standard setting to recall and informational activities. CPSC's use of product recalls and corrective action programs has significantly increased; from FY 1980 to FY 1989, the annual number of recalls grew from 132 separate actions to 260 such actions (Dewees et al., 1996).

Surveillance, Research, and Standards Development

CPSC's surveillance, research, and standards development activities are conducted within the office responsible for hazard identification and analysis and hazard reduction. These activities were funded at about $13 million in FY 1996. Most of these funds are devoted to surveillance and standards development.

CPSC maintains two surveillance systems, one for fatal injuries, and one for injuries requiring emergency treatment, which captures nonfatal injuries. Deaths caused by product-related injuries are monitored through the purchase and analysis of state death certificates and through CPSC's Medical Examiner and Coroner Alert Project. Surveillance of product-related injuries requiring emergency treatment is captured by CPSC's National Electronic Injury Surveillance System (NEISS).

Under NEISS, data are collected at a probability sample of 101 hospital emergency departments, enabling CPSC to generate national estimates of the frequency and severity of product-related injuries. The approximately 330,000 annual reports in this database cover demographic data, the cause of injury, the type of product, and the body part injured, among other information. CPSC uses NEISS and other data collection systems to set priorities, develop standards, ban and recall products, evaluate the effectiveness of previous standards, and formulate information and educational campaigns.

In a recent report, the General Accounting Office (GAO) contends that CPSC's surveillance of injury-related morbidity and mortality underestimates the full extent of product-related hazards because it omits cases not treated in emergency departments and fails to capture information on vulnerable populations and those with chronic conditions. The GAO recommends an assessment of the feasibility, cost, and design of new data systems (GAO, 1997).

Research conducted or sponsored by the CPSC has traditionally encompassed two general activities: (1) the testing and evaluation of consumer products to ascertain the nature and cause of any safety hazard and (2) applied research to explore the possibility of developing innovative product designs to reduce existing safety hazards, and to explore the feasibility of new performance requirements. At the present time, the agency's limited resources for research are devoted almost entirely to the first of these activities. Product testing and evaluation are conducted intramurally or by small contracts. The CPSC maintains two laboratories, one in chemistry and the other in engineering, to test and assess the safety of consumer products.[7] The FY 1997 budget for contracts to supplement the agency's internal capability was $250,000. CPSC does not support any extramural research grants.

Public Education

In recent years, CPSC has intensified its educational activities to inform the public about product-related injuries. A noteworthy feature is that the educational activities are frequently undertaken through partnerships. Such partnerships enable CPSC to leverage its resources, given its relatively modest budget in relation to its broad jurisdiction. Two partnerships, highlighted in the CPSC publication *Success Stories*, are Baby Safety Showers and preventing infant suffocation (CPSC, 1996b). Baby Safety Showers is a national grassroots campaign inaugurated in 1995 to educate prospective parents about injury prevention at home. Predicated on the traditional baby shower, the program offers educational tips for prospective parents and encourages guests to give safety-related gifts instead of traditional gifts. CPSC promotes the program along with other federal partners and national safety and medical groups, while the program's chief financial supporter, Gerber Products Company, prints and distributes for parents, thousands of "how to" kits and checklists for safety. CPSC has sent out over 420,000 kits and checklists since the campaign began.

---

[7]Because of the small scale of the laboratory program (approximately $200,000 annually), CPSC does not routinely peer-review individual research projects unless they are highly complex.

To prevent infant suffocation, CPSC contributes to a public-private venture that encourages care givers to put infants to sleep on their backs or sides instead of on their stomachs. CPSC research, conducted in the wake of 35 infant deaths associated with bean bag cushions, found that rebreathing carbon dioxide trapped in bean bags and other soft bedding may contribute to approximately 30 percent of deaths previously determined to be, and probably misdiagnosed as, Sudden Infant Death Syndrome (SIDS) (CPSC, 1996b). Through safety alerts, press conferences, and public health campaigns with the American Academy of Pediatrics, the National Institute of Child Health and Human Development, and the SIDS Alliance, CPSC has sought to warn the public about soft bedding and the importance of placing infants on their backs or sides.

Assessment and Recommendation

In contrast to many other federal regulatory agencies, including OSHA, the CPSC has been criticized more for weakness than for overregulation (see, e.g., Viscusi [1984]; Christoffel and Christoffel [1989]). For the first decade of its existence, the prevailing view among economists was that the CPSC's regulatory actions had little or no effect in reducing product-related injuries, imposing costs on manufacturers and consumers without achieving any significant benefits (Viscusi, 1984). As a result, the agency faced the possibility of elimination. Since 1981, CPSC has suffered from chronic underfunding; its budget has decreased almost 50 percent in inflation-adjusted dollars, and the number of agency staff is less than half of what it was in 1980.

More recently, however, peer-reviewed scientific studies of specific regulatory actions by the CPSC have usually found that product-related injuries were substantially reduced at reasonable cost. Examples include child-resistant packaging of oral prescription drugs (Rodgers, 1996), bicycle safety standards (Magat and Moore, 1996), performance standards for walk-behind power lawnmowers (Moore and Magat, 1996), and the 1988 consent decree for all-terrain vehicles (Rodgers, 1993; Moore and Magat, 1997). Even one of the agency's most persistent critics has ranked CPSC regulation of unvented space heaters as one of the most cost-effective examples of risk regulation (Viscusi, 1992) and has found that behavioral adaptations do not offset the safety benefits of CPSC performance standards for child-resistant cigarette lighters (Viscusi and Cavallo, 1994).

Studies of regulatory success have begun to reshape the reputation of the CPSC. Once considered an ineffectual agency targeted for elimination, it now appears to represent a model of regulatory efficiency. This reputation has been reinforced over the past several years by the agency's efforts to leverage its resources through partnerships with manufacturers and consumer organizations. The committee believes that the CPSC is on the right course, relying heavily upon cooperative efforts with industry to raise prevailing standards of safety, all occurring in the shadow of the agency's regulatory authority. However, the committee believes that the agency's capacity to carry out this strategy needs to be strengthened by increasing its resources for injury surveillance, hazard analysis, and applied research. The key to successful regulation is better information.

Surveillance

Surveillance of product-related injuries is the foundation of CPSC's regulatory activities, including hazard identification, hazard analysis, and priority setting. The backbone of the CPSC surveillance system is NEISS. A recent GAO report questioned the adequacy of NEISS on the grounds that it is incomplete (omitting injuries treated outside emergency rooms) and lacks detail about the injury incidents (GAO, 1997). However, the committee agrees with CPSC that NEISS is adequate to serve the purposes for which it is used by CPSC. The real question raised by the GAO criticism is whether expansion of NEISS to cover other types of injuries would assist the injury field as a whole. From this perspective, the committee believes that the feasibility of expanding NEISS to cover all injury-related emergency department visits should be explored (see Chapter 3).

Additionally, the committee agrees with the GAO suggestion that CPSC's capacity to conduct more internal analysis, in order to identify product hazards, should be strengthened. Data needs identified by the GAO include exposure data and incident-based information bearing on consumer vulnerability. These suggestions should be considered in the context of a broader review of data needs bearing on residential and recreational injuries, conducted collaboratively by CPSC and NCIPC.

Research

When it established CPSC, Congress recognized that research was an important component of the agency's mission. Section 5(b) of the Consumer Product Safety Act authorizes CPSC to "conduct research studies and investigations on the safety of consumer products and on improving the safety of such products." Despite the fact that CPSC is the only government agency that conducts in-depth product hazard research, the agency has limited capacity to carry out this important responsibility. As noted above, CPSC currently uses most of its limited technical resources to test and evaluate specific products and to support development of safety performance requirements. When the agency decides to take corrective action or to develop safety standards, it must present adequate evidence to demonstrate the existence of a safety hazard and the efficacy of proposed regulatory actions. Unfortunately, a few regulatory initiatives can fully deplete the agency's resources, especially if the products utilize newly developed technologies. As a result, the agency rarely has the resources to conduct applied research on generic safety problems that require more extensive study. If "research" is given its customary definition, which would exclude the testing and evaluation of specific products, CPSC's research expenditures, which amounted to more than $6 million in FY 1980, have nearly been extinguished.

CPSC has difficulty funding even some of its basic needs. For example, its guidelines for determining the age-appropriateness of various types of toys are almost 15 years old and should be updated. These guidelines are used for enforcing CPSC's toy regulations and for assessing hazards associated with toys. Since these guidelines were developed, there have been major changes in the design, use, and marketing of different toy types. The agency will have to spread the cost of obtaining this extremely important information over many years, simply because it does not have sufficient funds to obtain new data.

Many significant consumer product hazards that have previously been considered impossible to address may now have potential solutions because of advanced technology. For example, the agency is currently evaluating sensor technology that may be able to detect a pre-fire condition on kitchen ranges and thereby prevent cooking fires, the number one cause of residential fires and fire injuries in the United States. Although this important applied research could save lives, it is being spread over several years because of limited resources. It is clear that CPSC requires upgraded laboratory resources and expanded technical capacity.

The consumer product market often fails to generate sufficient incentives for firms to compete over safety and to invest in research and development of safer product designs. Whatever incentives might otherwise be generated by the market are sometimes weakened by manufacturers' concerns that safety innovation could open the door to liability suits for earlier generations of less safe products (Huber and Litan, 1991). A strong applied research capability at the CPSC is needed to compensate for the weaknesses of market-generated incentives for safety innovation. By exploring new product designs and performance requirements for identified hazards, the agency can encourage further innovation by industry and can stimulate the development of voluntary standards.

The committee recommends that CPSC's capacity to conduct product safety research be significantly strengthened.

Additional resources for research are needed to enhance the CPSC's capacity to study safety problems and stimulate product innovation; examine the feasibility and efficacy of safer product designs and proposed safety standards; and develop and test methodologies for setting performance standards and for monitoring compliance with such standards.

OCCUPATIONAL SAFETY AND HEALTH ADMINISTRATION

The Occupational Safety and Health Administration of the Department of Labor was created by the Occupational Safety and Health Act of 1970 (P.L. 91-

596). This legislation separated regulation from research by also creating a research agency, the National Institute for Occupational Safety and Health (NIOSH), within the Department of Health and Human Services. The two agencies are formally linked by the statutory authority encouraging NIOSH to make recommendations to OSHA on the basis of occupational research. OSHA, in turn, contributes both formally and informally to the development of NIOSH research priorities.

OSHA's statutory mission is to "assure so far as possible every working man and woman in the nation safe and healthful working conditions" (Section 2(b)). This mission is carried out by setting mandatory standards, enforcing standards, and offering compliance assistance,[8] training, and education. Surveillance activities, which are also discussed below, are carried out by a sister agency within the Department of Labor. OSHA activities are conducted in 25 states and the District of Columbia, whereas the other 25 states—which contain about 40 percent of the labor force—operate their own occupational safety and health programs that are approved by OSHA. The Occupational Safety and Health Act permits states to implement their own programs as long as they are "at least as effective" as OSHA "in providing safe and healthful employment" (section 18 (c)(2)).

When OSHA was formed, it adopted existing federal safety standards, most of which were promulgated under the Walsh–Healy Act of 1936, and it adopted 20 consensus standards of the American National Standards Institute. Since then, OSHA has issued about five dozen safety standards and two dozen health standards, with many more in various stages of development (OTA, 1985).

OSHA holds the dubious distinction of being one of the most criticized regulatory agencies in the federal government (OTA, 1985). Being a focal point for criticism is a natural outgrowth of a mission that often divides employees and employers in terms of their values, perceptions of risk, and economic interests, amidst a historical backdrop of rancor and distrust. OSHA's rule making is subject to intense scrutiny and frequent court challenges. It is not uncommon for a rule to require more than five years from inception to final rule making, if it even proceeds to the final stage.

As it strives to reduce the burden of workplace fatalities and injury, OSHA has been compelled to adapt to strong historical forces—political, technological, and demographic in origin. Among these are a tide of antiregulatory sentiment ushered in during the 1980s, the transformation of U.S. industries from manufacturing to service orientation, entry into a global economy, expansion in the number of U.S. workers, and technological advances that have brought unanticipated health and safety concerns to the workplace. Another major impetus for change at OSHA is the Government Performance and Results Act (GPRA) of 1993. This

---

[8]Provided at no cost to employers that request help in establishing and maintaining a safe and healthful workplace.

legislation requires federal agencies to improve their performance and increase their results through the development of strategic plans, annual performance plans, and annual reports on how well performance targets have been met. Under this legislation, OSHA issued in 1997 a performance report for FY 1996 and its first-ever strategic plan for FY 1998–2002 (OSHA, 1997a,d). The strategic plan establishes clear benchmarks for reductions in injury and illness rates, along with the intent to evaluate performance.

Resources and Structure

In FY 1997, OSHA had a budget of $325 million and 2,238 FTEs. Staffing was at its highest level in 1980 (2,951 FTEs), and there has been a gradual decline since then. OSHA has its administrative headquarters in Washington, D.C., while maintaining a presence in 10 regional offices. OSHA and its state partners together have 2,100 inspectors with jurisdiction over 6.5 million employers employing more than 100 million people nationwide (OSHA, 1997a). Injury standard setting is housed in OSHA's Directorate of Construction and Directorate of Safety Standards Programs, two of its seven directorates. These directorates have the scientific and engineering expertise to identify workplace safety hazards, to develop standards, to propose solutions after an assessment of alternatives, and to offer technical assistance. (OSHA administratively separates acute injury from chronic injury; these are handled by the Directorate for Safety Standards and the Directorate for Health Standards, respectively.) Before the issuance of regulations, their economic impact is assessed by a separate office, the Office of Policy. Compliance with existing OSHA regulations is carried out by the Directorate of Compliance Programs.

Regulation

OSHA administers 695 separate rules (OSHA, 1997a), the majority of which relate to safety. Safety rules cover a wide variety of workplace conditions, ranging from concrete masonry construction safety, to electrical safety, to fire prevention, to safety at grain-handling facilities. Rule making, according to the Occupational Safety and Health Act, can be triggered by an interested party, employers or employees, standard-setting organizations, NIOSH, or states. In practice, most regulations have been propelled by labor organizations, NIOSH recommendations, and congressional mandate. Since 1992, 15 final rules have been adopted in the area of safety, while another 8–10 have been proposed (J. Martonik, OSHA Directorate of Safety Standards Programs, personal communication, 1997).

OSHA regulations are fervently contested, typically on the basis of cost of compliance, inappropriateness, ineffectiveness, and rigidity (Dewees et al.,

1996). Because of the extensive reach of the OSHA regulations and the health and economic issues at stake, rule making is required by statute to be rigorous and to ensure extensive opportunity for public comment. OSHA's rule-making requirements are "arguably . . . among the most demanding of all of Federal agencies with health, safety, and environmental regulatory responsibilities" (OTA, 1985). As a result of statutory requirements, court decisions, executive orders, and OSHA policy, several criteria govern the development of regulations once OSHA demonstrates a "significant" risk. A significant risk with respect to safety is usually defined qualitatively and supported, where possible, by quantitative risk assessment. After the finding of a significant risk, OSHA proceeds to (1) confirm that the required actions are technologically feasible; (2) demonstrate that the new costs incurred in compliance are economically feasible for the effective sectors; and (3) demonstrate that the standard is cost-effective relative to alternative solutions (OTA, 1985). These are the essential elements of OSHA rule making, which the Office of Technology Assessment (OTA) evaluated in a 1985 report. Based on a retrospective analysis of several cases, OTA found that OSHA relies on credible methods for rule making and that its assessments and forecasts are generally accurate. OTA's chief criticism was that OSHA pays insufficient attention to estimating the potential for technological innovation to address hazards.

More recently, OSHA has announced a new policy of pursuing "common sense" regulations (OSHA, 1997c). Under the rubric of regulatory reform, this policy declares OSHA's intent to change its approach to regulation by tackling the most pressing priorities through a priority-planning process with stakeholders; by streamlining and updating past regulations; and by pledging to interact more with business and labor in the development of rules.

Enforcement

OSHA's traditional enforcement activities include unannounced inspections and the levying of penalties. Past priorities for investigations have been (in order of importance) imminent danger, catastrophe and fatality investigations, employee complaints, special inspection programs, and programmed inspections (OTA, 1985). OSHA's enforcement has drawn fire for a host of reasons, including unnecessary overzealousness and excessive red tape—from the point of view of employers—and insufficient numbers of inspectors and insufficient penalties for violators to act as deterrents—from the point of view of labor. In 1992, the GAO revealed that penalties were substantially below the maximum allowed by law (GAO, 1992).

Under the philosophy that traditional OSHA enforcement has been "driven too often by numbers and rules, not by smart enforcement and results," OSHA recently announced a new enforcement policy that calls for more focused inspections for industries with higher injury rates. It also calls for giving employers a choice as to how they wish to be regulated—through partnerships with OSHA or through traditional enforcement (OSHA, 1997c). This policy expands on one actually begun in the 1980s, the Voluntary Protection Program, an incentive program that recognized and promoted employers who established successful safety and health programs in partnership with OSHA. Employers who created effective programs became exempt from routine inspections, as long as they met OSHA criteria for quality. OSHA has built on this concept by now offering regulatory relief and penalty reductions to firms that join this program. The additional benefits, according to OSHA, are enhanced worker productivity and motivation, reduced workers' compensation costs, and community-wide recognition.

In addition, OSHA has begun to nationalize a program inaugurated with the State of Maine in 1993. This program—entitled the Maine 200 program, for the 200 firms that first participated—focuses on firms with the highest numbers of injuries. It gives them the choice of forming a partnership with OSHA to forge an effective health and safety program or of encountering enhanced enforcement. An evaluation of the Maine 200 program found that injury or illness rates of participating companies declined from 1991 to 1996 by 30 percent (OSHA, 1997b).

Surveillance

For injury surveillance, OSHA has, until recently, relied on another agency of the Department of Labor, the Bureau of Labor Statistics (BLS). BLS collects and analyzes annual data on the number of workplace fatalities, injuries, and illnesses through two surveys: the Census of Fatal Occupational Injuries and the Survey of Occupational Injuries and Illnesses (see Chapter 3). The BLS census is considered the most reliable because it uses diverse sources to identify and verify fatalities (Leigh et al., 1997); the survey compiles questionnaire data from approximately 250,000 private firms. These firms are a sample of more than 5 million establishments, which are required under the Occupational Safety and Health Act to maintain records of injuries and illnesses. In 1995, for example, employers reported 500,000 injuries and illnesses that resulted in 21 or more days away from work (BLS, 1997). Sprains, cuts, and fractures account for most of the injuries reported by employers. However, the BLS survey is widely considered to underreport injuries and illnesses by as much as 70 percent because of economic incentives on the part of employers (NRC, 1987; Leigh et al., 1997). Furthermore, the survey does not cover the self-employed, government workers, and farms with fewer than 11 employees. Since 1992, the survey also has collected demographic and detailed case characteristics on a sample of injuries and illnesses that resulted in days away from work (BLS, 1997).

OSHA has recently acquired surveillance capacity of its own with the publication of a final rule that requires employers to notify OSHA of their reportable injury and illness rates (*Federal Register*, 1997). This information is similar to that required by the BLS; however, the new rule requires incidence rates rather than just absolute values and also requires that the employer be identified. BLS reporting is, on the other hand, confidential. OSHA sought this surveillance capacity in order to target its enforcement actions to the most hazardous work sites.

Training

Through its Office of Training and Evaluation, OSHA had a training budget of $2.4 million in FY 1997. This office administers training grants to safety and health organizations, employer associations, labor groups, and educational institutions. Grants are geared to employers and employees who are in industries or establishments with significant injuries or hazards. In addition, OSHA offers safety and health courses through the OSHA Training Institute and Education Centers. The Training Institute has outreach education centers in each OSHA region of the United States. The Training Institute fulfills part of OSHA's responsibility to oversee all aspects of health and safety programs for federal employees.

Assessment

OSHA's broad standard-setting authority leaves the agency with a great deal of discretion. Not surprisingly, the agency's approach has varied with changes in presidential administrations, and the efficacy and cost-effectiveness of OSHA health and safety standards have been subject to considerable debate. Critics have claimed that the existing standards tend to regulate trivial risks with unnecessary specificity in a one-size-fits-all mode, with little significant impact on injury rates. They argue that OSHA regulations should be subject to cost-benefit analysis (Viscusi, 1983; Mendeloff, 1979) or that safety standard setting should be abandoned in favor of an "injury tax," leaving it to employers to take safety precautions to minimize their tax liability (Nichols and Zeckhauser, 1977). OSHA's defenders argue that neither of these proposals will adequately protect worker safety and that OSHA should be strengthened so that it has adequate resources to regulate more effectively (McGarity and Shapiro, 1993).

Outcome studies of OSHA regulation have been inconclusive. Overall, the most reasonable assessment is that OSHA safety regulation has probably had a modest effect in reducing workplace injuries against the general backdrop of a long-term decline (Dewees et al., 1996). Evaluation of OSHA reform proposals lies outside the scope of the present study. However, a key element of any reform strategy is to strengthen the information systems on which employers and the agency rely to identify hazards and make decisions about conducting inspections, proposing corrective action, and standard setting. The challenge is to strengthen employers' incentives to maintain reliable data on all injuries, counteracting the tendency to underreport that may be generated by OSHA enforcement policies.

From this perspective, the committee supports OSHA's balanced approach, which is structured to offer collaborative assistance to employers with elevated injury rates, but still reserves the option to undertake aggressive enforcement and fines. For example, under its Cooperative Compliance Program, OSHA offers employers with the highest injury (and illness) rates the option of working with the agency to improve rates, rather than facing an increased possibility of "wall-to-wall inspection." Although the program has had the support of employee organizations and many employers, it faces a judicial challenge on the ground that it "coerces" participation by employers with high injury rates who otherwise face a near-certain inspection. Whatever the judicial fate of the cooperative compliance program, the committee urges OSHA to continue to develop regulatory strategies that emphasize collaborative efforts between the agency, employers, and employees to achieve reasonable reductions in injury rates based on employer size, current injury rates, industry needs, and safety experience.

NATIONAL INSTITUTE FOR OCCUPATIONAL SAFETY AND HEALTH

The National Institute for Occupational Safety and Health is a research agency of the CDC devoted solely to work-related safety and health. NIOSH was created by the Occupational Safety and Health Act of 1970. NIOSH investigates potentially hazardous working conditions at the behest of employers or employees; evaluates and identifies chemical and safety hazards in the workplace; conducts research to prevent occupational disease, injury, and disability; supports training of health professionals; and develops educational materials and recommendations for worker protection. In FY 1997, NIOSH acquired research responsibility in the area of mine safety through the transfer of several research programs formerly within the Bureau of Mines of the U.S. Department of Interior. NIOSH's vision statement is "delivering on the nation's promise: safety and health at work for all people, through research and prevention" (NIOSH, 1998a).

Resources and Structure

NIOSH's total budget in FY 1998 was $153 million. Injury-related funds were spent on research (intramural and extramural), training, prevention, and public education. The majority was devoted to the activities of NIOSH's Division of Safety Research, one of its seven divisions. Most of its research and surveillance activities are performed intramurally, but about 21 percent are conducted in conjunction with state health departments through cooperative agreements. Within the division are three branches: (1) the Surveillance and Field Investigations Branch is responsible for injury surveillance and descriptive epidemiology studies (see below); (2) the Analysis and Field Evaluations Branch is responsible for in-depth epidemiological studies; and (3) the Protective Technology Branch develops and evaluates new technologies to protect workers against injuries.

NIOSH administers occupational injury-related grants through the Office of Extramural Coordination and Special Projects. These are traditional investigator-initiated grants. All grants are competitively awarded after a peer-review process conducted by a study section made up of researchers outside the federal government.

Research Priority Setting

NIOSH's intramural and extramural research is being guided by a pioneering national research agenda, the National Occupational Research Agenda (NORA). NORA was spawned by an innovative priority-setting process. It is designed to set the course for national occupational safety and health research, coordinated across the public and private sectors (NIOSH, 1998b; Rosenstock et al., 1998). The development of NORA priorities was performed in partnership with about 500 organizations that represent workers, employers, health officials, health professionals, and the public. The priorities were selected by consensus according to the following criteria: the seriousness of the hazard, the magnitude of the risk, the potential for risk reduction, and the possibility that research will make a difference, among other criteria. Several of the 21 top priorities relate to injury, including traumatic injuries, intervention effectiveness research, emerging technologies, organization of work, and special populations at risk. Within these major priorities, teams of experts from the public and private sectors forge a detailed research agenda. The team on traumatic injuries, for instance, recently released a research agenda, *Traumatic Occupational Injury Research Needs and Priorities* (NIOSH, 1998c). Plans are under way to track NORA's implementation and to evaluate its impact on research.

Training Grants

The scope of NIOSH training grants is restricted by federal law to occupational injury training for health professionals. The competitively awarded grants are largely for training at the master's, doctoral, and/or resident level. In FY 1997, approximately 18 educational institutions received NIOSH training grants in occupational safety (with "safety" defined programmatically as injury, safety, and ergonomics). About half of these occupational safety grants went to multidisciplinary programs that are part of larger, university-based research and training grants called Education and Research Center Grants, whereas the other half supported single-discipline academic programs. Together, these two types of training grants totaled about $1.2 million in FY 1997. In addition, NIOSH supported occupational medicine training at about 28 medical schools and schools of public health. Injury was one of a host of covered topics.

Education

NIOSH places high priority on educational materials for worker protection. As a result of the decade-long trend favoring occupational education over regulation (Dewees et al., 1996), NIOSH has come to rely on a variety of documents to disseminate findings and recommendations to the affected industries and the public. These include *Alerts* and *Current Intelligence Bulletins* for the general public, and occupational and public health professional communities. An *Alert* is a brochure for public consumption that describes a threat to worker safety and offers recommendations for prevention. It carries a one-page tear sheet that can be posted readily. NIOSH tailors its dissemination strategy to ensure that *Alerts* reach the most appropriate audience. For example, the tear page from an *Alert* on adolescent worker safety was sent to every secondary school principal in the United States.

Beyond publications, NIOSH supports a host of educational activities that include research literature evaluations and community-based projects. An example of the latter is the Young Worker Community-Based Health Education Project, launched in 1995 to promote adolescent worker safety. This community-based project was prompted by surveillance data revealing disturbing evidence of adolescent deaths and injuries in the workplace, mostly in the construction, farm equipment, and food service industries (NIOSH, 1995). Through this project, cooperative agreements were awarded for three community-based health education projects to develop and test interventions that increase community awareness of adolescent worker safety in order to change the knowledge, attitudes, and behavior of organizations delivering services to teens.

Assessment and Recommendation

The committee applauds NIOSH in its paradigmatic approach to research priority setting through NORA. The contemporary scientific community values planning as a tool for setting broad priorities and integrating diverse research programs (NIH, 1994a; IOM, 1998). The key is to set priorities in a way that does not dictate individual research projects, that encourages innovation, and that ensures stakeholder investment in the outcome.

NORA promulgates national priorities for occupational safety and health research for both the public and private sectors (Rosenstock et al., 1998). One shortcoming, however, is that NORA's 21 priorities are themselves not priori-tized. NORA's widespread support appears to depend on these key procedural elements: a participatory and consensus-building approach to planning in part-nership with stakeholders; criteria for setting priorities; refining of priorities as circumstances change; and plans to evaluate the impact of priority setting. The inclusion of other federal agencies, such as NIH and OSHA, as partners in the priority-setting process is another important milestone. NORA gives OSHA a formal opportunity to fulfill its regulatory needs by influencing the research agenda of a sister agency. Through research planning, NIOSH remains respon-sive to regulatory demands, while preserving its scientific integrity and commit-ment to high-quality science.

Congress recognized the importance of NORA by appropriating an addi-tional $5 million to NIOSH in FY 1998 for implementation of research priorities relating to occupational dermatitis, musculoskeletal disorders, and asthma. NIOSH leveraged these resources with an additional $3 million from several NIH institutes to issue a joint announcement seeking research proposals from the extramural community (NIOSH, 1998a). The total allotment of $8 million repre-sents the largest-ever single infusion of research funds for investigator-initiated occupational safety and health research (NIOSH Budget Office, personal com-munication, 1998).

Traumatic injury research priorities recently developed by the multidiscipli-nary NORA team assigned to this topic also warrant special consideration by Congress. The NORA team specified detailed research priorities under the gen-eral topics of surveillance, analytic injury research, prevention and control, communication and technology transfer, and evaluation (NIOSH, 1998b). Trau-matic occupational injuries, which received only about 8 percent of NIOSH's budget, have not attained sufficient priority in light of the magnitude and costs of occupational injuries. A recent study found that the mortality, morbidity, and costs of occupational injuries considerably overshadowed those of occupational diseases (Leigh et al., 1997). The study estimated that 6,500 deaths and 13.2 million occupational injuries occur annually at cost of $145 billion, compared with an annual cost of $26 million for occupational diseases. Therefore, more funding should be accorded to research on traumatic injury in the workplace.

The committee recommends that NIOSH, working in collaboration with other federal partners, implement the NORA research priori-ties for traumatic and other injury-related occupational injuries, and give higher priority to injury research.

NIOSH also deserves credit for heightened public awareness of occupa-tional safety and health. It initiated an improved dissemination strategy for pub-lications and other educational materials. The strategy targets materials to ap-propriate audiences, especially employers and workers at risk. For example, NIOSH's *Alert* of September 1994, *Preventing Injuries and Deaths of Fire*

Fighters, which identified four critical factors for prevention, was distributed to every fire department in the nation (NIOSH, 1994). Other influential *Alerts* were *Preventing Homicide in the Workplace* and *Preventing Deaths and Injuries of Adolescent Workers* (NIOSH, 1993, 1995). NIOSH received a special, $5 million earmarked appropriation in FY 1996, a major portion of which was devoted to the establishment of a research and education center to prevent child agricultural injuries at the National Farm Medicine Center in Wisconsin.

NATIONAL INSTITUTES OF HEALTH

The National Institutes of Health ranks as the world's leading institution for biomedical research and training. Originating as a one-room Laboratory of Hygiene in 1887, the 21 institutes and centers that today comprise NIH started to take shape after World War II, under the authority of the Public Health Service Act. Many NIH institutes and centers are organized around specific diseases, such as cancer, neurological diseases, and alcoholism. The monumental scope and reach of NIH is captured in its budget of about $13 billion in FY 1997 (NIH, 1998). This budget is estimated to support 50,000 researchers at 1,700 institutions nationwide (NIH, 1993). NIH's mission is "science in pursuit of fundamental knowledge about the nature and behavior of living systems and the application of that knowledge to extend healthy life and reduce the burdens of illness and disability" (NIH, 1997). The mission is accomplished through a profusion of research, training, public and professional education, and technology transfer activities.

Injury is not the primary focus of any single institute at NIH; rather, there are several discrete programs on injury located within a few institutes, and individual projects are funded across virtually all NIH institutes and centers. The collective effort, totaling less than $200 million, is relatively small by NIH standards (see below). More than 30 years ago, the NRC report *Accidental Death and Disability* recommended the creation of a separate institute, a proposed "National Institute of Trauma," but it never materialized (NRC, 1966). In 1985, the Institute of Medicine (IOM) considered, but rejected, placement of an injury center or institute at NIH; this report noted that the establishment of a sizable injury center or institute would not be accorded high priority because NIH is generally disinclined to establish new institutes (NRC, 1985). Instead, the 1985 report turned to the CDC for an administrative location in which to place an injury center. However, in light of CDC's resource constraints, and a host of unmet needs in basic and clinical research that only NIH can fulfill, many continue to advocate a stronger role for NIH in injury research and training (Mickel, 1990). By the early 1990s, Congress foresaw the need for a larger commitment by NIH in trauma research by authorizing a new research program, but funds were not allocated.

Resources

The total level of injury-related funding at NIH was about $194 million in FY 1995 (NCIPC, 1997a). Injury funding constitutes less than 2 percent of the NIH budget. NIH supports three relatively small programs with injury or rehabilitation as the sole focus. These three programs, which are described below, represent about two-thirds of the total NIH injury expenditures. They are located within three separate institutes: the National Institute of General Medical Sciences (NIGMS), the National Institute of Neurological Disorders and Stroke (NINDS), and the National Institute of Child Health and Human Development (NICHD). Even though the remaining institutes and centers at NIH sponsor some small degree of injury research related to their particular mission, these three institutes have the most concentrated and identifiable programs. All are extramural programs, meaning that the research and training are conducted via grants and other funding instruments awarded mostly to universities, medical centers, and other academic institutions after a peer-review process. The competitive peer-review process is considered responsible for NIH's reputation for scientific excellence.

NIGMS has the most broad-based program. Its program on trauma and burns, funded at approximately $48 million in FY 1998, supports investigator-initiated grants, center grants, and training grants that span the spectrum of basic and clinical research, including treatment of acute trauma.[9] The NINDS program on trauma, regeneration, and pain—funded at approximately $60 million annually—is almost exclusively focused on neurotrauma. Finally, a center within the NICHD—the National Center for Medical Rehabilitation Research—funds about $20 million annually in rehabilitation research. Yet not all rehabilitation research is injury related, because injury is but one of a constellation of diseases and conditions responsible for functional disability. These three extramural programs (within NIGMS, NINDS, and NICHD) are administered by a total of 3–5 FTEs.

Training

NIH's largest research training program in injury.is supported by NIGMS. Under this institute's trauma and burn program, an estimated $3 million is spent annually on about 19 training grants to institutions nationwide. These grants pay

---

[9]The NIGMS program focuses on the following topics: organ, tissue, cellular, and molecular responses to injury; mechanisms of cellular and organ failure; pathophysiologic changes following injury and factors or therapies influencing recovery; factors involved in wound healing, tissue repair, and wound infection; mechanisms of electrolyte and solute transport across cell membranes and mechanisms of resuscitation therapy; cryopreservation of cells and organs; and behavioral consequences of trauma and burn injury (among other areas).

for the tuition and stipends of about 60 postdoctoral candidates, most of whom are M.D.s. Predoctoral candidates are not eligible to receive funds under these grants. The grants are for training in basic and clinical research "to improve the understanding of the body's systemic responses to major injury and to foster the more rapid application of this knowledge to the treatment of trauma and burn-injured victims" (NIGMS, 1998).

Assessment and Recommendation

Injury research is not a high priority at NIH, despite NIH's pivotal significance to the injury field. NIH is the only source of funding for certain types of basic and clinical injury research. It also is one of the few sources of funding for research training programs. However, the total level of funding for injury research is not commensurate with the magnitude of the injury problem (see Chapters 2 and 9), nor is the level of funding commensurate with that accorded by NIH to other cardinal contributors to disease and disability. As important, NIH lacks a focal point and a mechanism to coordinate its disparate injury research projects and programs.

Congress has previously recognized that NIH needs to accord trauma research greater priority. Under P.L. 103-43 (1993),[10] Congress authorized a major new trauma research program and a coordinating mechanism for its implementation. In response, NIH convened a special task force of trauma experts nationwide to develop a research plan. The final research plan, *A Report of the Task Force on Trauma Research*, contained recommendations for a comprehensive trauma research program (NIH, 1994b). The report outlined significant opportunities in such areas as basic research, clinical trials, clinical research, health systems research, and translational research (Chapter 6). To implement the program, the report recommended doubling the current number of trauma research centers, without explicitly stating the costs. The research plan was not implemented because the necessary resources were not allocated (although some elements of the plan may have been implemented through the normal course of peer review). Under this legislation, the NIH director was required to "assure the availability of appropriate resources to carry out the program. . . ." The failure to secure funding suggests that a supplementary congressional direction or appropriation is needed.

To fulfill the critically important research opportunities described in the trauma research plan, the committee envisions in its recommendations below an expanded research and training program located within NIGMS. An expanded program also serves to enhance the stature and visibility of injury as a field of inquiry, to promote collaborations, and to attract more researchers. The committee chose NIGMS as the administrative site at which to build a more prominent

---

[10]Section 300d-61.

program because it already has the most broad-based injury program at NIH. Placement within an existing institute capitalizes on prevailing resources and avoids creating an additional bureaucracy. Further, the committee recommends the elevation of NIGMS's current trauma and burn program to its own division. The trauma and burn program is currently located within the NIGMS Division of Pharmacology, Physiology, and Biological Chemistry, one of three NIGMS divisions. The trauma and burn program is among the 12 research programs administered by this division. Any increase in funding must be accompanied by appropriate increases in staff. Since NIH remains under personnel ceilings set by the Office of Management and Budget, increasing the staff level continues to be an NIH-wide problem.

With additional funding, a newly created Division of Trauma and Burns could be charged with conducting the following activities: serving as a focal point for injury research at NIH; implementing the NIH Trauma Task Force Report of 1994 (NIH, 1994b); maintaining a comprehensive extramural research and training program that includes individual grants, center grants, and institutional training grants; ensuring that research gaps and opportunities are filled; and conducting planning and evaluation activities.

An expanded program at NIGMS also would be instrumental for training researchers. Existing NIGMS training grants are very important for basic and clinical research in trauma and burns, but they are only for postdoctoral training. Chapter 6, which discusses trauma care systems, describes the multidisciplinary nature of the research needed to advance injury treatment. This research cannot be accomplished without a cadre of researchers with special training in injury research. Trainees also should include predoctoral candidates who are now excluded from receiving funds under NIGMS's institutional training grants.

The committee supports a greater focus on trauma research and training at NIH and recommends that the National Institute of General Medical Sciences elevate its existing trauma and burn program to the level of a division.

To accomplish this goal, the committee recommends the expansion of research and training grants, the formation of an NIH-wide mechanism for sharing injury research information, and for promoting collaborations spearheaded by NIGMS.

MATERNAL AND CHILD HEALTH BUREAU

The Maternal and Child Health Bureau (MCHB) of the Health Resources and Services Administration has a long and distinguished history of promoting the health of mothers and children. Although injury is a far more recent component of its programs, MCHB began as the Children's Bureau in 1912. Funds were later authorized to the bureau to provide states with direct funding for personal health services under the Sheppard–Towner Act of 1922. This landmark legislation was the first to establish the practice of giving states the funds to implement their own public health programs (NRC, 1988). In 1935, the role of MCHB was expanded with the enactment of Title V of the Social Security Act, which mandated that the bureau administer both maternal and child health service programs covering a broad spectrum of public health topics. The programs under Title V were converted and consolidated (under the same title) into the federal MCH Block Grant Program in 1981, a transformation that gave states more latitude in the expenditure of funds. The purpose of the block grant ($681 million in FY 1997) is to enable states to develop service systems in maternal and child health that reduce infant mortality, provide preventive and primary care services and immunizations, reduce adolescent pregnancy, and prevent injury and violence, among other goals (HRSA, 1997).

Under the MCH block grant, states are given funds on a formula basis (related to population and poverty indices) and are required to match 3 dollars for every 4 dollars they receive in federal appropriations. As a result of legislation in 1989, states are required to earmark funds for broad categories such as preventive and primary care services for children. Injury is subsumed under each major category, but not directly specified by the legislation. MCHB is committed to injury prevention and treatment through its Injury and Violence Prevention Program, which strives to reduce injury and violence among children and their families through a relatively modest portfolio of discretionary grants and contracts authorized under Title V and other authorities.

Discretionary grants and contracts constitute about 15 percent of the Title V block grant appropriation, but they cover a host of other maternal and child health topics besides injury. Title V grants and contracts fall under two authorities: the Special Projects of Regional and National Significance (SPRANS) and the Community Integrated Service Systems (CISS) (HRSA, 1997). In addition to these discretionary resources, the bureau and a related office within HRSA administers two other categorical grant programs that more directly address state and local injury prevention and control: the Emergency Medical Services for Children (EMS-C) and the Traumatic Brain Injury (TBI) programs.

Resources and Structure

MCHB spent a total of about $17.6 million in FY 1997 for injury prevention through four separate programs (described in the next section). In FY 1997, programs under Title V distributed about $2.3 million in injury-related grants and contracts. Another $12.5 million and $2.8 million were awarded under the EMS-C and the TBI programs, respectively. Funds were awarded for service delivery, research, demonstrations, training, and public education under four different grant and contract programs. All four programs, which make awards after a competitive process, are described in more detail in the following section. MCHB has no internal research or surveillance capacity for injury prevention and control. Given its limited resources and the breadth of its purview (i.e., all facets of occupational and non-occupational injury related to children and families), the bureau strives to stretch its resources through partnerships with many other federal, state, and private sources.

Injury-Related Grants and Contracts

Special Projects of Regional and National Significance

This discretionary grant and contract program has a broad mandate to improve state- and community-based maternal and child health. Grants and contracts are distributed mostly to state and local governments, universities, and nonprofit groups and can take the form of research, demonstrations, and training grants. Of the 500 projects supported under this program, about 20 were injury related in 1997. Although injury projects covered such diverse areas as domestic violence training and playground safety, the largest—and most widely recognized—cluster of grants was awarded to each of the organizations that comprise the Children's Safety Network (CSN).

CSN is a group of organizations that serve to strengthen the state infrastructure for injury and violence prevention and to support policy development at the national and state levels. The CSN acts as a resource for, and provides technical assistance to, state and local public health departments, especially MCH agencies, by helping them assess the injury problem, identify and overcome barriers to implementation of injury prevention programs, evaluate prevention programs, and link with others in the field. CSN also develops and distributes publications and facilitates the development of training and continuing education programs for national organizations and professional groups.

This network evolved from a resource center previously funded by the Carnegie Corporation of New York. It was inaugurated in 1991 with the award of two grants from the federal MCHB, one to the Education Development Center in Newton, Massachusetts, and the other to the National Center for Maternal and Child Health at Georgetown University, Washington, D.C. Currently, the network consists of four national centers: the lead center is responsible for addressing all aspects of child and adolescent injury and violence prevention, and three other centers focus on injury data, rural and agricultural injury, and the costs of injury. The four centers work collaboratively to meet the needs of injury practitioners, to help integrate injury and violence prevention into existing MCH programs and policy, and to conduct research and policy activities that improve the state of the art of injury and violence prevention.

Community Integrated Service Systems (CISS)

Authorized in 1989, CISS is a grant program aimed at reducing infant mortality and improving maternal and child health via integrated services at the local level. With a special focus on rural areas and families with special needs, CISS seeks to build service systems. Its grants promote public–private partnerships between community-based organizations.

Emergency Medical Services for Children

The EMS-C program was authorized in 1985 under Section 1910 of the U.S. Public Health Service Act. Its overall purpose is to reduce child and youth mortality and morbidity sustained through severe illness or trauma. More specifically, the program strives to ensure state-of-the-art emergency medical care for children with serious illnesses or injuries; to ensure that pediatric services are integrated into an emergency medical services system; and to ensure that children and adolescents receive a constellation of emergency services, including primary prevention, acute care, and rehabilitation. The program was propelled by research that found that, relative to adults, children suffered disproportionately high rates of morbidity and mortality under emergency circumstances. Emergency medical services had overlooked the needs of children and were ill prepared to deal with children's distinct anatomies, physiological responses, vital signs, body proportions, and deficiencies in communication (IOM, 1993). Over the course of the program, 52 states and territories have received grant assistance. NHTSA has also joined the program and supports a variety of grants, especially those targeted at curriculum development. The EMS-C program funds diverse projects ranging from systems development, research, and demonstrations to training, curriculum development, resource centers, and public education. Evaluation components are now routinely integrated into grants (HRSA, 1996). The first broad evaluation of the EMS-C grant program was undertaken by Solloway and colleagues (1996), using case studies of EMSC grants in seven states. The evaluation found the program to be highly successful in enabling states to develop, implement, and sustain EMS-C programs. Grants were most successful at training and education, enabling hundreds of prehospital providers to be specially trained by a cadre of instructors who can continue to train others. The report also made recommendations to improve and refine the program, many of which were anticipated and had already been adopted by MCHB before publication of the evaluation report.

In 1995, MCHB and NHTSA jointly published a five-year plan (1995–2000) to improve EMS-C services nationwide. The plan not only articulates broad objectives, but also lays out concrete action-oriented steps for federal, state, local, and private organizations (HRSA, 1995). The plan was an outgrowth of broad-based recommendations contained in the 1993 IOM report that defined the underlying characteristics of an EMS-C system, the types of data needed for planning and evaluation, and the role of public agencies (IOM, 1993).

Traumatic Brain Injury Demonstration Grants Program

As a result of legislation passed in 1996, MCHB has been mandated to establish and implement a TBI State Demonstration Grant Program. HRSA was one of three federal agencies charged with developing TBI programs under this legislation (P.L. 104-166). The demonstration projects are intended to improve statewide systems for the delivery of coordinated services to TBI victims. The bureau plans to award planning grants and implementation grants, once it establishes the program's goals and objectives with the aid of a specially convened TBI State Demonstration Grant Program Task Force, with membership from national organizations across the service delivery system.

Assessment

MCHB deserves credit for the quality of its programs and quality of its collaborations with other federal agencies. Although they operate with only a handful of staff, MCHB programs have a remarkable impact on building state and local capacity in injury prevention. MCH is adept at developing enduring relationships with state and local health departments and at disseminating information. Its vital role in emergency medical services for children is described more fully in Chapter 6, which recommends an even greater role for HRSA in trauma systems development and evaluation.

OFFICE OF JUSTICE PROGRAMS

The Office of Justice Programs is a large administrative entity of the Department of Justice headed by an Assistant Attorney General. The mission of the OJP is to develop the nation's capacity to prevent and control crime, administer justice, and assist crime victims. Within this broad mandate, OJP ventures into novel areas of crime prevention and control under the Violent Crime Control and Law Enforcement Act of 1994 (Crime Act), which provided for new programs in community policing, violence against women, sentencing and corrections, and drug courts.

Composed of 10 bureaus and offices,[11] OJP had an FY 1997 budget of $2.7 billion (U.S. DOJ, 1997b). The funds are largely awarded through formula,

---

[11]The Bureau of Justice Assistance, National Institute of Justice, Office of Juvenile Justice and Delinquency Prevention, Bureau of Justice Statistics, Office for Victims of

block, and discretionary grant programs to states, territories, and tribal units for local crime prevention programs.[12] Local crime prevention programs consist mostly of service delivery and demonstration programs. These programs are highly complex and variable in scope, eligibility, and legislative requirements, and the committee was unable to determine whether state and local health departments can avail themselves of funding. Given the magnitude of funding, it would be desirable for public health departments to tap into these funding streams for violence prevention programs.

Research and evaluation are beginning to be accorded higher priority by OJP in the wake of the 1994 Crime Act's statutory requirements for program evaluation. Many OJP bureaus have transferred funds to their sister agency, the National Institute of Justice (NIJ), to design and implement program evaluations. Since NIJ is the only unit of the U.S. Department of Justice that is devoted exclusively to research, the following section focuses on this institute and its potential to advance research and evaluate promising violence prevention programs.

National Institute of Justice

The National Institute of Justice was formed by the Omnibus Crime Control Act of 1968. Its mission is to conduct and support research on the causes and prevention of crime; on the improvement of law enforcement and the administration of justice; on the development of new technologies to prevent crime and enhance criminal justice; and on criminal justice surveillance. The mission is carried out mostly through an extramural grant program, although there is a small intramural research program. NIJ also has a modest training program, described later in this section. NIJ has no regulatory responsibilities but is authorized to make recommendations to federal, state, and local governments (U.S. DOJ, 1997a).

Resources and Structure

With an FY 1998 budget of approximately $50 million, NIJ is one of the smallest administrative bureaus within OJP. Yet its core appropriation is overshadowed by funding transfers from other federal crime prevention programs created by the 1994 Crime Act. The act's requirements for program evaluation generated an infusion of funds to NIJ in the form of transfers from other DOJ

Crime, Corrections Program Office, Drug Courts Program Office, Executive Office for Weed and Seed, Violence Against Women Grants Office, and Violence Against Women Office.

[12]For further description of these funding instruments, see Sherman et al. (1997).

offices (NIJ, 1997). By FY 1998, these transfers amounted to $85 million. Therefore, NIJ's total FY 1998 budget was approximately $135 million, about half of which was spent on evaluation of crime prevention programs.

The NIJ is organized into three major offices. The Office of Research and Evaluation supports grants in the social sciences relating to the causes and prevention of crime. The Office of Science and Technology supports investigator-initiated grants for the development, testing, and evaluation of technologies to deter crime and enhance criminal justice operations. It also funds six regional National Law Enforcement and Corrections Technology Centers that provide technical assistance on research and development to help state and local criminal justice agencies. The Office of Development and Dissemination transmits information through publications and conferences geared to practitioners (i.e., judges, prosecutors, police, corrections officials, and victims' advocates).

Research

NIJ supports research in the following areas: criminal behavior, crime control and prevention, and the criminal justice system. The preponderance of NIJ's budget is awarded for extramural projects conducted by academic researchers and researchers at private nonprofit institutions. Grants average about $250,000 per year over a two-year period. All extramural funds are awarded through a competitive selection process carried out by independent peer-review panels in a process similar to that conducted by NIH. The major differences are that NIJ study sections are not standing study sections, and they require that at least one reviewer be a practitioner (i.e., a judge, prosecutor, policeman, correction official, or victim advocate). Investigator-initiated projects are awarded as a result of an open solicitation process, but this avenue represents a minor component of NIJ's extramural grant program (U.S. DOJ, 1997a). The majority of NIJ's research funds, including transfers from other offices, is awarded after a directed solicitation for research proposals targeted to specific topics, many of which are prescribed by the Crime Act of 1994.

One of the few programs of investigator-initiated grants relates to violence against women. The research program began in FY 1998 through the receipt of $7 million in earmarked appropriations to NIJ. It is being undertaken in collaboration with CDC's NCIPC over a five-year period (NIJ, 1998). The purpose of the joint program is to implement the research agenda propounded by the NRC in its 1996 report *Understanding Violence Against Women* (NRC, 1996). The development of this research agenda was mandated by the Violence Against Women Act of 1994 (Title IV of the Crime Act). The report recommends research on prevention (including longitudinal research), improving research methods, developing the research infrastructure, and the acquisition of new knowledge on all facets of the problem, especially as it affects women of color, disabled women, lesbians, immigrant women, and institutionalized women

(NRC, 1996). The joint program also is guided by the research recommendations of *Violence in Families: Assessing Prevention and Treatment Programs* (NRC, 1998).

Training

NIJ does not administer a program of training grants to institutions but does expend funds for a Graduate Research Fellowship Program and a Visiting Fellows Program. The former consists of individual research fellowships for graduate students working on dissertations in the criminal justice field, whereas the latter allows university researchers to join the NIJ staff to pursue collaborative intramural projects. NIJ's training budget is approximately $300,000 annually.

Assessment and Recommendation

The committee commends NIJ for its commitment to rigorous evaluation of the local crime prevention programs of the Department of Justice. NIJ is in an opportune position to evaluate these massive programs. Through a series of extended internal negotiations beginning in 1994, NIJ began to secure funds from other DOJ offices for program evaluation. The need for stronger program evaluation is abundantly clear. In two recent assessments, DOJ's crime prevention programs have been criticized for insufficient attention to evaluation (GAO, 1998; Sherman et al., 1997). These assessments, although differing somewhat in scope, each concluded that the effectiveness of most federal crime prevention programs is not known.

The report by Sherman and colleagues (1997) from the University of Maryland was most comprehensive and pertinent to DOJ, having been commissioned by NIJ under a mandate from Congress for an independent review of program effectiveness. The report found existing evaluations of DOJ's local crime prevention programs to be inaccessible to researchers and beset by methodological problems, statutory encumbrances, and inadequate funding. It praised the efforts of NIJ, but noted that NIJ has insufficient discretion in the selection of which prevention programs to evaluate. It recommended new legislation that would earmark for rigorous evaluation at least 10 percent of all DOJ local assistance funds for crime prevention (Sherman et al., 1997). The committee agrees with the need for more discretion (see below) and the need for a congressionally authorized set-aside for program evaluation. A congressionally mandated set-aside would provide continuity for evaluation research—a better system than the existing mechanism, which transfers evaluation funds to NIJ and must be renegotiated on a year-by-year basis.

Furthermore, NIJ discretion in program evaluation is imperative because not every promising intervention warrants an evaluation. The determination of which programs to evaluate was the focus of a set of five guiding principles established in a recent report (NRC, 1998). The use of principles such as these is vital, given the daunting array of DOJ programs that could be evaluated. NIJ needs greater flexibility to identify, in a carefully orchestrated manner, those programs that warrant evaluation.

The expansion of NIJ's role in program evaluation has implications for research training. To meet the growing demand for skilled evaluation researchers, more and more individuals from many disciplines require training at the predoctoral and postdoctoral levels. NIJ provides a modest degree of support for individual trainees, but it does not award full-fledged training grants to institutions. Institutional, as opposed to individual, training grants can create a critical mass of trainees at a given institution, draw young people into a career path, augment the field's research capacity, and sustain the field for the future. The Institutional National Research Service Awards established by the NIH provide a model for an institutional training grant.

NIJ should give its highest priority in crime prevention research and program evaluation to studies bearing on prevention of violence, especially lethal violence. While the terms "violence prevention" and "crime prevention" are often used interchangeably, Zimring and Hawkins (1997) have shown that thinking of violence simply as a subset of "the U.S. crime problem" fundamentally distorts our understanding of the problem and confuses our responses to it. Rates of death and life-threatening injury from assaultive behavior in the United States are 4–18 times higher than those in other developed nations, even though rates of property crime are about the same. Zimring and Hawkins argue that the uniquely higher rate of lethal violence in America is attributable to differences in the social environment, not differences in either the volume of crime or the number or characteristics of offenders. They also argue that the usual tools of criminal justice are not adequate to the task of reducing lethal violence and that undifferentiated emphasis on the prevention and control of "crime" or even "violence" misallocates resources, diffuses the focus of attention, and fails to address the specific factors most likely to reduce lethal violence. Thus, emphasis should be placed on the prevention of lethal violence (i.e., that subset of violent events that present a risk of serious injury or death).

> **The committee recommends that NIJ continue to give explicit priority to the prevention of violence, especially lethal violence, within its overall activity in crime prevention research and program evaluation, and that NIJ establish new institutional training grants for violence prevention research at academic institutions.**

NIJ also is to be credited with its collaborative approach to research support. As described earlier, NIJ sponsored a joint solicitation with NCIPC for extramural research proposals on the topic of violence against women. It also collaborated with NIH, NCIPC, and other federal agencies on a grant solicitation on the topics of violence against women and violence within the family. Another noteworthy example of research collaboration is to be found in the National Consortium on Violence Research. The consortium is a nationwide, multidisciplinary group of 50 violence researchers from many institutions. The group is brought together under the auspices of Carnegie Mellon University, the recipient of a large federal grant to form the consortium. Most of the approximately $2.4 million in annual funding comes from the National Science Foundation, with contributions from NIJ and the Department of Housing and Urban Development. The consortium is a unique program that organizes collaborative research projects on factors contributing to serious violence. It solicits and funds research proposals developed largely by its members and coinvestigators. The scope of the consortium's research solicitations is targeted by an internal steering committee and an advisory committee that engage in peer review of proposals. Members of the consortium also are provided access to a Data Center with linkable data sets and associated software. The consortium bears watching as an innovative model for bringing together outstanding yet dispersed researchers. It is to be evaluated by the National Science Foundation in 1999.

A formal interagency coordinating mechanism is needed to promote and facilitate research collaborations on violence prevention. Some of the above-mentioned interagency collaborations were the outgrowth of a previous Interagency Working Group on Violence Research. This working group was created in 1995 by the Department of Justice and the Department of Health and Human Services (DHHS), but it has not met for more than a year. A similar type of group needs to be reinstated and expanded to include all federal departments and agencies with an interest in violence prevention. The purpose of such a committee would be to develop systematic and coordinated research strategies for evaluating violence prevention programs. The committee urges the creation of an interagency coordinating committee for violence prevention research. NIJ should take the initiative to establish such a committee in concert with other federal agencies

NATIONAL CENTER FOR INJURY PREVENTION AND CONTROL

The National Center for Injury Prevention and Control (NCIPC) traces its origins to a 1985 NRC report *Injury in America.* This report prompted Congress to establish a new pilot program at the CDC to address the problem of injury. Placement at CDC was recommended by virtue of its research rather than regulatory emphasis, its strong relationships with state health departments, and its capacity to disseminate new information and technology (NRC, 1985). After three years of operation with funds transferred from the Department of Transportation, the NRC reviewed the program's progress and recommended in a 1988 report that it be made permanent (NRC, 1988). Congress responded with a significant milestone, the Injury Control Act of 1990, which authorized the program within CDC and paved the way for direct appropriations. In 1992, CDC elevated what was then called the Division of Injury Epidemiology and Control to the status of a center.

The mission of NCIPC is "to provide leadership in preventing and controlling injuries, i.e., reducing the incidence, severity, and adverse outcomes of injury" (NCIPC, 1996a). This mission is accomplished through a spectrum of public health activities in research, surveillance, implementation and evaluation of programs, and public education. NCIPC has no regulatory authority. It concentrates on non-occupational injuries to distinguish its role from that of NIOSH (described earlier).

Resources and Structure

In FY 1997, NCIPC commanded a budget of $49.2 million. Its 123 FTEs were divided among three divisions and two staff offices serving the director. The divisions are the Division of Unintentional Injury Prevention; the Division of Violence Prevention; and the Division of Acute Care, Rehabilitation Research, and Disability Prevention. One staff office is responsible for statistics and analyses of injury surveillance data and the other for administration of grants and cooperative agreements (described below).

Research Grants

NCIPC supports a nationwide extramural grant program to universities and other research entities. The grant program awards funds for peer-reviewed research in a manner almost identical to that of the NIH[13]; it sponsors a 21-member study section composed of extramural researchers whose function is to evaluate prospectively the technical merit of submitted applications and recommend funding levels. NCIPC's study section is one of two administered by CDC, with the other serving NIOSH. NCIPC supports three major types of projects: (1) individual investigator grants (discrete projects by a principal investigator); (2) program projects (a series of related individual projects that have an interdisciplinary study design); and (3) centers. Centers, as the most comprehensive type of grant, perform research in the three core phases of injury prevention and treatment (prevention, acute care, and rehabilitation), and also support public information and some training activities.

---

[13]The overall process begins with an internal staff review of submitted applications (for completeness and responsiveness), followed by the primary review for technical merit by an external study section and a secondary review by the NCIPC's Advisory Committee on Injury Prevention and Control..

When the research grant program began in 1987, there was a deluge of applications, but only 8 percent were awarded funding. As the realities of funding became apparent, fewer applications were submitted. Nonetheless, the grant program remains extremely competitive, with only 13 percent of new applications having been awarded in FY 1997. The extramural grant program distributes approximately $15 million per year, about $7 million of which is awarded to 10 injury research centers.

Cooperative Agreements

A cooperative agreement is a mechanism for joint funding of research and demonstrations,[14] and may also be used for public education and training. Cooperative agreements amounted to $19 million in FY 1997, representing 39 percent of NCIPC's budget. NCIPC employs cooperative agreements to build state and local programs for injury prevention. Areas covered by some recent cooperative agreements include bicycle head injury prevention, firearm injury surveillance, head and spinal cord injury, and playground safety.

Each year, NCIPC's cooperative agreements fund approximately 50 projects in 28 states. Most projects address either surveillance or public health interventions with annual budgets of about $120,000 to $300,000. More than half of the recipients are state and local health departments; the remainder are community-based organizations and universities. NCIPC defines the scope and purpose of cooperative agreements, solicits proposals, and then makes awards to the best proposals after a competitively reviewed process. CDC's role in a cooperative agreement, which generally accounts for about 50 percent of the total work load, is usually to advise on data collection and methodology, to devise evaluation criteria, and to disseminate findings. The partner's role is generally to tailor the project to the needs of the community it serves and to collect and analyze data.

The injury researchers at NCIPC administer cooperative agreements and provide technical assistance to states and local organizations (outside of a formal cooperative agreement). NCIPC researchers do engage in intramural research, such as analysis of injury data sets, but their own research represents a small fraction of their time. The devotion of their energies mostly to cooperative agreements and technical assistance, rather than to their own research pursuits, is a distinguishing feature of the NCIPC. NCIPC does not have a formal intramural research program of its own, like that at NIH, where institutes have dedicated intramural research budgets expressly designed to enable their researchers to conduct research full-time.

---

[14] A cooperative agreement is formally defined by CDC as an "assistance mechanism" in which "CDC anticipates considerable interaction with the recipient and substantial programmatic involvement by CDC staff" (CDC, 1993).

Before the widespread use of cooperative agreements in the mid-1990s, NCIPC awarded other types of grants to states that gave them more latitude in program development and implementation. There previously had been three general types of grants: capacity-building grants,[15] surveillance grants, and incentive grants for intervention projects (Hersey et al., 1995). In 1994, however, NCIPC made a policy decision to exercise greater participation in the building of state and local injury programs. Instead of awarding capacity building grants, NCIPC began to utilize the more focused cooperative agreements on the grounds that the agency's limited funds should be used to provide more guidance to states for introducing into practice, and monitoring the impact of, proven interventions like smoke detectors and bicycle helmets. During the same period, Congress began to earmark a large percentage of NCIPC's budget for program development and related activities at the state and community level. The overall impact of these changes was that NCIPC increasingly came to rely on cooperative agreements to carry out areas of emphasis defined by Congressionally earmarked appropriations.

Review and evaluation of cooperative agreements occur before and during the project. An RFP in the *Federal Register* announces the availability of funds. Each announcement culminates a mostly internal planning process to formulate and refine research priorities. Submitted proposals are reviewed by NCIPC according to published review criteria through ad hoc review panels.[16] A new external review procedure, analogous to a time-limited NIH study section, has been introduced in lieu of the ad hoc review panel when there is insufficient internal expertise to review proposals (U.S. DHHS, 1994). Once an award is made, projects are subjected to annual reviews by NCIPC to ensure that milestones are being met. An evaluation component is routinely incorporated into the cooperative agreement once it begins. The evaluation typically asks, Did this project succeed at accomplishing its objectives? Evaluation criteria are often developed by NCIPC (as indicated earlier), and evaluation findings are required in the final report to NCIPC. Approximately 20–25 percent of submitted applications are approved.

---

[15]Such grants were known as State and Community-Based Injury Control Programs. In FY 1994, these grants were distributed to 15 states and metropolitan areas (about $200,000–300,000 per grant) with the goal of developing, expanding, or improving injury control programs.

[16]These panels, which are made up of CDC and other federal employees, rank proposals by merit and recommend funding. In about 20 percent of RFPs, a second review by a similarly constituted panel is invoked by the NCIPC director when more than one ad hoc review panel ranks proposals or when NCIPC's research priorities and/or geographic distribution requirements are not satisfied by the first review. To avoid conflict of interest, none of the reviewers for any of the review panels is from the NCIPC division supporting the cooperative agreement.

Training

Due to budget limitations, NCIPC has a meager investment in the training of practitioners and researchers. Practitioner training generally refers to educational activities for clinicians or for professionals in state and local health departments, whereas research training generally refers to training of the pre- and postdoctoral students at universities. Practitioner and research training is conducted to a modest degree by NCIPC-supported Injury Control Research Centers, but because of the funding limitations described below, training is subordinated to research activities.

Assessment and Recommendations

The committee's evaluation of NCIPC covers the following crosscutting topics: research accomplishments, priorities for future research, training, building state and community infrastructure, and nuturing the field.

Research Accomplishments

The premier accomplishment of NCIPC is the development and support of the science base of injury prevention. Since its inception, NCIPC has sought to forge a research niche in injury prevention. Consequently, NCIPC's research on unintentional and intentional injuries has emphasized surveillance, risk factors, etiology, and evaluation of prevention programs. A prevention orientation also underlies NCIPC's program on acute care, rehabilitation, and disability. For example, with respect to traumatic brain injuries, the leading cause of death and serious long-term disabilities from injuries, NCIPC focuses on surveillance, whereas other DHHS agencies focus on treatment research and service delivery.

NCIPC has succeeded in generating important new knowledge through its support for high-quality research on injury prevention. NCIPC's contributions to research have been noted in comprehensive evaluations (Hersey et al., 1995) and in more focused evaluations of research programs in rehabilitation and disability, motor vehicle, and firearm research by its advisory committee (NCIPC, 1995, 1996b, 1997b). The committee wishes to draw particular attention to NCIPC's noteworthy development of a strong extramural program of investigator-initiated grants, including its support for injury centers and areas of research largely unaddressed by other agencies (discussed below). This discussion serves as a backdrop for the committee's recommendation for an expansion of NCIPC extramural research in several priority areas.

Extramural research. NCIPC is to be commended for its commitment to extramural research in areas essential to scientific progress in the field, but largely unsupported by other federal agencies. Examples are research on injury biomechanics, trauma system design and performance, and residential and recreational injury prevention. For instance, for more than a decade, NCIPC has funded several biomechanics research programs at universities, a commitment totaling about $2 million to $3 million annually. Grant recipients have used NCIPC funds to leverage support from the private sector. Without NCIPC's consistent support, biomechanics as a field of inquiry would have languished, even though it is critical for understanding injury causation (Chapter 4). Biomechanics and other important areas could easily have been forfeited in favor of fields enjoying stronger constituency support. Instead, NCIPC has sustained and nurtured these fields, despite persistent budget limitations.

NCIPC has cultivated a strong extramural program of investigator-initiated grants. These grants consist of individual investigator grants, program project grants, and center grants. NCIPC's extramural grant program has devised a careful process of independent peer review to fund research of high quality. Unfortunately, the program has suffered from chronically low funding. The extramural program's current funding level, about $15 million annually, is woefully insufficient to address NCIPC's vitally important mission. Competition for grants is so great that only 13 percent of applications were awarded funding in FY 1997. By contrast, research programs at NIH typically experience success rates of 20–30 percent. With increased funding over the long term, NCIPC should be able to establish and sustain a critical mass of injury prevention investigators and attract researchers from related fields. Increased funding should be allocated to all types of grants administered by NCIPC. With respect to center grants, the size of each grant should be increased, as discussed below.

Injury Control Research Centers (ICRCs). ICRCs have advanced injury research by bringing together biomedical scientists, epidemiologists and statisticians, social and behavioral scientists, engineers and specialists in biomechanics, policy experts, economists, and lawyers. Cultivation of ICRCs must be considered one of the major advances in the field of injury prevention since the publication of *Injury in America* (NRC, 1985). Before this program, there were no broad-based research centers dedicated to injury prevention. Although some strong research programs already had been established at individual universities (e.g., Wayne State University's pioneering program in biomechanics research and Johns Hopkins University's program to train injury researchers), no individual center could have achieved the catalytic role and breadth of the current program. In light of the highly important role of ICRCs, the current funding level of each center grant, about $750,000 annually, is not sufficient to cover the full range of activities for which each grant was intended: research, policy formation, and training and technical assistance for state and local injury prevention agencies. A center with a similarly comprehensive mission supported by the NIH for cancer or heart disease frequently receives more than $1 million annually. The

ICRCs' research and practitioner training activities have been especially circumscribed because of curtailed funding.

Priority Areas for Future Research

To advance the injury field, the committee believes that NCIPC needs more resources for extramural research in selected areas. The committee predicated its selection of priority areas on the following criteria: the magnitude of the problem, trends in surveillance, gaps in knowledge, and the degree of support from other federal agencies. On the basis of the foregoing discussion in this chapter and in Chapter 4, the committee urges NCIPC to support an expanded research portfolio in the following areas: biomechanics, residential and recreational injuries, suicide prevention, and violence prevention.

The elucidation of more detailed research priorities within each of these general areas should be undertaken by NCIPC, in close coordination with its stakeholders and federal partners, through a systematic priority-setting process described later.

Biomechanics. Injury biomechanics is a seminal discipline for the study of injury causation (Chapter 4). Biomechanics reproduces patterns of injury under well-controlled laboratory conditions and examines structural and biologic responses. As noted above, NCIPC has provided consistent support for investigator-initiated research in injury biomechanics. This support must continue and should be expanded to ensure advances in our understanding of injury causation. Advances in biomechanics will be especially important in understanding nonfatal injuries that lead to long-term disability including brain injury and arthritis and are likely to lead to improved treatment. It is important to continue to expand the research effort in the study of injuries to the study of children, short women, and the elderly.

Residential and recreational injuries. Residential and recreational injuries are a serious problem. Although there appears to have been some decline in prevalence since 1985, more recent trends suggest a leveling off (Chapter 4). Within these broad trends are more alarming ones, such as apparent increases in unintentional poisonings (Fingerhut and Cox, 1998) and falls in the elderly. Mortality rates for falls in the elderly increased slightly from 1985 to 1995 (Fingerhut and Warner, 1997). Because such falls frequently lead to hospitalization, they represent a costly societal problem (Chapter 2).

It is incumbent on NCIPC to monitor surveillance trends in order to focus research on the most important problems related to residential and recreational injuries. NCIPC's support for these areas of research amounted to $7.5 million in FY 1997 (NCIPC Budget Office, personal communication, 1997). Apart from NCIPC, no other federal agency supports a research program in the prevention of residential and recreational injuries. CPSC has a very small research budget that is restricted to consumer products in particular, rather than the broader category of residential and recreational injuries.

Suicide prevention. The design and evaluation of suicide prevention programs should be a high priority for NCIPC. NCIPC has played a critical role in raising awareness of suicide as a national problem for which prevention research is essential. It has drawn attention to the lack of evidence for effective suicide prevention programs. NCIPC spent approximately $400,000 on suicide research and demonstrations in FY 1997 (NCIPC Budget Office, personal communication, 1997). NCIPC should be given additional funds to establish a suicide prevention research center similar in function to, but more circumscribed in focus than, the ICRCs that it now supports. The expansion of suicide prevention research at NCIPC should not affect the commitment of the National Institute of Mental Health (NIMH) to its program of high-quality research on suicide etiology and treatment, because NCIPC's orientation to suicide surveillance, risk-factor identification, and prevention program development and evaluation complements rather than duplicates that of NIMH. Yet the two agencies must closely coordinate their suicide prevention research portfolios. NIMH expended an estimated $12 million in FY 1997 on extramural research in suicide (NIMH, 1998).

Violence prevention. Since its inception, NCIPC has played a leadership role in galvanizing attention to violence as a public health problem. NCIPC was virtually the only source of support for research on violence prevention until the passage of the Crime Act in 1994. This act led to a rapid expansion of violence prevention research by NIJ (see earlier discussion). NCIPC and NIJ are now the two federal agencies with the greatest emphasis on violence prevention research. For reasons discussed earlier in this chapter, the committee believes that research on the prevention of lethal violence—violence that results in serious injury or death—should merit explicit priority from both agencies. NCIPC and NIJ must coordinate their research portfolios to ensure that each pursues the facets of the problem for which it is best suited or is obligated to pursue (by virtue of intra-agency transfers or congressional mandates). The problem of lethal violence is sufficiently multifaceted, serious, and refractory to simple solutions that duplication of effort is unlikely as long as close coordination occurs.

Research priority-setting process. The committee already has taken the first step by identifying in the preceding section several prominent priority areas in which NCIPC should expand its research investment: biomechanics, residential and recreational injuries, suicide prevention, and violence prevention. The committee recommends these priorities on the basis of the magnitude of the problem, trends in surveillance, gaps in knowledge, and degree of support from other federal agencies.[17] Other major areas may have to be identified, and within each priority area, detailed priorities have to be elucidated.

In the past, NCIPC has not systematically incorporated its stakeholders in the ongoing process of setting priorities for its intramural and extramural research programs. Stakeholders include federal research partners; representatives of state, local, and private organizations; public health professionals and practitioners; academic researchers; and the public. The value of a participatory research priority-setting process is that it coordinates diverse research programs, responds to regulatory needs, encourages synergies, and maximizes the use of limited resources. The inclusion of stakeholders and the public helps to enhance the knowledge base for priority decisions and leads to more widely accepted decisions (IOM, 1998). NCIPC is to be commended for having undertaken from 1991 to 1993 a consensus-building planning activity that set forth an agenda for research and programs (NCIPC, 1993), but this activity was time limited and has not been monitored or evaluated in terms of implementation, impact, or cost-effectiveness.

NCIPC might wish to consider developing a priority-setting process similar to the award-winning one employed by NIOSH—the National Occupational Research Agenda (discussed above). The inclusion of federal research partners was one of the hallmarks of NORA. Their inclusion led to the single largest infusion of investigator-initiated research funds for occupational safety and health research. NIOSH's contribution of $5 million to this joint endeavor came from a special congressional appropriation in recognition of the value of NORA. At least two separate NCIPC advisory committee reports on firearms and motor vehicle research recommended that research planning be performed in conjunction with federal research partners (NCIPC, 1995, 1997b). Federal regulatory partners such as CPSC also must be included. CPSC has a substantial regulatory interest in preventing residential and recreational injuries caused by consumer products. NCIPC is the primary source of federal funding for research on residential and recreational injuries, including those in which consumer products are implicated. CPSC has only limited funds to conduct research, and the research is restricted to consumer products, which are not the only causes of residential and recreational injuries. Therefore, these areas of research need priority attention by the NCIPC.

The committee recommends that NCIPC establish an ongoing and open process for refining its research priorities in the areas of biomechanics, residential and recreational injuries, and suicide and

---

[17]Although NCIPC deserves credit for its support of trauma systems research, the committee believes that this area should be moved to HRSA, to ensure its expansion and linkage to a broader range of federal trauma systems development activities discussed in Chapter 6.

violence prevention, in close coordination with its stakeholders and federal partners.

Training

Because of funding limitations, NCIPC has been unable to launch a formal grant program for research training. The need for comprehensive training programs was underscored by *Injury in America* and reiterated in *Injury Control* (NRC, 1985, 1988). The lack of formal research training programs by NCIPC has inhibited the development of the injury field. (Problems with the paucity of training programs for injury practitioners are discussed at greater length in Chapter 7.)

Research training serves as a vital investment in the future of a field. It channels young people into a career pathway, ensures a pipeline of capable researchers, and sustains future progress of a field. Formal training grants either to individuals or to institutions are the hallmarks of NIH's approach to building research careers. Such grants have been employed by NIH for decades to create a critical mass of young researchers, to create curriculum, and to ensure innovation. The establishment of formal training grants represents a defining feature of a field (see Chapter 4 for recommendation regarding support of training and research careers).

Today, young researchers cannot look forward to a career in injury research because the funding and award structures are unreliable. In comparison, young people gravitate to careers in cancer and heart research where resources are plentiful for training and for the pathway that ordinarily follows—the receipt of grants for research. In these areas, students can envision a career trajectory as long as they have good ideas. NIH, as described previously, does fund mostly institutional training grants for clinical and basic research in trauma. Yet these training grants are geared mostly to M.D.s at academic medical centers for treatment-related research. There simply are no comparable types of training grants geared to pre- and postdoctoral students in the elements of injury prevention, including epidemiology, biostatistics, biomechanics, behavioral sciences, and program evaluation. NCIPC should establish a program of individual and institutional training grants to schools of public health and other institutions.

Furthermore, as fully discussed in Chapter 7, training opportunities are scarce for injury practitioners. The 1993 agenda-setting report *Injury Control in the 1990s: A National Plan for Action* identified the need for training of injury professionals as one of its critical recommendations (NCIPC, 1993).

The committee reasserts the need for training of injury professionals and strongly recommends that NCIPC expand training opportunities for injury prevention practitioners and researchers.

To ensure the success of this recommendation, the committee suggests that the NCIPC work with other relevant federal agencies (e.g., NHTSA, MCHB, NIOSH, CPSC) to implement the training recommendations of the National Plan (NCIPC, 1993). Additionally, to ensure a trained work force to conduct injury research, NCIPC should initiate a formal program of individual and institutional training grants for pre- and postdoctoral candidates.

Building State and Community Infrastructure

NCIPC has fallen short of expectations for building state and local injury prevention programs. The formation of such programs nationwide was a major force behind the placement of an injury center within CDC. In its 1988 report, the NRC recommended CDC as an opportune location for a federal injury program because of its long-standing and durable relationships with state and local health departments. The NRC envisioned a constellation of programs in every state and community, with the CDC as a focal point for financial and technical assistance. CDC was seen as pivotal to moving injury prevention research into practice (NRC, 1985, 1988). More broadly, the need for vigorous federal efforts to shore up state and local health programs was described in a landmark report (IOM, 1988).

NCIPC's shortcomings in cultivating state and local programs are a function of three factors: resource constraints, its policy decision (noted earlier) to steer away from capacity building and towards more focused injury surveillance and interventions (through cooperative agreements); and greater reliance by Congress on earmarked funding for state and local activities. NCIPC estimates that $15 million of the $19 million it disbursed through cooperative agreements in FY 1997 was directly or indirectly related to Congressional earmarks over the past several years (M. Scally, NCIPC, personal communication, 1998). From the point of view of the state and local programs, NCIPC's role does not sufficiently satisfy their needs for technical assistance and is overly prescriptive.

With respect to technical assistance, NCIPC has no formal office serving state programs. Most other federal agencies seeking to build state programs have entire offices whose mission is devoted to state and local assistance. The technical assistance should transcend the technical aspects of program design and implementation. It should also entail assistance in identifying and accessing funding from NCIPC as well as other federal and private sources. This report outlines the daunting array of possible funding sources in multiple government agencies. The complexity can be overwhelming even to aficionados of federal injury programs. It is imperative for state and local programs to receive help in identifying an array of potential sources of funding, in both the public and the private sectors, with which to build comprehensive injury programs.

The conversion to cooperative agreements is a relatively new development. The transformation of more flexible grants into more circumscribed cooperative agreements has been especially problematic for states without established injury programs. These states are at a disadvantage in the competitive process to attain funding, a process that favors states with more established programs. Yet states lacking established programs are the very states in need of federal assistance. They see themselves as falling further and further behind, whereas states with an injury infrastructure are seen as more and more successful. They point to an evaluation by Battelle, under contract to NCIPC, that found NCIPC's grants to states from FY 1989 to FY 1993 to have been so valuable that it recommended their expansion to all 50 states. According to the final report, "Efforts should be instituted to bring those states currently without adequately funded injury control programs at least up to a minimal level" (Hersey et al., 1995).

NCIPC, to its credit, responded to state concerns by inaugurating a new program on Basic Injury Program Development in FY 1997 (Chapter 7). This new program is a step in the right direction, but it is not sufficiently ambitious in size or scope to address current needs. In summary, NCIPC should restructure its financial assistance to states to give them more latitude and more technical assistance in building their infrastructure (see recommendation in Chapter 7).

The committee recommends that the NCIPC support the development of core injury prevention programs in each state's department of health, and provide greater technical assistance to the states.

Nuturing the Injury Field

The authors of *Injury in America* envisioned that the NCIPC would become the locus of an intensified federal effort in injury prevention and treatment (NRC, 1985). Since its inception, the NCIPC has been the main advocate for the public health paradigm of injury prevention and treatment. As described in Chapter 1, this paradigm has enriched the entire injury field—from traffic safety to criminology. Although NCIPC's relationship with other federal agencies requires clarification (see below), its role as a support for public health practitioners and researchers in the injury field should not be diminished, and it should continue to be responsible for and accountable to those constituents.

The NCIPC's responsibility for nurturing the field entails a variety of activities, including

• assembling, synthesizing, and disseminating information concerning current knowledge, programs, policies, and activities and identifying current needs and opportunities in the field (as an example of this clearinghouse function, the NCIPC prepared an inventory of current federal injury research funded in 1995 [NCIPC, 1997a]);

• stimulating and facilitating investments and activities that are needed to fill gaps in research and program support identified by NCIPC in collaboration with foundations, states and communities, businesses, and other federal agencies to leverage available resources;

• promoting communication and exchange among scientists and practitioners (NCIPC's sponsorship or cosponsorship of periodic injury conferences is an important contribution to this objective); and

• assisting communities, researchers, and other interested groups; identifying potential funding for worthy projects; and facilitating coordination among them.

The committee recommends that the NCIPC continue to nurture the growth and development of the public health effort in injury prevention and treatment through information exchange, collaboration with injury practitioners and researchers, and leveraging available resources to promote the effectiveness of programs and research.

COORDINATION AND LEADERSHIP

The crosscutting nature of the injury problem, as well as of injury research and interventions, has been highlighted throughout this report. Through collaboration and coordination, federal agencies can work jointly to combat related and sometimes overlapping problems and to overcome fragmentation. They can link activities and pool resources, which take the form of expertise, funds, databases, access to patient populations, and technology. They also can avoid unnecessary duplication of effort, although duplication does not currently appear to be a major problem across federal injury programs (U.S. DHHS, 1992; GAO, 1994). Although the committee is not naive about the difficulties facing federal agencies when attempting collaboration and coordination, there are effective mechanisms that may ensure success, such as memoranda of understanding, interagency task forces and committees, and funding for joint projects.

In 1985, *Injury in America* recommended that an injury center at the CDC be established to serve as a "lead agency among federal agencies and private organizations" (NRC, 1985). By using this formulation, the 1985 report appears to have envisioned that the CDC would provide leadership in two ways: (1) by nurturing the public health community's commitment to and interest in the injury field and (2) by coordinating the efforts of the multiple federal agencies involved in injury prevention and treatment. The committee believes that the NCIPC should continue to be a focal point for the public health commitment to the injury field (see above). However, when Congress enacted the Injury Control Act in 1990, it properly recognized that no single agency could "lead" such a diverse federal effort, and instead authorized the CDC to create a program to "work in cooperation with other Federal agencies, and with public and nonprofit private entities, to promote injury control" (P.L. 101-558). Congress envisioned a cooperative effort because, as a practical matter, an agency in one cabinet department has no authority to direct other agencies in the same department, much less in other departments.

It became apparent to the committee during numerous discussions and meetings with individuals representing diverse perspectives,[18] that characterization of the NCIPC as "the lead Federal agency" should be redefined by the NCIPC in collaboration with other relevant federal agencies, as it has led to unrealistic expectations about what NCIPC can accomplish with its resources. It also has impeded collaboration by spawning institutional rivalries and resentments, especially from federal agencies whose funding is similar to, or greater than, that of NCIPC. Although there are certainly stellar examples of coordination—for example, between NHTSA and HRSA on the Emergency Medical Services for Children program, and between CPSC and NCIPC on the expansion of emergency department injury surveillance—these examples are more the exception than the rule.

An effective federal response to injury requires many agencies to play a leadership role in their areas of strength and jurisdiction. Playing a leadership role means taking the initiative to persuade and induce others to join in collective action toward a common goal. NHTSA, for example, naturally plays a lead role in highway and traffic safety; CPSC naturally plays a lead role in the surveillance and prevention of product-related injuries and product design research; NIOSH naturally plays a lead role in occupational safety research and education; and NCIPC naturally plays a lead role in prevention research related to residential and recreational injuries. Yet playing a lead role is not an exclusive role; it involves collaboration with other agencies to reduce injuries, promote synergies, and harness limited resources. For example, NCIPC and NIMH should both exert leadership on suicide prevention by collaborating with one another and with other groups. NIJ and NCIPC should do the same for violence prevention research and program evaluation by providing joint leadership for the criminal justice and public health communities. In summary, leadership, or playing a lead role, requires each agency to forge partnerships with other federal agencies in a collaborative manner to meet the overall objective of preventing injuries and improving safety.

The committee recommends that federal agencies with injury-related programs create mechanisms (e.g., memoranda of understanding between federal agencies, working groups, interagency committees, task forces, funding for collaborative projects) to promote coordination and interagency collaboration. NCIPC recently proposed a new mechanism for coordination that would be

---

[18]The committee met with numerous federal, state, and local government representatives, researchers, practitioners, and public and private organizations during the course of the study.

overseen at a higher level of DHHS by the Assistant Secretary for Health. The new forum is viewed as the primary mechanism within DHHS for promoting the exchange of injury information and activities. The proposal also calls for invited membership from other federal agencies outside DHHS. New mechanisms of this kind should help to facilitate interagency coordination.

REFERENCES

BLS (Bureau of Labor Statistics). 1997. Lost-worktime injuries: Characteristics and resulting time away from work, 1995. *Bureau of Labor Statistics News* June 12, 1997.

CDC (Centers for Disease Control and Prevention). 1993. *Guide for Preparation of Assistance Requests*. Atlanta, GA: CDC Grants Management Branch, Office of Program Support.

Christoffel T, Christoffel KK. 1989. The Consumer Product Safety Commission's opposition to consumer product safety: Lessons for public health advocates. *American Journal of Public Health* 79(3):336–339.

CPSC (Consumer Product Safety Commission). 1996a. *1997 Budget Request*. Submitted to the Congress and the Office of Management and Budget. March 1996. Washington, DC: CPSC.

CPSC (Consumer Product Safety Commission). 1996b. *Success Stories: Saving Lives Through Smart Government*. Washington, DC: CPSC.

Dewees D, Duff D, Trebilcock M. 1996. *Exploring the Domain of Accident Law*. New York: Oxford University Press.

Federal Register. 1997. Reporting occupational injury and illness data to OSHA. Final Rule. *Federal Register* 62(28):6433–6442.

Fingerhut LA, Cox CS. 1998. Poisoning mortality 1985–1995. *Public Health Reports* 113(3):218–233.

Fingerhut LA, Warner M. 1997. *Injury Chartbook. Health, United States, 1996–97*. Hyattsville, MD: National Center for Health Statistics.

GAO (General Accounting Office). 1992. *Occupational Safety and Health: Penalties for Violations Are Well Below Maximum Allowable Penalties*. Washington, DC: GAO. GAO/HRD-92-48.

GAO (General Accounting Office). 1994. *Agencies Use Different Approaches to Protect the Public Against Disease and Injury*. Washington, DC: GAO. GAO/HEHS-9-85BR.

GAO (General Accounting Office). 1997. *Consumer Product Safety Commission: Better Data Needed to Help Identify and Analyze Potential Hazards*. Washington, DC: GAO. GAO/HEHS-97-147.

GAO (General Accounting Office). 1998. *At-Risk and Delinquent Youth: Multiple Programs Lack Coordinated Federal Effort*. Washington, DC: GAO. GAO/T-HEHS-98-38.

Graham JD. 1993. Injuries from traffic crashes: Meeting the challenge. *Annual Review of Public Health* 14:515–543.

Hersey JC, Abed J, Butler MO, Diver AR, Mitchell K. 1995. *Reducing the Burden of Injury: An Evaluation of CDC Injury Grant Programs. Final Report*. Arlington, VA: Battelle. Report to the Centers for Disease Control and Prevention, National

Center for Injury Prevention and Control and the Office of Program Planning and Evaluation.

HRSA (Health Resources and Services Administration). 1995. *Five-Year Plan: Emergency Medical Services for Children.* 1995–2000. Washington, DC: Emergency Medical Services for Children National Resource Center.

HRSA (Health Resources and Services Administration). 1996. *Emergency Medical Services for Children.* FY 1996 Report. Rockville, MD: HRSA.

HRSA (Health Resources and Services Administration). 1997. *HRSA* [World Wide Web document]. URL http://www.os.dhhs.gov/hrsa/mchb/mchb.html (accessed November 1997).

Huber P, Litan R, eds. 1991. *The Liability Maze: The Impact of Liability Law on Safety and Innovation.* Washington, DC: Brookings.

IOM (Institute of Medicine). 1988. *The Future of Public Health.* Washington, DC: National Academy Press.

IOM (Institute of Medicine). 1993. *Emergency Medical Services for Children.* Washington, DC: National Academy Press, 1993.

IOM (Institute of Medicine). 1998. *Scientific Opportunities and Public Needs: Improving Priority Setting and Public Input at the National Institutes of Health.* Washington, DC: National Academy Press.

Leigh JP, Markowitz SB, Fahs M, Shin C, Landrigan PJ. 1997. Occupational injury and illness in the United States. Estimates of costs, morbidity, and mortality. *Archives of Internal Medicine.* 157(14):1557–1568.

Magat WA, Moore MJ. 1996. Consumer product safety regulation in the United States and the United Kingdom: The case of bicycles. *RAND Journal of Economics* 27(1):148–164.

Mashaw JL, Harfst DL. 1990. *The Struggle for Auto Safety.* Cambridge, MA: Harvard University Press.

McGarity TO, Shapiro SA. 1993. *Workers at Risk: The Failed Promise of the Occupational Safety and Health Administration.* Westport, CT: Praeger Press.

Mendeloff J. 1979. *Regulating Safety: An Economic and Political Analysis of Occupational Safety and Health Policy.* Cambridge, MA: MIT Press.

Mickel HS. 1990. Critical need for a National Institute of Emergency Medicine. *Annals of Emergency Medicine* 19(11):1340–1341.

Moore MJ, Magat WA. 1996. Labeling and performance standards for product safety: The case of CPSC's lawn mower standards. *Managerial & Decision Economics* 17(5):509–516.

Moore MJ, Magat WA. 1997. The injury risk consequences of the all-terrain vehicle consent decrees. *International Review of Law and Economics* 17(3):379–393.

NCIPC (National Center for Injury Prevention and Control). 1993. *Injury Control in the 1990s: A National Plan for Action. A Report to the Second World Conference on Injury Control.* Atlanta, GA: Centers for Disease Control and Prevention.

NCIPC (National Center for Injury Prevention and Control), Special Panel on Firearm Injury. 1995. *Report of the Special Panel to Evaluate the Quality of Research on Firearm Injury Prevention that Has Been Supported by the National Center for Injury Prevention and Control.* Atlanta, GA: NCIPC.

NCIPC (National Center for Injury Prevention and Control). 1996a. *National Center for Injury Prevention and Control 1996 Fact Book.* Atlanta, GA: NCIPC.

NCIPC (National Center for Injury Prevention and Control), Rehabilitation Research and Disability Prevention Team. 1996b. *Programmatic Review: Disability and Rehabilitation Team.* Atlanta, GA: NCIPC.

NCIPC (National Center for Injury Prevention and Control). 1997a. *Inventory of Federally Funded Research in Injury Prevention and Control, FY 1995.* Atlanta, GA: NCIPC.

NCIPC (National Center for Injury Prevention and Control), Motor Vehicle-Related Injury Prevention Team. 1997b. *Programmatic Review: Motor Vehicle-Related Injury Prevention Activities.* Atlanta, GA: NCIPC.

NHTSA (National Highway Traffic Safety Administration). 1991. *Moving America More Safely: An Analysis of the Risks of Highway Travel and the Benefits of Federal Highway, Traffic, and Motor Vehicle Safety Programs.* Washington, DC: NHTSA.

NHTSA (National Highway Traffic Safety Administration). 1994. *Strategic Plan.* Washington, DC: NHTSA. Publication No. DOT HS 808 181.

NHTSA (National Highway Traffic Safety Administration). 1995. *The Highway Safety Assessment: An Interim Report.* Washington, DC: NHTSA Office of Strategic Planning and Evaluation.

NHTSA (National Highway Traffic Safety Administration) 1996. *Traffic Safety Facts 1995.* Washington, DC: NHTSA. Publication No. DOT HS 808 471.

NHTSA (National Highway Traffic Safety Administration). 1997. *Safe Communities: Annual Report.* Washington, DC: NHTSA. Publication No. DOT HS 808 585.

Nichols A, Zeckhauser R. 1977. Government comes to the workplace: An assessment of OSHA. *The Public Interest* 49:39.

NIGMS (National Institute of General Medical Sciences). 1998. *NIGMS Research Training and Fellowship Award Mechanisms.* [World Wide Web document]. URL http://www.nih.gov/nigms/funding/trngmech.html (accessed June 1998).

NIH (National Institutes of Health). 1993. *Investment for Humanity.* Bethesda, MD: NIH.

NIH (National Institutes of Health). 1994a. *Report of the External Advisory Committee of the Director's Advisory Committee.* Bethesda, MD: NIH. Nov. 17, 1994.

NIH (National Institutes of Health). 1994b. *A Report of the Task Force on Trauma Research.* Bethesda, MD:NIH.

NIH (National Institutes of Health). 1997. *NIH Almanac* [World Wide Web document]. URL http://www.nih.gov/welcome/almanac97/overview.htm (accessed June 1998).

NIH (National Institutes of Health). 1998. *NIH Budget* [World Wide Web document]. URL http://www.nih.gov/od/ofm.htm (accessed April 1998).

NIJ (National Institute of Justice). 1997. *Criminal Justice Research Under the Crime Act—1995 to 1996.* Washington, DC: NIJ.

NIJ (National Institute of Justice). 1998. *Research and Evaluation on Violence Against Women* [World Wide Web document]. URL http://ncjrs.org/txtfiles/s1000279.txt (accessed June 1998).

NIMH (National Institute of Mental Health). 1998. *NIMH Suicide Research Consortium.* [World Wide Web document]. URL http://www.nimh.nih.gov/research/suicide.htm (accessed July 1998).

NIOSH (National Institute for Occupational Safety and Health). 1993. *Preventing Homicide in the Workplace.* Cincinnati, OH: NIOSH. DHHS (NIOSH) Publication No. 93-109.

NIOSH (National Institute for Occupational Safety and Health). 1994. *Preventing Injuries and Deaths of Firefighters.* Cincinnati, OH: NIOSH. DHHS (NIOSH) Publication No. 94-125.

NIOSH (National Institute for Occupational Safety and Health). 1995. *Preventing Deaths and Injuries of Adolescent Workers.* Cincinnati, OH: NIOSH. DHHS (NIOSH) Publication No. 95-125.

NIOSH (National Institute for Occupational Safety and Health). 1998a. *NIOSH* [World Wide Web document]. URL http://www.cdc.gov/niosh/homepage/html (accessed June 1998).

NIOSH (National Institute for Occupational Safety and Health). 1998b. *National Occupational Research Agenda, Update. July, 1998: 21 Priorities for the 21st Century.* Cincinnati, OH: NIOSH. DHHS (NIOSH) Publication No. 98-141.

NIOSH (National Institute for Occupational Safety and Health). 1998c. *Traumatic Occupational Injury Research Needs and Priorities: A Report By the NORA (National Occupational Research Agenda) Traumatic Injury Team.* Cincinnati, OH: NIOSH. DHHS (NIOSH) Publication No. 98-134.

NRC (National Research Council). 1966. *Accidental Death and Disability: The Neglected Disease of Modern Society.* Washington, DC: National Academy Press.

NRC (National Research Council). 1985. *Injury in America: A Continuing Public Health Problem.* Washington, DC: National Academy Press.

NRC (National Research Council). 1987. *Counting Injuries and Illnesses in the Workplace: Proposals for a Better System.* Washington DC: National Academy Press.

NRC (National Research Council). 1988. *Injury Control: A Review of the Status and Progress of the Injury Control Program at the Centers for Disease Control.* Washington, DC: National Academy Press.

NRC (National Research Council). 1996. *Understanding Violence Against Women.* Washington DC: National Academy Press.

NRC (National Research Council). 1998. *Violence in Families: Assessing Prevention and Treatment Programs.* Washington DC: National Academy Press.

OSHA (Occupational Safety and Health Administration). 1997a. *OSHA's Mission* [World Wide Web document]. URL http://www.osha.gov/oshainfo/mission.html (accessed October 1997).

OSHA (Occupational Safety and Health Administration). 1997b. *Performance Report FY 1996.* Washington, DC: OSHA Office of Statistics.

OSHA (Occupational Safety and Health Administration). 1997c. *The New OSHA: Reinventing Worker Safety and Health.* [World Wide Web document]. URL http://www.osha.gov/reinvent/reinvent.html (accessed October 1997).

OSHA (Occupational Safety and Health Administration). 1997d. *Strategic Plan: Occupational Safety and Health Administration, United States Department of Labor FY 1997– FY 2002.* Washington, DC: OSHA.

OTA (Office of Technology Assessment). 1985. *Preventing Illness and Injury in the Workplace.* Washington, DC: OTA. OTA-H-256.

Rodgers GB. 1993. All-terrain vehicle injury risks and the effects of regulation. *Accident Analysis and Prevention* 25(3):335–346.

Rodgers GB. 1996. The safety effects of child-resistant packaging for oral prescription drugs. Two decades of experience. *Journal of the American Medical Association* 275(21):1661–1665.

Rosenstock L, Olenec C, Wagner GR. 1998. The National Occupational Research Agenda: A model of broad stakeholder input into priority setting. *American Journal of Public Health* 88(3):353–356.

Sherman LW, Gottfredson D, MacKenzie D, Eck J, Reuter P, Bushway S. 1997. *Preventing Crime: What Works, What Doesn't, What's Promising.* [World Wide Web document]. URL http://www.ncjr.org/works/index.html (accessed November 1997).

Solloway M, Gotschall CS, Barta LJ, Avery A. 1996. *Emergency Medical Services for Children: An Evaluation of Sustainability in Seven States.* Prepared for the Maternal and Child Health Bureau, HRSA (contract number 282-92-0040).

TRB (Transportation Research Board, National Research Council). 1990. *Safety Research for a Changing Highway Environment.* Transportation Research Board Special Report, No. 229. Washington, DC: TRB.

U.S. DHHS (U.S. Department of Health and Human Services). 1992. *Injury Control.* Washington, DC: U.S. DHHS Office of the Inspector General. OEI-02-92-00310.

U.S. DHHS (U.S. Department of Health and Human Services). 1994. *Disease, Disability, and Injury Prevention and Control Special Emphasis Panel Charter.* Washington, DC: DHHS.

U.S. DOJ (U.S. Department of Justice). 1997a. *Building Knowledge About Crime and Injustice: The 1997 Research Prospectus of the National Institute of Justice.* Washington, DC: NIJ. NCJ 163708.

U.S. DOJ (U.S. Department of Justice). 1997b. *Office of Justice Programs Fiscal Year 1997 Program Plans.* Washington, DC: U.S. DOJ.

U.S. DOT (U.S. Department of Transportation). 1997. *Investing in Transportation's Future: An Examination of the University Transportation Centers Program.* Cambridge, MA: DOT Research and Special Programs Administration.

Viscusi WK. 1983. *Risk by Choice: Regulating Health and Safety in the Workplace.* Cambridge, MA: Harvard University Press.

Viscusi WK. 1984. *Regulating Consumer Product Safety.* Washington, DC: American Enterprise Institute.

Viscusi WK. 1992. *Fatal Tradeoffs.* New York: Oxford University Press.

Viscusi WK, Cavallo GO. 1994. The effect of product safety regulation on safety precautions. *Risk Analysis* 14(6):917–930.

Zimring FE, Hawkins G. 1997. *Crime Is Not the Problem: Lethal Violence in America.* New York: Oxford University Press.

9

Challenges and Opportunities

Since 1985, significant strides have been taken to implement the vision outlined in *Injury in America* (NRC, 1985). The national investment in injury research has increased, albeit not as markedly as the report recommended. The field of injury science has developed and matured, attracting the interest of investigators from a wide range of disciplines. Important advances have been made in delivering emergency services and treatment to injured patients, saving lives, and reducing disability. Recent research is beginning to provide information about how cells respond to injury and how their normal functioning can be preserved. Important advances have also been made in demonstrating the efficacy and cost-effectiveness of preventive interventions in the field so that they can be successfully implemented on a wide scale.

One of the most impressive achievements over the past two decades has been a "political" one—through communication, advocacy, and constituency building, a national "community of interest" in promoting safety and preventing injury has emerged. Although injury prevention has achieved higher visibility in government at all levels, most of the energy for social action has come from the private sector and through the recruitment of individuals, businesses, foundations, community groups, and other organizations interested in preventing injuries and implementing safety programs (see Chapter 7). Future advances in the injury field depend on the continued development of the infrastructure of the field through public and private partnerships.

Progress has been made not only in developing a scientific field and generating social investment in injury prevention, but also in reducing injury. Over the past 25 years, injury rates have declined most substantially where the social investment in prevention, including regulatory initiatives, has been strongest.

• Motor vehicle fatality rates have declined markedly over the past 25 years (see Chapter 5). The improvement is attributable to reduction in drunk driving and increased use of occupant restraints, together with a continuation of longer-term influences (improved highway design, increased urbanization, improvement in emergency medical services, and safer vehicle designs) (Graham, 1993).

• Long-term downward trends in occupational fatalities appear to have accelerated in recent years. Although the long-term trends are probably attributable largely to changes in work-force composition and technological improvements, it seems likely that occupational safety initiatives have played a contributing role (McGarity and Shapiro, 1993)

• Residential fire death rates have also fallen substantially during this period, at least in part due to improvements in building codes, product safety improvements, and increased use of smoke detectors (U.S. Fire Administration, 1997).

• By contrast, the suicide rate has remained essentially unchanged for the past 20 years, and the homicide rate is the same as it was 20 years ago, although it has fluctuated considerably over this period (Baker et al., 1992; Kachur et al., 1995; Fingerhut and Warner, 1997).

The main challenge for the nation, in the view of the committee, is to consolidate the gains that have been made over the past 25 years, and particularly over the past decade, and to secure the foundation for further advances in injury science and practice. This challenge can be met by adhering to the following plan:

• *Improving coordination and collaboration:* Coordinating the diverse efforts currently devoted to injury prevention and treatment, promoting collaboration among interested agencies and constituencies, and clarifying the roles of the main federal agencies.

• *Strengthening capacity for research and practice:* Strengthening the infrastructure of the injury field for developing knowledge and for translating knowledge into practice.

• *Integrating the field:* Infusing the injury field with a common sense of purpose and a shared understanding of its methods and perspectives, and promoting new channels of communication.

• *Nurturing public understanding and support:* Broadening public understanding of the feasibility and value of efforts to prevent and ameliorate injuries and promoting investment in injury prevention by managed care organizations.

• *Promoting informed policy making:* Improving the information systems used for identifying and evaluating injury risks and setting priorities for research and intervention.

COORDINATION AND COLLABORATION

It did not take very long for the committee to realize that "injury prevention and control" is a large field, even if "the field" is understood to encompass only people and organizations who embrace this identity. As discussed in Chapter 1, the injury field is defined by its allegiance to the public health perspective and particularly by its use of the tools and methods of public health to prevent or ameliorate injuries. So defined, the injury field is part of a broader array of people and agencies devoted to promoting safety, whose methods and perspectives differ from those of public health, including the tort system, criminal justice, alcohol control, and fire protection. One of the greatest challenges facing the leaders of the injury field is to develop creative and effective ways of coordinating their own efforts and promoting collaboration with agencies and constituencies outside the field.

Public–Private Partnerships

Many reports in human services and public health in recent years have touted the value, indeed the necessity, of creating "strategic partnerships" between public and private organizations to harness private energy and leverage public resources. Many examples of successful public–private partnerships are mentioned in this report, involving state and local governments, foundations, and advocacy organizations, as well as regulatory agencies and regulated industries. These efforts must be replicated throughout the field. An area that is ripe for public–private cooperation, through public education and advocacy, is raising the salience and visibility of injury prevention and demonstrating program cost-effectiveness to health care payers, including self-insured employers.

Roles of Federal Agencies

It is also important to clarify the roles of federal agencies and to facilitate coordination among them. Injury prevention and treatment cover a vast terrain. Numerous federal agencies play important roles in supporting injury science or carrying out the national agenda in injury prevention and treatment. This potpourri of federal responsibilities emerged piecemeal over several decades rather than as components of a coordinated national plan. This is not to say that the federal response has been weak or wasteful. To the contrary, the key federal agencies have accomplished a great deal over the past three decades in building a new scientific field and reducing the burden of injury. The problem is one of missed opportunities due to lack of focus, cohesion, and coordination. The committee believes that the federal response could be strengthened significantly by several key refinements of the present organizational architecture of injury prevention and treatment.

In 1966, the National Research Council (NRC) report *Accidental Death and Disability: The Neglected Disease of Modern Society* recommended creation of a National Institute of Trauma to sponsor a program of injury treatment research at the National Institutes of Health (NIH); this recommendation has never been implemented. What is needed at this time is a mechanism for coordinating, rationalizing, and strengthening these diverse activities. The most sensible step in this direction is to create a new division within the National Institute of General Medical Sciences and to assign this division the responsibility for conducting trauma care and treatment research. Primary responsibility for trauma systems development and for outcomes research should be assumed by the Health Resources and Services Administration.

For injury prevention practice and research, spheres of responsibility emerge rather clearly from statutory arrangements and historical practices. The National Highway Traffic Safety Administration (NHTSA) bears primary responsibility for program support and regulation in highway safety, but responsibility for research in this area has been shared by NHTSA and the National Center for Injury Prevention and Control (NCIPC) in order to take advantage of the stronger scientific tradition of the Centers for Disease Control and Prevention (CDC). In the committee's view, NHTSA's role in supporting safety research should be strengthened through the introduction of peer-reviewed research, while the NCIPC continues to evaluate community safety interventions unaddressed by NHTSA and supports research in biomechanics as one of its highest priorities. Coordination of activities and cooperation between these two agencies is imperative.

The federal role in occupational safety and the responsibilities of the Occupational Safety and Health Administration (OSHA) and the National Institute for Occupational Safety and Health (NIOSH) are well defined by the Occupational Safety and Health Act of 1970. There is little overlap between the missions of these agencies and other federal agencies; however, opportunities to translate knowledge from the occupational setting to other settings, and vice versa, should be improved (e.g., the work of NIOSH and OSHA in violence prevention).

The statutory relationship between NIOSH and OSHA provides a useful model for enhancing cooperation between the NCIPC and the Consumer Product Safety Commission (CPSC). Although CPSC needs the capability provided by its National Electronic Injury Surveillance System (NEISS) to identify, and respond to, product hazards within its regulatory jurisdiction, the agencies should continue their collaborative efforts to study the feasibility of expanding the NEISS system into an all-injury emergency department surveillance system.

The federal investment in preventing lethal violence and suicide should be strengthened through cooperative arrangements between the agencies involved in these areas. Specifically, the National Institute of Justice (NIJ) and NCIPC should coordinate their efforts in violence prevention research, identifying the areas in which each has a comparative advantage. NIJ should be assigned primary responsibility for evaluating the violence prevention initiatives supported by multiple federal agencies. Similarly, a coordinated research program for suicide prevention should be planned by NCIPC and the National Institute of Mental Health.

Overall, the committee believes that greater cooperation and coordination among the many federal agencies involved in injury prevention is an indispensable condition for advancing the field. Unfortunately, cooperative relationships between the NCIPC and other federal agencies involved in injury prevention have too often been impeded by competition and institutional rivalries. To change this pattern, federal agencies involved in injury prevention and treatment should establish partnerships that reflect joint understandings of the missions of the respective agencies and their strengths and limitations.

STRENGTHENING CAPACITY FOR RESEARCH AND PRACTICE

Resources devoted to injury prevention and treatment have increased significantly since 1985, especially when all of the public and private investment is taken into account. However, some important gaps and inadequacies remain. The three main needs are (1) training for injury researchers and practitioners; (2) opportunities for investigator-initiated research in biomechanics, trauma, and injury prevention to build and maintain the research base of the field; and (3) building and maintaining an adequate infrastructure in public health departments to develop and implement injury prevention programs and to collaborate with partners in other agencies and organizations.

Training

There seems to be agreement that education is the area in which the field of injury has made the least progress. In 1985, *Injury in America* identified the shortage of trained injury prevention professionals and scientists as a major impediment to the development of the field (NRC, 1985). Despite repeated recommendations, these training needs have not yet been adequately addressed by the pertinent federal agencies. The two exceptions to this general statement appear to be NIOSH's training grants and education and research centers and NIH's training grants in trauma and burn programs. The committee recommends that NCIPC, NIOSH, NHTSA, NIH, and other federal agencies significantly increase their support for training of practitioners and researchers.

Investigator-Initiated Research

Numerous reports have pointed out that support for injury research has been seriously inadequate when measured against the magnitude of the injury problem. We do so once again.

In *Scientific Opportunities and Public Need*, an Institute of Medicine committee on priority setting at the NIH recommended that NIH develop a more systematic process for taking into account the social burden of various diseases and conditions in setting research priorities (IOM, 1998). By any measure of social burden (deaths, years of potential life lost, disability or disability-adjusted life years, and economic costs), injuries exact a major toll. Although other factors, including scientific opportunity and portfolio diversification, must also be considered, the NIH investment in injury research appears to take inadequate account of the magnitude of the problem (see Table 9.1).

In 1996, unintentional injury was third leading cause of years of life lost before age 75, after heart disease and malignant neoplasms. With few exceptions, the rank ordering of YPLL for injury follows the ordering for leading causes of injury deaths. Thus, maintenance of an extramural research community is vital and will require adequate funding for investigator-initiated, peer-reviewed research grants. It is also necessary to ensure viable careers for the country's best young researchers and to sustain experienced investigators. Investigator-initiated research should be encouraged to ensure the emergence of innovative approaches to injury research.

TABLE 9.1 Leading Causes of Death and Disability in the United States: Estimates of NIH Research Support in Relation to Years of Potential Life Lost (YPLL)

Leading Causes of Death and Disability	NIH Support in FY 1996 ($ millions)	Age-Adjusted YPLL Before Age 75, 1996 (per 100,000 population	NIH Support ($millions) FY 1996 per YPLL Before Age 75 (per 100,000 population)
Cancer	2,570.6	1,554.2	1.65
HIV infection and AIDS	1,410.9	401.9	3.51
Heart diseases	851.6	1,222.6	0.70
Diabetes	298.9	153.5	1.95
Injury [a]	194.4[b]	1,919.0	0.10
Chronic liver disease and cirrhosis	169.8	145.7	1.17
Stroke, cerebrovascular diseases	120.3	210.2	0.57
Chronic obstructive pulmonary diseases	62.4	161.1	0.39
Pneumonia and influenza	61.9	114.5	0.54

SOURCES: IOM (1998), NCHS (1998).

[a]Includes unintentional injuries, suicide, and homicide and legal interventions.
[b]NIH support in FY 1995. SOURCE: NCIPC (1997).

State Public Health Infrastructure

Successful efforts undertaken in occupational and traffic safety are characterized by a strong infrastructure for implementing safety programs. To strengthen the nation's capacity to promote residential and recreational safety and to prevent suicide and violence, an adequate infrastructure must be established within public health departments.

Most effective interventions require state and local initiatives. Unfortunately, however, many states lack the capacity to undertake these initiatives. A major priority for all federal agencies involved in reducing the injury burden, especially for NCIPC, is to help states establish the necessary public health infrastructure for effective injury prevention and treatment. This can be accomplished by redistributing and leveraging existing resources, as well as by seeking additional resources from federal, state, and private coffers. In the process, public agencies unaccustomed to working together may discover unforeseen efficiencies and the advantages of pooling resources. Resource limitations make it even more imperative for federal leadership in injury prevention and treatment to transcend a strictly federal orientation and assume a broader commitment to the injury field.

INTEGRATING THE FIELD

Although remarkable progress has been made in developing the injury field over the past decade, continued efforts are needed to establish a common understanding of the mission and perspectives of the field, to promote greater cohesion, and to facilitate scientific interchange.

Mission

Recognition of the common causal pathway of injury—excessive or unregulated energy transfer—has facilitated the conceptual and scientific integration of injury epidemiology, biomechanics, behavioral science, and treatment. Injury epidemiology is a recognized field of specialization that underpins injury-related research and program development. Scientific study of the pathophysiology, mechanisms, and risk factors of injury facilitates improvements in the design of products, environments, and programs to prevent or ameliorate the severity of injuries. Emergency and trauma care have been consolidated as specialized fields of clinical research and service delivery. The unfinished business in the evolution of the injury field is consolidation of the field around a common understanding of the implications of the transition from accident prevention to injury prevention.

Leaders in medicine and public health have proclaimed that violence is a public health problem. A growing cadre of public health researchers have turned their attention to the study of the causes and prevention of violence and suicide. However, these initiatives have stimulated an intense debate about the proper role of public health in violence prevention and about the policy implications of studies undertaken by public health researchers, particularly in relation to fire-arms. In the committee's judgment, application of the scientific paradigm of the injury field to suicide and violence represents an important intellectual advance that should be explicitly embraced by the leaders of the field and by its private and public sponsors.

Scientific Communication

Scientists who work in complex interdisciplinary fields such as injury pre-vention and treatment face a difficult challenge of maintaining credibility and sophistication within their "home" disciplines as well as within the injury field. Established channels of scientific communication exist within the constituent disciplines, including annual conferences, journals, and electronic networks. Similar channels are developing for the specialized spheres of interest within the injury field, promoting communication among specialists in biomechanics, injury epidemiology, emergency medicine, and other fields. Still missing, however, are channels of scientific communication for injury scientists, highlighting the most sophisticated research being conducted in the entire array of disciplines. Oppor-tunities for cross-fertilization and collaboration are now being missed (see Chapter 8). These problems could be successfully addressed by establishing a new organization of injury researchers (a society for injury research) analogous to scientific organizations that have emerged in other interdisciplinary areas (e.g., the College of Problems of Drug Dependence). Such an organization could hold an annual scientific meeting, establish communication links, and represent the voice of injury science in the political process and in public policy debate.

NURTURING PUBLIC SUPPORT

Ultimately, the level of social investment in the injury field depends on public recognition of the value and potential payoff from the investment. One positive sign is that focused initiatives (e.g., prevention of drunk driving, spinal cord injury research) have achieved public visibility. However, uncoordinated efforts by component constituencies will not yield a stable public investment. Forces should be joined to promote the common agenda of the field, preventing and ameliorating injury through research and implementation of cost-effective interventions. The American public is increasingly safety conscious, and the time appears right for a sustained media campaign to heighten public awareness of injury problems, to educate the public on the lifesaving and injury-ameliorating potential of prevention interventions, and to highlight the cost-effectiveness of these interventions.

Various national organizations engaged in injury prevention activity should explore the feasibility and usefulness of establishing an umbrella organization to pursue their common agenda, including the formulation and implementation of a long-term media strategy for communicating key messages regarding the preventability of injuries and the cost-effectiveness of preventive interventions. The value of discrete messages about safer storage of firearms, drunk driving, bicycle helmets, and smoke detectors might be enhanced by framing them as part of a broader safety message (that injuries are preventable and that taking steps to reduce risks is worth the effort and the investment). This umbrella organization should also develop a strategy for identifying opportunities to incorporate prevention into evolving health care financing and delivery systems (Mechanic, 1998). In fact, large self-insured employers who are already pursuing preventive approaches would be valuable members of the umbrella coalition.

PROMOTING INFORMED POLICY MAKING

Improving Surveillance Systems

Ideally, regulatory decisions, policy making, and priority setting in injury prevention should be based on sound, readily accessible epidemiological information concerning the incidence and severity of various types of injuries. Too often, however, the available data relate only to fatalities, and fatality rates are not necessarily good proxies for injury rates in general or for rates of serious injuries, significant medical costs, or severe disabilities. A recurrent theme of this report is that attention should be directed to the development of better information on the epidemiology, treatment, and outcomes of nonfatal injuries. As more lives are saved due to more effective prevention and regionalization of care, attention is shifting from a singular focus on survival as the criterion for success to a detailed consideration of nonfatal outcomes as well. Improving data systems for nonfatal injuries is a precondition for informed policy making and must be one of the highest priorities of the field.

Protecting Science

Freedom of scientific inquiry is a powerful engine for advancing knowledge and promoting technological innovation. Science must be accountable to the public, of course, but political interference with the customary process of scientific inquiry should be avoided. Peer review has traditionally served as the main mechanism for ensuring accountability, even when public funding is at stake.

The merit of a controversial study must be judged by whether it is good science, not whether it is good politics. Whether public policy based on contested research is adopted (e.g., funding for needle exchange programs or sex education programs) is properly a political judgment, but whether research does or does not show that these programs reduce HIV (human immunodeficiency virus) transmission (and whether the question is studied at all) should be primarily scientific questions, not political ones. By this measure, case-control studies on the risks associated with the presence of firearms in the home or the effect on injuries of restrictions on the possession of weapons, for example, should be judged by the yardstick of scientific excellence, not according to preconceived positions on the virtues or vices of gun ownership.

Priority Setting for Research and Social Action

The committee has already noted the comparatively lower priority assigned to injury in the overall federal investment in health-related research and the comparatively lower priority assigned to prevention in public expenditures for health and public safety. Prevention and amelioration of injury should be given a higher priority in the allocation of monies for research and in the array of programs funded by public health and public safety agencies. Whatever the overall level of public investment, however, priorities for research and social action must be set. Questions are raised not only about *who* should be setting priorities, but also *what* the priorities should be. The challenge facing the field is developing criteria for setting these priorities.

In such a diverse field, completely centralized priority setting would not be desirable even if it were achievable. Federal initiatives regarding program implementation should allow substantial leeway for priority setting at the state and community levels. Although research priorities should be set at a national level, criteria for setting priorities at NIH might properly differ from those used at CDC, NHTSA, or other mission-oriented agencies, because of their different areas of expertise, statutory missions, and constituencies. Priorities for regulatory action might sensibly differ among regulatory agencies, particularly in light of differences in the statutory framework. However, even if priorities differ among communities, among federal agencies, and across spheres of activity, they still must be set. Priorities will emerge by happenstance if they are not established by planning and choice. In all of these contexts, the priority-setting process should be transparent and subject to public participation and review.

The committee was struck by the lack of attention given to the criteria for guiding priority setting in the injury field—for research funding, for program support and choice of interventions, and for regulatory action. Regulatory agencies have been criticized for weaknesses in their respective priority-setting processes (Mashaw and Harfst, 1990; Office of the Vice President, 1993; GAO, 1997), and NIH has been urged to open up its process to greater public participation (IOM, 1998). Among federal agencies that support injury research, public involvement and explicitness of criteria for setting priorities have varied widely. The recent undertaking by NIOSH provides a useful model of how to engage public and private partners to set research priorities based on explicit criteria. Through the National Occupational Research Agenda, NIOSH was able to examine broadly perceived needs and systematically address those topics that were most likely to yield gains to protect workers. NCIPC has also facilitated public involvement through its own efforts, although mechanisms for follow up have not been established.

Despite differences in context and emphasis, many common questions arise in setting priorities for research and social action in the injury field. How should the severity of particular injury problems be measured (deaths, disability) and taken into account? Under what circumstances should recent trends (rises or declines in incidence or rates) affect priority setting? Of what significance is the proportion of the population exposed to any given risk? Of what significance are various factors associated with increased risk, such as the voluntariness of exposure or the vulnerability of the population affected? When priorities are being set for interventions, including regulatory action, how should cost and cost-effectiveness be measured and taken into account? Although consideration of these issues is beyond the mandate of this committee, they should receive more systematic attention by federal agencies and their public and private partners than they have thus far. Exploration of common problems in priority setting for research and social action provides an important opportunity for a collaborative venture.

Finally, this report has presented the committee's considered recommendations for further developing the field of injury prevention and treatment and for reducing the burden of injury in America. We trust that our findings will take their place alongside other IOM-NRC reports that have highlighted the need to strengthen the injury field and to assist public and private agencies as they develop their priorities. We commend the diverse array of public and private agencies who embrace the mission of injury prevention and treatment, and applaud the many accomplishments the field has achieved. We are confident that the field will continue to make great strides in reducing the burden of injury.

REFERENCES

Baker SP, O'Neill B, Ginsburg MJ, Li G. 1992. *The Injury Fact Book.* New York: Oxford University Press.

Fingerhut LA, Warner M. 1997. *Injury Chartbook. Health, United States, 1996–97.* Hyattsville, MD: National Center for Health Statistics.

GAO (General Accounting Office). 1997. *Consumer Product Safety Commission: Better Data Needed to Help Identify and Analyze Potential Hazards.* Washington, DC: GAO. GAO/HEHS-97-147.

Graham JD. 1993. Injuries from traffic crashes: Meeting the challenge. *Annual Review of Public Health* 14:515–543.

IOM (Institute of Medicine). 1998. *Scientific Opportunities and Public Needs: Improving Priority Setting and Public Input at the National Institutes of Health.* Washington, DC: National Academy Press.

Kachur SP, Potter LB, James SP, Powell KE. 1995. *Suicide in the United States, 1980–1992.* Atlanta, GA: NCIPC. Violence Surveillance Summary Series, No. 1.

Mashaw JL, Harfst DL. 1990. *The Struggle for Auto Safety.* Cambridge, MA: Harvard University Press.

McGarity TO, Shapiro SA. 1993. *Workers at Risk: The Failed Promise of the Occupational Safety and Health Administration.* Westport, CT: Praeger Press.

Mechanic D. 1998. Topics for our times: Managed care and public health opportunities. *American Journal of Public Health* 88(6):874–875.

NCHS (National Center for Health Statistics). 1998. *Health, United States, 1998 with Socioeconomic Status and Health Chartbook.* Hyattsville, MD: NCHS. DHHS Publication No. (PHS) 98-1232.

NCIPC (National Center for Injury Prevention and Control). 1997a. *Inventory of Federally Funded Research in Injury Prevention and Control, FY 1995.* Atlanta, GA: NCIPC.

NRC (National Research Council). 1966. *Accidental Death and Disability: The Neglected Disease of Modern Society.* Washington, DC: National Academy Press.

NRC (National Research Council). 1985. *Injury in America: A Continuing Public Health Problem.* Washington, DC: National Academy Press.

Office of the Vice President. 1993. *Improving Regulatory Systems. Accompanying Report of the National Performance Review.* Washington, DC: Office of the Vice President.

U.S. Fire Administration. 1997. *Fire Death Rate Trends: An International Perspective.* Washington, DC: Federal Emergency Management Agency, U.S. Fire Administration, National Fire Data Center.

Appendixes

A

Acknowledgments

The committee would like to thank the following persons who shared their expertise.

Whitney Addington
American College of Physicians

Marilena Amoni
National Highway Traffic Safety
  Administration

Lee Annest
National Center for Injury
  Prevention and Control

Jean Athey
Health Resources and Services
  Administration

Bernard Auchter
Department of Justice

Elaine Auld
Society for Public Health
  Education

Diane Baer
Washington State Department of
  Health

Linda Bailey
Department of Health and Human
  Services

Susan Baker
Johns Hopkins University School
  of Hygiene and Public Health

Jerry Barancik
Brookhaven National Laboratory

Barbara Barlow
Harlem Hospital Injury Prevention
  Program

Charles Barrett
Indiana Department of Health

William Baxt
University of Pennsylvania
    Medical Center

Mary Beachley
Maryland State Trauma Program

Catherine Becker
Pennsylvania Department of Health

Larry Bedard
American College of Emergency
    Physicians

Georges Benjamin
Maryland Department of Health
    and Mental Hygiene

Jack Bergstein
Medical College of Wisconsin

Alan Berman
American Association of
    Suicidology

Henry Betts
Rehabilitation Institute of Chicago
    Foundation

Paul Blackman
National Rifle Association

F. William Blaisdell
University of California at Davis
    Medical Center

Allen Bolton
Greater Dallas Injury Prevention
    Center

Sandra Bonzo
National Center for Injury
    Prevention and Control

Christine Branche
National Center for Injury
    Prevention and Control

Susan Brink
Health Mark Associates

Marvin Brooke
Tufts University School of
    Medicine

Ann Brown
U.S. Consumer Product Safety
    Commission

Bruce Browner
University of Connecticut

Stephen Camp
University of Virginia

B.J. Campbell
University of North Carolina

Charles Carrico
Southwestern Medical School

Howard Champion
University of Maryland, Baltimore

Roger Chapman
Iowa Department of Public Health

Barbara Chatterjee
Madison, Wisconsin

Tom Christoffel
University of Illinois at Chicago

Jeffrey Cohen
University of Pittsburgh

Larry Cohen
Education Development Center

Lisa Cohen
Centers for Disease Control and
    Prevention

Arthur Cooper
Columbia University College of
    Physicians and Surgeons

Edward Cornwell
University of Southern California
    Medical School

JoEllen Courtney
Dupage County Health Department

Andrea Craig
Trauma Foundation

Cherie Crowe
Missouri Office of Injury Control

Margo Cullen
Institute of Medicine

Thomas Danenhower
Montana Department of Health

Elizabeth Datner
University of Pennsylvania
    Medical Center

Erich Daub
Maryland Department of Health
    and Mental Hygiene

Steve Davidson
Georgia Division of Public Health

Miriam Davis
Silver Spring, Maryland

Linda Degutis
Yale School of Medicine

Edwin Deitch
New Jersey Medical School

Carol Delaney
Health Resources and Services
    Administration

Barbara DeLateur
Johns Hopkins University

Robert Demling
Harvard Medical School

Patricia Dischinger
University of Maryland

John Downey
Columbia University College of
    Physicians and Surgeons

Donna Duncan
Institute of Medicine

Jane Durch
Institute of Medicine

Buff Easterly
Arkansas Department of Health

A. Brent Eastman
Scripps Memorial Hospital

Howard Eisenburg
University of Maryland School of
    Medicine

Mickey Eisenburg
University of Washington Medical
    Center

Barbara Elliott
University of Minnesota–Duluth
    School of Medicine

Richard Ellis
Washington State Department of
Health

Doris Evans-Gates
Arizona Department of Health
Services

Timothy Fabian
University of Tennessee

Jeffrey Fagan
Columbia University

John Ferguson
National Institutes of Health

Philip Fine
University of Alabama at
Birmingham

Sherry Fines
South Dakota Department of
Health

Lois Fingerhut
National Center for Health
Statistics

Marilyn Fingerhut
National Institute for Occupational
Safety and Health

Adam Finkel
Occupational Safety and Health
Administration

Michael Finkelstein
Michael Finkelstein and Associates

John Finklea
Centers for Disease Control and
Prevention

Baruch Fischoff
Carnegie Mellon University

Leslie Fisher
Delmar, New York

Gary Fleischer
Children's Hospital of Boston

Lewis Flint Jr.
Tulane University Medical Center

Ginger Floerchinger-Franks
Idaho Office of Health Promotion

William Foege
Emory University

Barbara Foley
ENA/ENCARE

Carolyn Fowler
Johns Hopkins University

Earl Fox
Health Resources and Services
Administration

Leroy Frazier
South Carolina Office of Injury and
Disability Prevention

Sharon Galloway
Institute of Medicine

Donald Gann
University of Maryland School of
Medicine

Bruce Gans
Rehabilitation Institute of Michigan

Jennifer Gao
University of California at
  Los Angeles

Mary Garrett-Bodel
Brain Injury Association

Thomas Gennarelli
Allegheny University of the
  Health Sciences

Pamela Gilbert
U.S. Consumer Product Safety
  Commission

Michelle Glassman
National Youth Sports Safety
  Foundation

Susan Glick
Violence Policy Center

Stephen Godwin
Transportation Research Board

John Graham
Harvard School of Public Health

Christopher Grande
International Trauma Anesthesia
  and Critical Care Society

Lazar Greenfield
University of Michigan

Elizabeth Grossman
Occupational Safety and Health
  Administration

Anara Guard
Children's Safety Network

Deborah Haack
Colorado Department of Public
  Health and Environment

Frank Haight
University of California at Irvine

Rodney Hammond
National Center for Injury
  Prevention and Control

Susan Hardman
New York State Department of
  Health

Stephen Hargarten
Medical College of Washington

Susan Hariri
Colorado State University

Linda Harner
Michigan Department of Public
  Health

Joan Harris
National Highway Traffic Safety
  Administration

James Hedlund
Ithaca, New York

Allen Heinemann
Rehabilitation Institute of Chicago

Jean Henze
Brain Injury Association

David Herdon
Shriners Burns Institute

Howard Hill
National Center for Injury
  Prevention and Control

James Holcroft
University of California at Davis
  Medical Center

Jennifer Holliday
Institute of Medicine
John Holmes
University of Pennsylvania

David Hoyt
University of California at San
  Diego

Thomas Hunt
University of California at San
  Francisco Medical Center

Nancy Isaac
Harvard School of Public Health

David Jacobsen
Florida Injury Prevention and
  Control Program

Lynn Jenkins
National Institute for Occupational
  Safety and Health

Mark Johnson
Alaska State Department of Health

B. Tilman Jolly
Association for the Advancement
  of Automotive Medicine

Jerry Jurkovich
Harborview Medical Center

Arthur Kellerman
University of Tennessee at
  Memphis

Alexander Kelter
California Department of Health
  Services

Tim Kerns
National Study Center for Trauma

Marie Kiely
New Hampshire Division of Public
  Health Services

Mark Kinde
Minnesota Department of Health

Albert King
Wayne State University

Marian Knapp
Institute for Healthcare
  Improvement

Thomas Kniesner
Harvard School of Public Health

Mary Knudsen
University of California at San
  Francisco

Jess Kraus
University of California at Los
  Angeles

Etienne Krug
Centers for Disease Control and
  Prevention

Victor LaCerva
New Mexico Department of Health

Virginia Lancaster
Arkansas Department of Health

David Lawrence
Louisiana Office of Public Health

Anna Ledgerwood
Wayne State University

Frank Lewis Jr.
Henry Ford Hospital

Jim Lieberman
Columbia University College of
    Physicians and Surgeons

Donna Livingston
Institute of Medicine

Stephen Luchter
U.S. Department of Transportation

Ronald Maier
Harborview Medical Center

Mark Mallangoni
MetroHealth Medical Center

Stephanie Malloy
Children's Safety Network

Patrick Malone
Vermont Department of Health

Donald Marion
University of Pittsburgh

Donald Martin
Transportation Research Board

Ricardo Martinez
National Highway Traffic Safety
    Administration

John Martonic
Occupational Safety and Health
    Administration

Kenneth Mattox
Baylor College of Medicine

Wendy Max
University of California at
    San Francisco

John May
Central Detention Facility Health
    Services

Fred Maynard Jr.
Metro Health Center for
    Rehabilitation

Kathleen McCormally
Institute of Medicine

Andrew McGuire
Trauma Foundation

Susan McHenry
National Highway Traffic Safety
    Administration

David Meaney
University of Pennsylvania

Ronald Medford
U.S. Consumer Product Safety
    Commission

Patrick Meehan
Georgia Division of Public Health

Gary Melton
University of South Carolina

James Mercy
National Center for Injury
    Prevention and Control

Anthony Meyer
University of North Carolina

Jeff Michael
National Highway Traffic Safety
  Administration

Angela Mickalide
National SAFE KIDS Campaign

Ted Miller
National Public Services Research
  Institute

David Milzman
District of Columbia General
  Hospital

Lois Mock
National Institute of Justice

Luis Montes
Los Angeles County Immunization
  Program

Ernest Moore Jr.
Denver General Hospital

Jane Moore
Association of State and Territorial
  Health Officials

Mark Moore
Harvard University

Jon Morgan
Wisconsin Bureau of Public Health

Mike Moser
Ohio Bureau of Health Promotion
  and Risk Reduction

Robert Mullen
American Public Health
  Association

Barry Myers
Duke University

Carol Mysinger
Alabama Department of Public
  Health

Keith Neely
Oregon Health Sciences University

Nancy Nelson
Department of Health and Human
  Services

Elena Nightingale
Institute of Medicine

Audrey Nora
Health Resources and Services
  Administration

Alex Ommaya
Agency for Health Care Policy and
  Research

Claude Organ
University of California at Davis

Tori Ozonoff
Massachusetts Bureau of Family
  and Community Health

Richard Pain
Transportation Research Board

Joe Parker
Governor's Highway Safety
  Program, North Carolina

Jane Pearson
National Institute of Mental Health

Corinne Peek-Asa
University of California at
  Los Angeles

Barry Pless
McGill University

Deborah Prothrow-Stith
Harvard School of Public Health

Basil Pruitt Jr.
University of Texas Health Science
  Center

Linda Quan
University of Washington School
  of Medicine

James Reswick
Department of Education

Valerie Reyna
University of Arizona Health
  Sciences Center

Dorothy Rice
University of California at
  San Francisco

Fred Rivara
Harborview Injury Prevention
  Center

Leon Robertson
Nanlee Research

Peter Rosen
University of California at San
  Diego

Mark Rosenberg
National Center for Injury
  Prevention and Control

Barbara Rosenfeld
U.S. Consumer Product Safety
  Commission

Linda Rosenstock
National Institute for Occupational
  Safety and Health

Ellen Rudy
University of Pittsburgh

Carol Runyan
University of North Carolina
  School of Public Health

Des Runyan
University of North Carolina
  School of Medicine

Rosanne Rutkowski
Kansas Department of Health and
  Environment

Mark Scalley
National Center for Injury
  Prevention and Control

David Schaeffer
Columbia University

C. William Schwab
University of Pennsylvania

Nancy Schwartz
National Fire Protection
  Association

George Sheldon
University of North Carolina
  School of Medicine

Erima Shields
Virginia Department of Health

282

George Thomas Shires
Texas Tech University Health
Sciences Center

Eileen Silver
Washington Department of Health

Jeff Simon
Children's Hospital of Philadelphia

Gary Slutkin
University of Illinois School of
Public Health

Andrew Smith
National Highway Traffic Safety
Administration

Richard Smith III
Indian Health Service

Rose Ann Soloway
American Association of Poison
Control Centers

Thomas Songer
University of Pittsburgh

Susan Sorenson
University of California at
Los Angeles

Dan Sosin
National Center for Injury
Prevention and Control

Carl Spurlock
Kentucky Injury Prevention Center

Ann St. Claire
Institute of Medicine

Lorann Stallones
Colorado State University

John Paul Stapp
New Mexico Research Institute

Edith Sternberg
Illinois Department of Health
Promotion

Judith Lee Stone
Advocates for Highway and Auto
Safety

Marion Storch
Connecticut Department of Health

Michael Stoto
Institute of Medicine

Nancy Stout
National Institute for Occupational
Safety and Health

Gerald Strauch
American College of Surgeons

Ellen Taliaferro
Parkland Memorial Hospital

Eric Tash
Hawaii Injury Prevention and
Control Program

Harry Teter Jr.
American Trauma Society

Erwin Thal
University of Texas Southwestern
Medical Center

Ann Thatcher
Rhode Island Injury Prevention
Program

Ian Thompson
Brooke Army Medical Center

Donald Trunkey
Oregon Health Sciences University

Timothy Van Wave
Delaware Department of Public
Health

Marla Vanore
University of Pennsylvania

Christine Vischer
Department of Justice

E. Elaine Vowels
District of Columbia General
Hospital

Elinor Walker
Agency for Health Care Policy and
Research

Julian Waller
El Cerrito, CA

William Waters IV
Doctors for Integrity in Policy
Research

Rich Waxweiller
National Center for Injury
Prevention and Control

John Weigelt
American College of Surgeons

Billie Weiss
County of Los Angeles Department
of Health Services

Genie Wessel
American School Health
Association

Robert Henry Wharton
Massachusetts General Hospital
Gale Whiteneck
Craig Hospital

Bill Wilkinson
Campaign to Make America
Walkable

Garen Wintemute
University of California at Davis

David Wisner
University of California at Davis
Medical Center

Joseph Wright
Children's National Medical Center

David Zane
Texas Department of Health

George Zitnay
Brain Injury Association

B

Timeline

1913	National Safety Council is chartered.
1924	First car with safety glass windows as standard equipment is offered by Cadillac.
1927	Interstate mailing of firearms through the U.S. Postal Service is banned.
1932	Maryland is the first state to introduce mandatory car inspections.
1934	National Firearms Act regulates the sale of fully automatic weapons, silencers, sawed-off shotguns, and other "gangster-type weapons."
1937	Godfrey publishes one of the first statements on the need for public health involvement in accident prevention in the *American Journal of Public Health*.
1938	Legislation is passed mandating the licensing of dealers and manufacturers involved in interstate firearm transactions; firearm sales to people convicted of certain crimes are prohibited.
1942	DeHaven describes structural environments as a primary cause of injury in falls from heights.

1943   American Public Health Association (APHA) Committee on Administrative Practice appoints a subcommittee on accident prevention; the subcommittee reports accident prevention programs in six state and two local health departments.

1945   Federal Children's Bureau, American Academy of Pediatrics (AAP), National Safety Council, and Metropolitan Life Insurance cosponsor national child safety campaign.

                                 APHA Subcommittee on Accident Prevention develops program guidelines for accident prevention; the subcommittee reports accident prevention programs in 9 state and 25 local health departments.

1948   W.K. Kellogg Foundation awards first home accident prevention demonstration grant.

1949   Gordon formalizes concept that epidemiology could be used as a theoretical foundation for accident prevention.

1950   AAP forms Committee on Accident Prevention.

                                 First International Committee on Alcohol, Drugs, and Traffic Safety Conference is held in Stockholm.

1951   W.K. Kellogg Foundation awards 3- to 6-year home accident prevention demonstration projects to 10 states

1953   First conference on home accident prevention is held at University of Michigan, School of Public Health; sponsors include National Safety Council, APHA, U.S. Public Health Service (U.S. PHS), and W.K. Kellogg Foundation.

                                 Human Factors in Air Transportation is published by McFarland.

                                 Flammable Fabrics Act and Federal Hazardous Substances Act are passed.

1955	McFarland publishes on epidemiological principles applicable to the study and prevention of childhood accidents, in the *American Journal of Public Health*.
	First annual Stapp conferences on the biomechanics of crashes is held.
	APHA surveys 1,556 state, local, and provincial health departments to assess the scope and effectiveness of health department programs in accident prevention; 33 state, 3 provincial, and 296 local health departments report having an accident prevention program; 62 report a full-time position in place for public health safety.
1956	Accident Prevention Program is initiated by the U.S. PHS.
1957	The American Association for Automotive Medicine (later, the Association for the Advancement of Automotive Medicine) is established.
1959	Insurance Institute for Highway Safety is founded.
1960	APHA public policy statement recommends that accident prevention be recognized as a major public health problem and that all units of APHA cooperate to improve accident prevention efforts at the local, state, and national levels.
	U.S. PHS Division of Special Health Services establishes the Division of Accident Prevention.
1961	Gibson publishes theory of injury produced by energy exchange.
	APHA publishes *Accident Prevention: The Role of Physicians and Public Health Workers*.
	The *Journal of Trauma* begins publication.
1964	Haddon, Suchman, and Klein publish *Accident Research: Methods and Approaches*.

Eleven schools of public health develop training programs in injury prevention, funded by the U.S. PHS.

The four major U.S. auto manufacturers install two front-seat lap belts as standard equipment.

1965   *A Guide to the Development of Accidental Injury Control Programs* is published by U.S. PHS.

Unsafe at Any Speed by Ralph Nader is published.

1966   Haddon matrix is published.

Accidental Death and Disability: The Neglected Disease of Modern Society is published by the National Research Council (NRC).

National Traffic and Motor Vehicle Safety Act establishes the National Highway Safety Bureau (later, National Highway Traffic Safety Administration [NHTSA]).

1968   APHA publishes *Accidents and Homicide* by Iskrant and Joliet.

Federal Gun Control Act places additional restrictions on who can own firearms.

American Trauma Society is established.

Lap belts in all seated occupant positions are installed as standard equipment by the four major U.S. auto manufacturers.

1969   *Accident Analysis and Prevention* journal begins publication.

Journal of Safety Research begins publication.

1970   Poison Prevention Packaging Act mandates use of safety caps on a variety of products.

Occupational Safety and Health Act of 1970 establishes the Occupational Safety and Health Administration and the National Institute for Occupational Safety and Health.

Highway Safety Act of 1970 establishes NHTSA.

Final Report on the National Commission on Product Safety is released.

1972   Consumer Product Safety Act establishes the Consumer Product Safety Commission.

Highway Loss Data Institute is founded.

1973   *Roles and Resources of Federal Agencies in Support of Comprehensive Emergency Medical Services* is published by the NRC.

National Center on Child Abuse and Neglect is established with the passage of the Child Abuse Prevention and Treatment Act (P.L. 93-247).

Emergency Medical Services Systems Act of 1973 is passed.

National Institute on Disability and Rehabilitation Research is founded at the Department of Education.

1974   General Motors produces first airbags.

Congress enacts the 55-mile-per-hour national maximum speed limit.

National Association of Governors' Highway Safety Representatives is established.

1975   Fatality Analysis Reporting System is established by NHTSA.

1977   Mine Safety and Health Administration is established to administer the provisions of the Federal Mine Safety and Health Act of 1977.

1978   National Coalition Against Domestic Violence is founded.

Emergency Medical Services at Midpassage is published by the NRC.

Tennessee is the first jurisdiction in the world to pass a child passenger safety law.

Remove Intoxicated Drivers (RID) is founded.

1979   Division of Maternal and Child Health funds injury prevention projects in Massachusetts, Virginia, and California for 3 years, including the first statewide comprehensive injury prevention program effort based in a state health agency.

Surgeon General issues the first national agenda for health promotion and disease prevention, *Healthy People: The Surgeon General's Report on Health Promotion and Disease Prevention*, which identifies the reduction of injuries as a major preventive health goal.

The Centers for Disease Control (CDC) establishes a violence epidemiology branch to track the incidence of interpersonal violence.

1980   *Handbook on Accident Prevention* is published by AAP.

First population-based and emergency-room-based injury surveillance system is implemented in the United States (Massachusetts and Ohio).

Mothers Against Drunk Driving (MADD) is founded.

1981   National Environmental Health Association conducts survey to evaluate injury prevention efforts (particularly within state health departments) nationwide; only 12 state health departments are found to have programs.

National Child Passenger Safety Association is established.

First National Conference on Injury Control, sponsored by the Johns Hopkins University and the CDC, is held in Baltimore.

1983

Developing Childhood Injury Prevention Programs: An Administrative Guide for Maternal and Child Health (Title V) Programs is published by the Division of Maternal and Child Health.

CDC hosts an invitational injury program management course for state health agency officials.

Center to Prevent Handgun Violence is founded.

1984

First U.S. seat-belt use law is enacted in New York.

Health Services, Preventive Health Services, and Home and Community Based Services Act (P.L. 98-555) establishes the Emergency Medical Services for Children (EMS-C) program.

Contra Costa County, California, issues isolation fencing ordinance for new pools.

Association of Schools of Public Health Conference on the Prevention of Injuries is held in Atlanta.

1985

Every state has passed legislation requiring the use of child safety seats.

Injury in America: A Continuing Public Health Problem is published by the NRC and the Institute of Medicine (IOM).

New England Network to Prevent Childhood Injuries establishes the first regional injury control network. Surgeon General's Workshop on Violence and Public Health is held in Leesburg, Virginia.

1986

Injury Prevention Act places an injury control program at CDC; Division of Injury Epidemiology and Control is established in the CDC Center for Environmental Health.

Minimum drinking age of 21 legislation is enacted by Congress.

National Council on Disability report *Toward Independence* is released.

First Maternal and Child Health demonstration is funded to address violence.

1987   National SAFE KIDS Campaign is launched.

Conference on Injury in America: A New Approach to an Old Problem, is held in Atlanta sponsored by CDC and NHTSA.

California enacts first legislation requiring bike helmets for children 4 years and under as passengers on bicycles.

CDC violence prevention program moves from Center for Health Promotion to Center for Environmental Health and Injury Control.

1988   *Injury Control: A Review of the Status and Progress of the Injury Control Program at the Centers for Disease Control* is published by NRC and IOM.

Second National Injury Control Conference, sponsored by CDC and NHTSA, is held in San Antonio, Texas.

Harvard Childhood Injury Prevention Resource Center survey report *Injury Prevention Programs in State Health Departments* is published.
Surgeon General's Workshop on Drunk Driving is held in Washington, D.C.

Advocates for Highway Safety is established.

1989   *Cost of Injury: A Report to Congress* is released.

Arizona, Rhode Island, and Washington are the first states to mandate E-coding for hospital discharges.

Injury Prevention: Meeting the Challenge is published as a supplement to the *American Journal of Preventive Medicine*.

First World Conference on Accident and Injury Prevention is held in Stockholm, Sweden.

1990   CDC releases report to Congress, *Childhood Injuries in the United States*.

CDC sponsors Forum on Youth Violence in Minority Communities—Setting the Agenda for Prevention—in Atlanta.

Carnegie Corporation of New York sponsors conference on the state of the art of evaluation in violence prevention programs for adolescents.

Trauma Care Systems Planning and Development Act of 1990 is passed.

Children's Safety Network is established by Maternal and Child Health Bureau (MCHB).

The Injury Control Act of 1990 (P.L. 101-558) is passed.

1991   First International Conference on Safe Communities, Safecomm-91, is held in Falkoping, Sweden, sponsored by the World Health Organization (WHO).

Intermodal Surface Transportation Efficiency Act is enacted, continuing state drunk-driving incentive grant programs.

Third National Injury Control Conference is held in Denver, Colorado, sponsored by CDC.

WHO Helmet Initiative begins.

NIMH and MCH sponsor conference on The Impact of Community Violence on African American Children and Families: Collaborative Approaches to Prevention and Intervention.

Disability in America: Toward a National Agenda for Prevention is published by IOM.

Child Health Day 1991—Looking Out: Understanding and Preventing Childhood Injuries is held.

A Data Book of Child and Adolescent Injury is released by Children's Safety Network.

1992   Americans with Disabilities Act is passed.

Surgeon General's Workshop—Keeping Kids Safe: Strategies for Preventing Violence and Injury, sponsored by MCHB, is held in Columbia, Maryland.

CDC Division of Injury Control (DIC) becomes the National Center for Injury Prevention and Control.

Department of Health and Human Services Office of Inspector General releases its report, *Injury Control.*

Handgun Epidemic Lowering Plan Network is established.

1993   *Understanding Child Abuse and Neglect* is published by NRC.

Injury Control in the 1990s: A National Plan for Action is published by CDC.

Second World Conference on Injury Control is held in Atlanta.

Understanding and Preventing Violence is published by NRC.

Emergency Medical Services for Children is published by IOM.

1994   First Symposium of the International Collaborative Effort on Injury Statistics is held in Bethesda, Maryland.

Brady Handgun Violence Prevention Act establishes a 5-day waiting period and background check for handgun purchases.

General Accounting Office report *Public Health Services: Agencies Use Different Approaches to Protect Public Against Disease and Injury* is published.

Third International Conference on Safe Communities is held in Harstad, Norway.

The Partnership Against Violence Network is created in response to a report to the President and the Domestic Policy Council by the Interdepartmental Working Group on Violence.

A Report of the Task Force on Trauma Research is published by NIH.

Violent Crime Control and Law Enforcement Act bans manufacture and sale of semiautomatic rifles and handguns with specific characteristics.

1995   *Injury Prevention* begins publication.

National Violence Prevention Conference—Bridging Science and Program is held in Des Moines, Iowa.

Fourth International Conference on Safe Communities is held in McMurray, Alberta, Canada.

All states but one have mandatory seat-belt use laws.

1996   International Conference on Bicycle Helmet Initiatives is held in Melbourne, Australia

Third International Conference on Injury Prevention and Control is held in Melbourne, Australia.

NRC publishes *Understanding Violence Against Women.*

National Occupational Research Agenda is published by NIOSH.

Final Report of the Poison Control Center Advisory Work Group is released.

Domestic Violence Offenders Gun Ban is passed, which prohibits gun purchase by individuals convicted of a domestic violence misdemeanor.

1997   Fourth National Injury Control Conference—*Safe America* is held in Washington, D.C.

Injury Chartbook. Health, United States, 1996–1997 is published by the National Center for Health Statistics.

Enabling America: Assessing the Role of Rehabilitation Science and Engineering is published by IOM.

1998   Fourth World Conference on Injury Prevention and Control is held in Amsterdam.

Safe Kids at Home, at Play, and on the Way is published by the National SAFE KIDS Campaign.

Dual airbags are standard equipment for all passenger cars.

Violence in Families: Assessing Prevention and Treatment Programs is published by NRC.

SOURCES

Baker SP. 1989. Injury science comes of age. *Journal of the American Medical Association* 262(16):2284–2285.
Waller JA. 1994. Reflections on a half century of injury control. *American Journal of Public Health* 84(4):664–670.

Contributors: Ann St. Claire, Leslie Fisher, Susan Ferguson, Susan Gallagher, Anara Guard, James Hedlund, Barry Pless, and Allan Williams.

C

Public Meeting Agenda

INSTITUTE OF MEDICINE
Committee on Injury Prevention and Control
July 30, 1997

Auditorium, National Academy of Sciences
2101 Constitution Avenue, N.W., Washington, D.C.

7:30–8:00 a.m.	**REGISTRATION**
8:00–8:15 a.m.	**OPENING REMARKS** Richard Bonnie, *Chairman*
8:15 a.m.–6:00 p.m.	**PUBLIC COMMENTS**
8:15–9:10 a.m.	**Transportation-Related Injury** Stephen Luchter, National Highway Traffic Safety Administration Barbara Harsha, National Association of Governors' Highway Safety Representatives B. Tilman Jolly, Association for the Advancement of Automotive Medicine Tim Kerns, University of Maryland at Baltimore National Study Center for Trauma Judith Stone, Advocates for Highway and Auto Safety Bill Wilkinson, Campaign to Make America Walkable
9:10–9:25 a.m.	**Question and Answer Session**

9:25–10:50 a.m.	**General Topics**

Consumer Product Injuries
> Ronald L. Medford, Consumer Product Safety
> Commission

Injuries at School
> Lisa Cohen, Centers for Disease Control and
> Prevention
> Richard Ellis, Washington State Department of
> Health
> Genie Wessel, American School Health
> Association

Sports Injuries
> Michelle Glassman, National Youth Sports
> Safety Foundation

Poison Control Centers
> Rose Ann Soloway, American Association of
> Poison Control Centers

Occupational Injuries
> John Finklea, Centers for Disease Control and
> Prevention

Suicide
> Alan Berman, American Association of
> Suicidology
> David Shaffer, Columbia University

10:50–11:05 a.m.	**Question and Answer Session**

11:05 a.m.–12:10 p.m.	**Acute Care**

> Larry Bedard, American College of Emergency
> Physicians
> Christopher Grande, International Trauma
> Anesthesia and Critical Care Society
> Audrey Nora, Health Resources and Services
> Administration
> Harry Teter, American Trauma Society
> John Weigelt, American College of Surgeons
> Joseph Wright, Children's National Medical
> Center

Rehabilitation
> Henry Betts, Rehabilitation Institute of Chicago
> Foundation

12:10–12:40 p.m.   **PLENARY SESSION**—General Discussion

12:40–1:15 p.m.   **LUNCH**

1:15–3:45 p.m.   **Violence Prevention**
                               Whitney Addington, American College of
                                 Physicians
                               Jack Bergstein, Medical College of Wisconsin
                               Paul Blackman, National Rifle Association
                               Mary Garrett-Bodel, Brain Injury Association
                               Larry Cohen, Children's Safety Network
                               Barbara Elliott, University of Minnesota School
                                 of Medicine
                               Susan Glick, Violence Policy Center
                               John May, Central Detention Facility Health
                                 Services, Washington, D.C.
                               C. William Schwab, Hospital of the University of
                                 Pennsylvania
                               Gary Slutkin, University of Illinois School of
                                 Public Health
                               Susan Sorenson, University of California at Los
                                 Angeles School of Public Health
                               Dan Sosin, Centers for Disease Control and
                                 Prevention
                               William Waters, Doctors for Integrity in Policy
                                 Research
                               Billie Weiss, County of Los Angeles Department
                                 of Health Services

3:45–4:15 p.m.   **Question and Answer Session**

4:15–4:35 p.m.   **Alcohol and Injury**
                               Linda Degutis, Yale School of Medicine
                               David Milzman, Providence Hospital

4:35–5:35 p.m.   **Infrastructure and Crosscutting Issues**

                           Infrastructure
                               Richard Smith, Indian Health Service
                           Data and Economic Issues
                               Ted Miller, National Public Services Research
                                 Institute

Crosscutting Issues
Elaine Auld, Society for Public Health Education
Allen Bolton, Greater Dallas Injury Prevention Center
Robert Mullen, American Public Health Association

5:35–6:00 p.m.   **PLENARY SESSION—General Discussion**

6:00 p.m.   **Adjourn**

Please Note: This meeting is being held to gather information to help the committee conduct its study. This committee will examine the information and material obtained during this, and other public meetings, in an effort to inform its work. Although opinions may be stated and lively discussion may ensue, no conclusions are being drawn at this time; no recommendations will be made. In fact, the committee will deliberate thoroughly before writing its draft report. Moreover, once the draft report is written, it must go through a rigorous review by experts who are anonymous to the committee; the committee then must respond to this review with appropriate revisions, and the report must adequately satisfy the Academy's Report Review committee and the chair of the NRC before it is considered an NRC report. Therefore, observers who draw conclusions about the committee's work based on today's discussions will be doing so prematurely.

D

Acronyms

AAP	American Academy of Pediatrics
ACS	American College of Surgeons
ADL	Activity of Daily Living
AHCPR	Agency for Health Care Policy and Research
AIS	Abbreviated Injury Scale
AJPH	American Journal of Public Health
ALS	Advanced Life Support
AP	Anatomic Profile
APHA	American Public Health Association
ATF	Bureau of Alcohol, Tobacco and Firearms
ATV	All-Terrain Vehicle
BAL	Blood Alcohol Level
BCCOA	Census of Agriculture—1992
BIA	Brain Injury Association
BJS	Bureau of Justice Statistics
BLS	Bureau of Labor Statistics
BRFSS	Behavioral Risk Factor Surveillance System
CDC	Centers for Disease Control and Prevention
CFOI	Census of Fatal Occupational Injuries
CODES	Crash Outcome Data Evaluation Systems
COI	Cost of Injury
CPS	Child Protective Services
CPSC	Consumer Product Safety Commission
CSN	Children's Safety Network

DALY	Disability-Adjusted Life Year
DAWN	Drug Abuse Warning Network
DEEDS	Data Elements for Emergency Department Systems
DHEW	Department of Health, Education, and Welfare (now DHHS)
DHHS	Department of Health and Human Services
DIC	Division of Injury Control (CDC)
DIEC	Division of Injury Epidemiology and Control (CDC)
DTEMS	Division of Trauma and EMS (HHS)
EMS	Emergency Medical Services
EMS-C	Emergency Medical Services for Children Program
EMT	Emergency Medical Technician
FARS	Fatality Analysis Reporting System
FBI	Federal Bureau of Investigation
FHWA	Federal Highway Administration
FIM	Functional Independence Measure
GES	General Estimates System
HCFA	Health Care Financing Administration
HCUP	Healthier Cost and Utilization Project
HIV	Human Immunodeficiency Virus
HRQOL	Health-Related Quality of Life
HRSA	Health Resources and Services Administration
ICD	International Classification of Diseases
ICE	International Collaborative Effort for Injury Statistics
ICECI	International Classification for External Causes of Injury
ICRC	Injury Control Research Center
IHS	Indian Health Service
IHSACS	Indian Health Service—Ambulatory Care System
IHSICS	Indian Health Service—Inpatient Care System
IIHS	Insurance Institute for Highway Safety
IOM	Institute of Medicine
ISS	Injury Severity Score
LEOKA	Law Enforcement Officers Killed and Assaulted
LOS	Length of Stay
MADD	Mothers Against Drunk Driving
MCHB	Maternal and Child Health Bureau
MTFS	Monitoring the Future Study

NAMCS	National Ambulatory Medical Care Survey
NAS	National Academy of Sciences
NASS	National Automotive Sampling System
NASSCDS	National Automotive Sampling System—Crashworthiness Data System
NASSGES	National Automotive Sampling System—General Estimates System
NCANDS	National Child Abuse and Neglect Data System
NCEH	National Center for Environmental Health
NCHS	National Center for Health Statistics
NCIPC	National Center for Injury Prevention and Control
NCVS	National Crime Victimization Survey
NEISS	National Electronic Injury Surveillance System
NFA	National Fire Administration
NFIRS	National Fire Incident Reporting System
NHAMCS	National Hospital Ambulatory Medical Care Survey
NHDS	National Hospital Discharge Survey
NHIS	National Health Interview Survey
NHTSA	National Highway Traffic Safety Administration
NIAAA	National Institute on Alcohol Abuse and Alcoholism
NIBRS	National Incident Based Reporting System
NIDA	National Institute on Drug Abuse
NIGMS	National Institute of General Medical Sciences
NIH	National Institutes of Health
NIJ	National Institute of Justice
NIMH	National Institute of Mental Health
NIOSH	National Institute for Occupational Safety and Health
NIS	National Incidence Study of Child Abuse and Neglect
NISS	New Injury Severity Score
NLM	National Library of Medicine
NMFS93	National Mortality Followback Survey—1993
NOPUS	National Occupant Protection Use Survey
NORA	National Occupational Research Agenda
NPTS	Nationwide Personal Transportation Survey
NRC	National Research Council
NTDB	National Trauma Data Bank
NTIS	National Technical Information Service
NTOF	National Traumatic Occupational Fatalities System
NVSSF	National Vital Statistics System—Final Mortality Data
NVSSS	National Vital Statistics System—Current Mortality Sample
OSHA	Occupational Safety and Health Administration
QALY	Quality-Adjusted Life Year

QWB	Quality of Well-Being Scale
RCT	Randomized Controlled Trial
RTS	Revised Trauma Score
SAE	Society of Automotive Engineers
SAMHSA	Substance Abuse and Mental Health Services Administration
SCI	Special Crash Investigation (program)
SIP	Sickness Impact Profile
SOII	Survey of Occupational Injuries and Illnesses
STIPDA	State and Territorial Injury Prevention Directors' Association
STOP	Steps to Prevent Firearm Injury
TIPP	The Injury Prevention Program (AAP)
TRISS	Trauma and Injury Severity Score
UCR	Uniform Crime Reporting (system)
UCRSHR	Uniform Crime Reporting System—Supplemental Homicide Reports
UHDDS	Uniform Hospital Discharge Data Set
WHO	World Health Organization
WIC	Women, Infants, and Children
YPLL	Years of Productive Life Lost
YRBSS	Youth Risk Behavior Surveillance System

Index

Abbreviated Injury Scale (AIS), 153, 154
Accident
    defined, 28
    perception of injury as, 199
    prevention, 21, 24, 28, 32–33
Accidental Death and Disability report, 18–19,
    138, 159, 227, 261
Acute care, 9, 20, 29, 30, 129, 140, 150, 152,
    165, 167, 240, 243
Administration for Children and Families, 206
Administration on Aging, 206
Adolescents. *See also* Age
    firearm-related injuries, 7–8, 132–133,
        134
    impulsivity, 26
    violence prevention programs, 184, 191
    worker safety, 225, 227
Advocacy, 36, 180, 185, 199–201
Age
    and deaths from injuries, 41, 46–48, 49–
        50, 86
    and emergency department visits, 51–52
    and falls, 48, 52
    and fire and burn injuries, 48, 52
    and firearm injuries, 47, 52, 100
    and homicides, 47
    and hospitalizations, 50–51
    minimum-age drinking laws, 47, 117–
        118, 123, 200
    minimum for firearm purchase, 126, 127
    and motor vehicle traffic-related injuries,
        46–47, 52, 100
    patterns of injury by, 49–52
    and poisonings, 48, 52
    and response to injury, 154

and risk-taking behavior, 100
    and suffocations, 48, 52
    and suicides, 47, 86
Agency for Health Care Policy and Research
    (AHCPR), 9, 148, 167, 206
Agent of injury, 93. *See also* Product safety
Airbags, 61, 75, 91, 208
Alcohol Incentive Grants, 208
Alcohol use, 26
    Blood alcohol level laws, 35, 36, 103, 209
    designated driver program, 198
    excise taxes and, 94–95, 198
    legal sanctions for, 91, 118, 122
    minimum-age drinking laws, 47, 72, 117–
        118, 123, 200
    and motor vehicle traffic-related deaths,
        46–47
    safe ride program, 198
    server intervention programs, 92
    socioeconomic environment and, 94, 95
    and violence, 89, 95
All-terrain vehicles, 34, 215
American Academy for the Certification of
    Brain Injury Specialists, 184
American Academy of Pediatrics, 179, 196,
    215
American Academy of Physical Medicine and
    Rehabilitation, 77
American Bar Association, 75
American Board of Medical Specialties, 145
American College of Surgeons, 76, 140, 141,
    144, 148
    Committee on Trauma, 77, 150
American Medical Association Committee on
    Medical Education, 145

305

American National Standards Institute, 218
American Pediatric Surgical Association, 142
American Public Health Association, 31, 179, 194
American School Health Association, 179
American Society for Criminology, 130
American Trauma Society, 21
Anatomic Profile, 153
Antilock brakes, 123
Apoptosis, 99
ASCOT, 154
Assaultive injuries, 24, 29, 86, 88, 89
    prevention, 8, 91, 92, 94, 132, 238
    research, 89-90, 129
Auto insurance, 91, 163
Aviation safety, 95-96

Baby Safety Showers, 214
Basic Injury Program Development, 189
Behavioral adaptation to safety improvements, 100-101, 122, 215
Behavioral interventions, 32-33
    incentives and deterrence, 91-92, 95
    self-protection, 92
    targeting high-risk groups, 92, 128, 133
Behavioral research, 6, 91, 99-101, 119-120, 128, 130, 208
Behavioral Risk Factor Surveillance System, 67
Biases in data, 48
Bicycle helmets, 84-85, 87, 92, 102, 122, 189, 190, 198, 215, 241, 242
Biofidelic models, 98
Biological sciences, research in, 99, 128, 130
Biomechanics, 20, 32
    interventions, 96, 179, 208
    research, 6, 96-98, 99, 106, 119, 129, 130, 208, 211, 244, 245, 247-248
Biomedical engineering, 185
Blood alcohol level (BAL) laws, 35, 36, 103, 209
Brady Handgun Violence Prevention Act, 127
Brain and spinal cord injury, 96-97, 99, 119, 122, 151, 155, 157, 158, 184, 187, 189, 228, 231, 241, 243, 245
Brain Injury Association (BIA), 184, 199
Buckle Up America!, 209
Bureau of Alcohol, Tobacco, and Firearms, 126, 127, 207
    Project LEAD, 125
Bureau of Justice Statistics, 207
Bureau of Labor Statistics, 66, 207, 221, 222
Bureau of Mines, 223
Bureau of the Census, 69

California, injury prevention plan, 187-188

California Wellness Foundation, 184
Canada
    motor vehicle safety, 123
    trauma care, 142, 151
Carbon monoxide in cooking gas, 26, 87-88
Carnegie Corporation of New York, 232
Case-control studies, 6, 102, 103
Case-crossover studies, 102-103
Case mix, 152-154
Case studies
    defined, 103
    firearm injuries, 124-135
    misuse of, 103
    motor vehicle injuries, 115-124
Cause of injury
    behavioral research, 101
    biomechanics research, 96
    E codes, 63-64, 65
    economic costs by, 54
    mortality rates by, 42-43, 47, 54, 132
    patterns of injury by, 52
    phases, 22, 29, 30
    years of potential life lost by, 53, 54
Census of Agriculture, 69
Census of Fatal Occupational Injuries, 53, 66, 72, 221
Center on Children and the Law, 75
Center to Prevent Handgun Violence, 197 n.3
Centers for Disease Control and Prevention, 19, 103, 189 n.2, 223, 240
    conferences, 31
    injury control research centers, 2, 20, 24, 31, 227, 249
    injury focus, 206, 239
    leadership role, 12, 251, 261
    surveillance systems, 67, 73, 125, 147
    trauma care funding, 160
    violence prevention, 236
Child protective services, 182
Child safety, 21
    biomechanical research, 97, 98
    child-resistant packaging, 84, 101, 215
    cigarette lighter standards, 93, 215
    evaluation of programs, 198
    gun safe-storage laws, 127, 132
    home visits for first-time mothers, 26, 84, 90, 92
    playground safety, 85, 232, 241
    seat restraints in motor vehicles, 91-92, 95, 119, 120, 179, 190
    state and local initiatives, 182, 185, 191, 192, 193
    surveillance systems, 68, 75
Children. *See also* Age
    agricultural injuries, 227
    arrests for weapons offenses, 133

causes of death, 142
death review teams, 75, 184
firearm injuries, 124, 130, 134
mortality rates, 49, 84, 86, 124, 132
poisonings, 48, 83–84, 101
trauma care for, 142
Children's Bureau, 206, 230
Children's National Medical Center, 185
Children's Safety Network, 194, 197, 232
Cigarette lighters, child-resistant, 93, 215
Clinical research, 32, 130, 148, 226, 227, 229, 230
Coalition building, 185, 190, 192, 193, 198, 201
Cochrane Collaboration, 198
Coding issues, 29
cause of injury, 63–64, 65, 77
location of injury occurrence, 63–64
nature of injury, 62–63
recommendations, 3
training, 3, 64, 71
Cohort studies, 6, 102, 103
Committee on Injury Prevention and Control, charge to, 20, 30, 37
Community Integrated Service Systems (CISS), 231, 233
Computer models of injury, 98
Conferences, 31, 192, 251
Constituency building, 199–200
Consumer Product Safety Act, 21, 212, 216
Amendments of 1981, 213
Consumer Product Safety Commission (CPSC)
achievements, 215–217
hotline, 212
mission and focus, 206, 212
public education, 214–215
recommended role, 3–4, 11, 13, 16, 217, 247, 249, 252, 261
regulatory activities, 21, 126, 207, 213
research, 11, 93, 214, 216–217, 246, 247
resources and structure, 212–213
standards development, 207, 213–214
surveillance activities, 3–4, 13, 67, 70, 7, 79, 125, 213–214, 216, 252, 261
training role, 249
Controversies
advocacy by researchers, 36
boundaries of injury field, 25
federal priority-setting role, 35–36, 266–267
firearms-related, 131–132
motor vehicle safety, 121–123
paternalistic interventions, 34–35
Cooperative Compliance Program, 223

Cost-benefit analysis of preventive interventions, 33, 220, 222
Costs of injury. *See also* Years of potential life lost
direct, 1 n.1, 18 n.1, 41 n.1, 55, 157, 158
economic, 41, 53, 54, 55, 56–57, 97, 154, 156–159
estimates, 1, 18, 41 n.1, 54
fatalities, 55
friction cost method, 56
human capital (cost-of-illness) method, 54–55, 56, 57
indirect, 1 n.1, 18 n.1, 41 n.1, 55, 56
occupational injuries, 48, 226
outcomes and, 157
quality of life, 53, 56, 57–58
revealed-preference method, 56
stated-preference method, 56
total lifetime, 55
trauma care, 9, 154, 156–159, 168
unreimbursed, 157
willingness-to-pay method, 56–57
worker productivity, 158
Counseling, injury prevention, 191, 196–197
Crash Injury Research and Engineering Network (CIREN), 32
Crash Outcome Data Evaluation Systems (CODES), 78
Criminal Justice Periodical Index, 105
Criminal justice system, violence prevention, 88–89
Criminology, 89, 130
Cutting and piercing injuries, 45, 49, 52

Data Elements for Emergency Department Systems (DEEDS), 77, 147
Databases, 105–106. *See also* Surveillance systems; *individual databases and systems*
Death certificate data, 65, 78
Death review teams, 75, 184
Deaths. *See* Cause of injury; Mortality
Demonstrating Your Program's Worth, 198
Department of Agriculture, 206
Department of Commerce, 206
Department of Defense, 206
Department of Education, 195, 206
Department of Energy, 206
Department of Health and Human Services (DHHS), 8, 68, 69, 88, 90, 134, 148, 206, 239, 243, 253
Department of Health, Education, and Welfare, Division of Child and Maternal Health, 21
Department of Housing and Urban Development, 207, 239

Department of Justice, 4, 8, 71, 74, 126, 128, 134, 207, 235, 237, 238, 239
Department of Labor, 207, 217, 218, 221
Department of the Interior, 223
Department of the Treasury, 207
Department of Transportation, 207, 239
Department of Veterans Affairs, 207
Disability-adjusted life year (DALY), 57–58
Domestic Violence Offenders Gun Ban, 127
Driver education and licensing, 118, 119, 120, 123, 161
Driver/occupant safety, 21. *See also* Highway safety; Motor vehicle safety
    airbags and, 61, 75, 91, 123, 208
    antilock brakes, 123
    Blood alcohol level laws, 35, 36, 103, 209
    center high-mounted brake lights, 93, 119
    child safety restraints, 91–92, 95, 119, 120, 179, 190
    crash testing, 98, 184
    enforcement of mandatory requirements, 122, 123
    grassroots organizations, 21, 120, 184
    minimum-age drinking laws, 47, 72, 117–118, 123, 200
    motorcycle helmet laws, 34, 78, 84–85, 92, 120, 122, 209
    safety-belt use laws, 34–35, 78, 91–92, 95, 119, 120, 122, 123, 209, 259
    speed limit, national maximum, 46 n.3, 82, 120, 121, 123
    zero-tolerance laws, 36
Drownings, 45, 48, 52, 76, 193
Drug Abuse Warning Network, 69
Drunk driving. *See also* Alcohol use
    injuries, 46–47, 91, 92, 94–95

E codes, 63–64, 70, 147, 187, 191
Ecologic study design, 103
Educating Professionals in Injury Control series, 196
Education and Research Centers (ERCs), 194, 196, 225, 227
Education Development Center (Newton, Mass.), 232
Education interventions, 3, 32. *See also* Training
    child safety seats, 179
    firearm injuries, 134
    focus of, 180
    funding, 197 n.3, 241
    helmet use, 85, 241
    of legislators and political leaders, 199–200
    occupational safety, 225, 226–227
    research, 240

state and community initiatives, 179, 180, 185, 190, 191, 199, 200
    techniques, 199
    traffic safety, 85, 92
    violence prevention, 85, 197 n.3
Elderly people. *See also* Age
    cause of injury deaths, 52, 245
    trauma care for, 143, 168, 245
Emergency department (ED) visits, 41, 48–49, 51–52, 165
    costs, 55
    number, 1, 18
    surveillance systems, 70, 71, 77–78, 147, 187, 209, 213
Emergency medical services. *See also* Trauma care systems
    cost containment, 166–167
    curriculum development, 196
    elderly, 143
    funding, 182
    helicopter medical transport, 158
    infrastructure, 182
    legislation, 142, 143, 144
    levels of providers, 140
    paramedic, 158
    pediatric, 142
    prehospital, 140, 152, 157, 158
    research by, 119, 120
    rural, 141–142
    training, 145–146
Emergency Medical Services for Children (EMS-C) Program, 13, 142, 144, 160, 231, 233–234, 252
Emergency Medical Services Systems Act of 1973, 143, 144
Emergency Medical Treatment and Active Labor Act of 1985, 164
Emergency Nurses Association, 146
Emergency nursing, 146
Emotional sequelae, 27
Enforcement of mandatory requirements, 7, 122, 123, 126, 133, 134, 190, 220–221, 222
Environmental interventions, 26, 33, 84
Epidemiology, injury, 32
    childhood, 142
    literature, 105
    research, 101–103, 128, 130, 211–212, 224
    surveillance systems, 76, 77–78
EuroQol, 57
Evaluation of interventions, 3, 24, 60
    behavioral research, 101
    child safety, 233
    factors considered, 90–91
    funding for, 189, 233, 238, 242, 243, 252

guidelines for, 198, 209
methodological problems, 88, 151
motor vehicle safety, 5, 97, 120, 209
occupational safety, 226
outcome measures, 101, 150–152
process, 95
product, 93
studies, 87, 198
support for, 5, 106, 120, 197, 226, 243
surveillance systems for, 74–75
technical assistance for, 197
trauma systems, 9, 146–147, 148, 149,
    150–152, 154–156, 168
violence prevention, 235, 237, 238

Falls
    age and, 52, 245
    mortality rates, 45, 46, 48, 52, 245
    nonfatal, 49
    prevention, 94
    research, 84, 85, 87, 245
    years potential life lost, 53
Fatal intentional injury surveillance system,
    72–74, 79
Fatality Analysis Reporting System (FARS),
    4, 68, 72, 79, 117, 209
Federal Aviation Administration, 207
Federal Bureau of Investigation, 67, 72, 125
Federal Emergency Management Agency, 207
Federal Hazardous Substances Act, 212 n.6
Federal Highway Administration, 68, 118,
    119, 207, 208
Federal Railroad Administration, 207, 211
Federal response. *See also individual depart-
    ments and agencies*
    agencies involved in injury field, 11–12,
        206–207
    coordination and leadership role, 12–13,
        251–253, 260–262
    interagency collaboration, 12–13, 192,
        251–253
    priority-setting role, 35–36, 200
    private-sector partnerships, 260
    state infrastructure building, 10, 189, 191,
        201
    technical assistance to states, 10, 197, 201
    training of injury prevention practitioners,
        194–195, 197
    trauma systems support, 8, 9, 147, 149,
        159–161, 168
Federal Transit Administration, 207
Financing/funding
    construction, tied to highway safety, 36,
        118, 123
    education, 197 n.3
    evaluation research, 189

federal sources, 8, 10, 18, 19, 103–105,
    106, 119, 130, 148, 160, 189
infrastructure building, 10, 189, 201
patient care, 161–163
private-sector sources, 179, 184
research, 7, 8, 18, 19, 103–105, 106, 119,
    104, 130, 148
state and community sources, 10, 179,
    180, 181, 182–183, 188–190, 201
for training, 6, 103–105, 106, 196
trauma care systems, 9, 138, 143, 149,
    159–163, 167, 168
violence prevention programs, 235
Fire and burn injuries, 45, 48, 52
    mortality rates, 259
    prevention, 61, 75, 84, 87, 93, 217, 226–
        227, 228–229
    research accomplishments, 84, 85, 87,
        228–229
    surveillance data, 75, 189
Fire Prevention Week, 185
Fire safety, 182, 185
Firearm Owner Protection Act, 127
Firearm-related injuries, 89
    access issue, 7, 132, 133
    age and, 47, 52, 100, 124
    child and adolescent vulnerability, 7–8,
        132–133, 134
    controversies, 131–132
    enforcement of regulations, 133
    federal role, 7, 130, 134–135
    gender and, 47
    homicides, 45, 47, 48, 73
    individual freedom issue, 7, 131
    instrumentality issue, 131
    measures of exposure, 129
    mortality rates, 7, 45, 46, 47, 48, 52, 103,
        115, 124, 132
    prevention, 2, 7–8, 24, 86, 89, 126–128,
        130, 132–134
    recommendations, 7, 8, 131, 134
    research, 7, 128–130, 134, 243, 247
    state and local programs, 130
    suicides, 8, 45, 47, 48, 73, 86
    surveillance systems, 7, 71, 73, 125–126,
        128, 134, 187, 241
    treatment, 129
    trends, 46, 124
    unintentional, 8, 124, 125, 129, 132
Firearms
    design interventions, 129, 133
    illegal commerce, 128, 132
    number in circulation, 7, 132
    regulation and legislation, 7, 126–128,
        132, 134
    safety and performance standards, 126

First National Conference on Injury Control, 31
Flammability standards, 87, 93
Flammable Fabrics Act, 212
Functional Independence Measure, 155
Future of Public Health report, 199

Gas Appliance Manufacturers Association, 185
Gender
    and deaths from injuries, 49–50
    and emergency department visits, 51–52
    and firearm-related suicides, 47
    and hospitalizations, 50–51, 52
    and occupational injuries, 53
    patterns of injury by, 49–52, 53
    and poisonings, 48, 52
General Accounting Office, 214, 216, 220
General Health Status Measure Short Form-36, 155
Glasgow Coma Scale, 151, 153
Government Performance and Results Act, 218–219
Governor's Highway Safety Program, 120, 189
Grassroots organizations, 180, 200, 214. *See also individual organizations*
Gun Control Act, 127
Guns. *See* Firearm-related injuries

Haddon matrix, 22, 23, 29, 33, 117
Handgun access laws, 35
Harlem Hospital Injury Prevention Program, 85–86
Harlem Hospital Pediatric Trauma Registry, 85
Head injury, 97, 153, 155, 158, 241. *See also* Brain and spinal cord injury
Head Injury Criterion (HIC), 97
Helicopter medical transport, 158
Health Care Cost and Utilization Project, 65, 69
Health Care Financing Administration, 68
Health insurance, private, 162, 163, 164, 165
Health-related quality of life measures, 154–155, 156
Health Resources and Services Administration, 9, 13, 77, 120, 160, 167, 185, 189, 206, 230, 234, 247 n.17, 252, 261
Health Services, Preventive Health Services, and Home and Community-Based Services Act, 144
Health-state classification system, 57
Health status measures, 154–155, 156
Health Utilities Index, 57
Healthy People 2000 goals, 200

High-risk groups, targeting interventions to, 92, 100, 133
Highway Loss Data Institute, 184
Highway safety
    construction funding tied to, 36, 118, 123
    engineered safety features, 94, 118
    legislation, 21, 118, 120, 144, 145, 179
    strategic planning, 187
Highway Safety Act, 21, 118, 120, 144, 145, 159, 208, 209
Homicide Research Working Group, 130
Homicides, 24
    age and, 47, 124
    domestic violence, 128
    firearm-related, 45, 47, 48, 73, 128, 132
    race/ethnicity and, 50
    rates, 45, 46, 88
    socioeconomic environment and, 94
    surveillance systems, 4, 72, 73, 74, 125
    workplace, 53, 227
Hospitalizations, 1, 18, 41, 48, 49
    costs of, 55
    lengths of stay, 150, 154, 158, 165–166
    number of, 143
    patterns of injury, 50–51, 52
    readmissions, 77
    surveillance systems, 65, 66, 75–76, 77–78
    transfers, 166

IDEA program, 211
Indian Health Service, 68, 194, 195, 206
Industrial safety, 21
Information systems. *See* Surveillance systems; *specific networks and databases*
Injury and Violence Prevention Program, 231
Injury control. *See also* Injury field
    defined, 29–30
Injury Control Research Centers, 2, 6, 19–20, 24, 31, 103, 148, 195, 196, 240–241, 243, 244–245
Injury Control Act of 1990, 12, 239–240, 251
Injury Control report, 2, 20, 30, 104, 195, 248
Injury field
    accomplishments, 13–14, 258–259
    adjacent fields, 32
    barriers to growth, 30, 194
    boundaries, 2–3, 23–24, 25, 27
    challenges, 15, 32, 198–199, 259
    coordination and collaboration in, 2, 6, 31–32, 79, 89, 130, 150, 223, 239, 259, 260–262
    core disciplines, 30
    databases, 105–106
    development of, 2, 30–36

integration of methods and perspectives, 2, 259, 264–265
investment priorities, 2–3
mission, 2–3, 23–27, 30, 33, 264–265
organization of report, 36–37
origins, 20–22, 284–295
policy making, informed, 266–268
public health perspective, 22, 23, 33, 260
public support for, 259, 265–266
scientific communication, 265
study background, 18–20
timeline, 284–295
vocabulary, 28–30
Injury in America report, 2, 12, 13, 19, 23, 24, 30, 104, 194, 239, 244, 248, 250, 251, 262
Injury Prevention report, 198
Injury science, 21, 22, 26, 32, 266–267
Injury Severity Score (ISS), 153
Institute of Medicine, 1, 2, 19, 20, 227
Institutional National Research Service Awards, 238
Insurance Institute for Highway Safety, 120, 184
Intelligent transportation systems, 211
Intentional injuries, 23–24. *See also* Homicides; Suicides
    defined, 28–29
    integration with unintentional injuries, 2, 25–26
    prevention, 86–90
    research on, 24
Interagency Working Group on Violence Research, 239
International Classification for External Causes of Injuries (ICECI), 64
International Classification of Diseases (ICD), 3, 28–29, 62–64, 70, 79, 153
International Collaborative Effort for Injury Statistics (ICE), 63
Internet, 105–106
Interventions. *See also* Evaluation of interventions
    agent, 93
    behavioral, 91–92
    categories of, 90
    biomechanical, 96
    development process, 5, 82
    effectiveness of, 86, 191
    environmental, 94
    and health care costs, 163
    implementation of programs, 9, 178–180
    incentive grants, 242
    intentional injuries, 86–95
    opportunities for, 22
    paternalistic, 33, 34–35

peer training, 92
prevention, 21, 82, 85–86, 90–95
research, 90–95
socioeconomic, 94–95
unintentional injuries, 83–86
John D. and Catherine T. MacArthur Foundation, 1, 20
Johns Hopkins University, 31, 244
    Center for Injury Research and Policy, 194
Journal of Emergency Medical Services, 149
Journals, 31, 149

"Kids Plate" vehicle license tags, 190

Law Enforcement Agency Data, 125
Law Enforcement Officers Killed and Assaulted, 67
Lawnmower performance standards, 215
Learn Not to Burn curriculum, 185
Legislation. *See also individual statutes*
    highway safety, 21, 118, 120, 144, 145, 179
    trauma care, 139–140, 143, 144, 145, 149, 159–161
Lifesavers Conference, 192
Lobbying, 200
Location of injury occurrence, 63–64

Magnitude of injury
    cost, 53–58
    morbidity, 48–49
    mortality rates, 44–48
    patterns, 49–53
Maine 2000 program, 221
Major Trauma Outcome Study, 151
Managed care, 150, 162, 163, 164–167, 168, 191
Maternal and Child Health Bureau
    accomplishments, 142, 185, 234
    Block Grant Program, 189, 231
    Community Integrated Service Systems, 231, 233
    Emergency Medical Services for Children (EMS-C) Program, 142, 144, 160, 231, 233–234
    grants and contracts, 232–234
    health performance measures, 191
    mission and focus, 206, 230–231
    recommended role, 10, 196, 249
    resources and structure, 231–232
    Special Projects of Regional and National Significance, 231, 232–233
    technical assistance, 194
    training initiatives, 10, 195, 196, 231, 232, 233, 249

Traumatic Brain Injury Program, 231
violence prevention program, 90, 194, 195, 231
Medical Examiner and Coroner Alert Project, 213
Medical examiner and coroner data, 4, 5, 48, 73, 75, 77, 78, 209
Medical Examiner and Coroner Information Sharing Program, 73, 74
Medical informatics, 105
Medicaid, 162, 164, 165, 166
Medicare, 162, 164
Mental health, 27, 86, 130
Metropolitan Life Foundation, 197 n.3
Minimum-age drinking laws, 47, 72
Model Trauma Care System Plan, 143, 144, 161
Molecular biology, 32
Monitoring the Future Study, 69
Morbidity, injury-related
    coding, 62, 63
    costs of, 18
    measures of, 152, 154
    by nature of injury, 49, 62, 63
    overall burden of, 48–49
Mortality, 18. *See also* Deaths; Years of potential life lost
    age-related, 41, 42–43, 46–47, 49–50, 84
    aviation-related, 96
    by cause of death, 42–43, 47, 54
    coding of data, 62–63
    consumer product-related, 212
    firearm-related injuries, 7, 45, 46, 47, 48, 52, 103, 115, 124, 132, 259
    gender and, 49–50
    by manner of death, 45–46, 86
    motor vehicle-related, 7, 45, 46, 48, 50, 52, 94, 95, 115–116, 121, 123, 141, 259
    number, 1, 18, 41, 44–45, 83
    occupational injuries, 48, 52, 226, 259
    race/ethnicity and, 49–50
    sex ratios, 50
    socioeconomic environment and, 94
    surveillance systems, 65, 66, 67, 72–74
    trends, 5, 46–48
Mothers Against Drunk Driving (MADD), 21, 120, 184, 199
Motor Vehicle Information and Cost Savings Act, 205
Motor vehicle and traffic-related injuries. *See also* Driver/occupant safety
    age and, 46–47, 52, 100
    alcohol-related, 46–47, 91, 92, 94–95
    cellular telephones and, 103
    controversies, 121–123

evaluation of interventions, 87, 97, 120, 209
hospital lengths of stay, 166
mortality rates, 7, 45, 46, 48, 50, 52, 94, 95, 115–116, 121, 123, 141, 179, 259
nonfatal, 49
number, 24
occupational, 52–53
perceptions of risk and, 100–101, 122
prevention, 6, 7, 84, 85–86, 87, 91–92, 93, 94–95, 99–100, 116–120, 191
public support for safety, 120
race/ethnicity and, 50
regulation and legislation, 118–119
research, 6, 83, 84, 99–100, 119–120, 123, 208, 243, 247
socioeconomic conditions and, 94
speed limit and, 46 n.3, 82, 119
state and local programs, 120, 209
surveillance data, 4, 65, 68, 71, 72, 78, 117–118
trends, 46
Motor vehicle safety
    design mismatches, 123
    inspections, 119
    literature, 105
    organizations, 184
    research, 208
    standards, 21, 118, 205
Motorcycle
    headlights, 121
    helmet laws, 34, 78, 84–85, 92, 120, 122, 209

National Ambulatory Medical Care Survey (NAMCS), 63, 65, 66
National Association of EMS Physicians, 146
National Automotive Sampling System (NASS), 68, 69, 72, 117, 209
National Center for Chronic Disease Prevention and Health Promotion, 206
National Center for Environmental Health (NCEH), 4, 73, 206
National Center for Health Statistics (NCHS), 4, 62, 65, 66, 67, 125
National Center for Injury Prevention and Control (NCIPC)
    accomplishments, 243–247, 250
    Basic Injury Program Development, 250
    cooperative agreements, 240, 241–242, 249–250
    educational activities, 240, 241, 243
    evaluation research, 120, 197–198, 242, 243, 252
    extramural research, 243–244, 245, 247

Injury Control Research Centers, 2, 6, 19–20, 24, 31, 103, 148, 195, 196, 240–241, 243, 244–245, 249
mission and focus, 206, 240
nurturing role, 12, 250–251
origins, 239–240
priority areas for research, 12, 242, 245–248, 268
recommended role, 4, 6, 9, 10, 12–13, 16, 104–105, 167, 190, 196, 245–249, 250–251, 252, 261–262
research grants, 240–241, 243–247
resources and structure, 240
state and community infrastructure building, 12, 128, 181, 188, 189, 190, 241, 242, 249–250, 251
suicide prevention, 246, 252, 262
surveillance activities, 4, 13, 70, 71, 147, 148, 240, 241, 242, 243, 245, 249, 252
technical assistance, 10, 12, 188, 197, 241, 249
training activities, 6, 10, 12, 104–105, 195, 196, 240, 241, 243, 244, 248–249, 262
trauma systems research, 9, 77, 120, 147, 148, 167, 247 n.17
violence prevention, 90, 128, 195, 236, 238, 246, 247–248, 252
National Center for Maternal and Child Health, 232
National Center for Medical Rehabilitation Research, 206, 228
National Center for Statistics and Analysis, 209
National Child Abuse and Neglect Data System (NCANDS), 68
National Children's Center for Rural and Agricultural Health and Safety, 197
National Committee on Vital and Health Statistics, 63
National Consortium on Violence Research, 128, 130, 239
National Council on Accident Prevention, 19
National Crime Victimization Survey, 66, 72, 88, 125
National Criminal Justice Reference Service, 105
National Directory of Injury Prevention Professionals, 31
National Drive Safely@Work Week, 209
National Electronic Injury Surveillance System (NEISS), 3–4, 67, 70, 71, 79, 125, 213–214, 216, 261
National Farm Medicine Center, 227
National Fire Administration, 69
National Fire Code, 185

National Fire Incident Reporting System, 69
National Fire Protection Association, 185
National Firearms Act, 127
National Health Interview Survey (NHIS), 63, 65, 66, 70
National Highway Safety Act of 1995, 36
National Highway Safety Bureau, 21, 118, 205
National Highway System Designation Act of 1995, 121 n.1
National Highway Traffic Safety Administration (NHTSA)
achievements, 47, 209–212
child safety initiatives, 12, 185, 233, 252
collaborative programs, 192
mission and focus, 21, 118, 205, 207
recommended role, 6, 10, 13, 16, 104, 196, 212, 249, 252, 261, 262
regulatory activities, 205, 207
research, 6, 21, 105, 119, 130, 198, 208, 212, 247
resources and structure, 207–208
Safe Communities program, 193
Special Crash Investigation (SCI) program, 61
Section 402 grants, 189, 208
surveillance systems, 4, 32, 69, 71, 73, 78, 209, 212
training activities, 6, 10, 194, 196, 212, 249, 262
trauma systems development, 13, 142, 145, 147, 148, 160, 188
workshops, 194
National Highway Traffic and Motor Vehicle Safety Act, 118
National Hospital Ambulatory Medical Care Survey (NHAMCS), 63, 65
National Hospital Discharge Survey (NHDS), 65, 66, 157
National Incident Based Reporting System, 67
National Incidence Study of Child Abuse and Neglect, 68
National Injury and Violence Prevention Resource Center, 194, 197
National Institute for Occupational Safety and Health (NIOSH)
accomplishments, 219, 225–226
educational activities, 198, 225, 226–227
mission and focus, 206, 218, 223, 261
motor vehicle safety research, 120
recommended role, 6, 10, 11, 16, 196, 226–227, 249, 252, 261
research priority setting, 11, 224. 225–226, 268
resources and structure, 223–224, 240
surveillance activities, 67, 223–224, 226
technical assistance, 197

training grants, 6, 10, 103–104, 194, 196, 224–225, 249, 262
violence prevention, 128, 227
National Institute of Arthritis and Musculoskeletal and Skin Diseases, 206
National Institute of Child Health and Human Development, 142, 206, 215, 228
National Institute of General Medical Sciences, 11, 16, 206, 228–230, 261
National Institute of Justice (NIJ)
    accomplishments, 237–238
    evaluation of programs, 237, 238
    mission and focus, 207, 235
    recommended role, 4, 11, 16, 73, 238–239, 252, 261–262
    research, 235, 236–237, 238, 246
    resources and structure, 235–236
    technical assistance, 236
    training activities, 11, 235, 237, 238
    surveillance system, 4, 73, 74, 125
National Law Enforcement and Corrections Technology Centers, 235
National Institute of Mental Health, 90, 128, 206, 246, 252, 262
National Institute of Neurological Disorders and Stroke, 206, 228
National Institute of Standards and Technology, 206
National Institute on Aging, 119, 206
National Institute on Alcohol Abuse and Alcoholism, 90, 119–120, 206
National Institute on Disability and Rehabilitation Research, 142, 147, 206
National Institute on Drug Abuse, 69, 90, 206
National Institute on Trauma, 19
National Institutes of Health
    accomplishments, 229–230
    center-based research, 244
    grant process, 240, 242
    institutional training grants, 238
    mission and focus, 206, 227
    recommended role, 11, 19, 227, 230, 261, 263, 267–268
    resources, 228
    trauma research, 11, 148, 226, 227, 230
    training, 11, 104, 228–229, 230, 262
    violence prevention, 238
National Library of Medicine, MEDLINE database, 105
National Mortality Followback Survey, 66
National Occupant Protection Use Survey, 69
National Occupational Research Agenda (NORA), 11, 224, 225–226, 247, 268
National Pediatric Trauma Registry, 142
National Personal Transportation Survey, 68
National Program for Playground Safety, 197

National Registry of Emergency Medical Technicians, 145
National Research Council, 145
    Transportation Research Board, 211
National SAFE KIDS campaign, 179, 185, 190, 193, 199
National Safety Council, 21, 185
National Science Foundation, 128, 207, 239
National Suicide Prevention Conference, 88
National Technical Information Service, 105
National Traffic and Motor Vehicle Safety Act of 1966, 205
National Transportation Safety Board, 207
National Trauma Data Bank (NTDB), 76, 147
National Traumatic Occupational Fatality Surveillance System, 67, 72
National Vital Statistics System, 65, 67, 117
Nationwide Personal Transportation Survey, 68
Nature of injury
    coding, 62–63
    morbidity trends, 49
    surveillance systems, 64
Network of Employers for Traffic Safety, 209
New Injury Severity Score, 153
9-1-1 systems, 138, 140, 149, 165
Nonprofit organizations, 180, 184–185, 199–200. *See also individual organizations*
Northern Manhattan Injury Surveillance System, 85, 86

Occupational injuries
    costs, 48, 226
    high-risk occupations, 53
    mortality rates, 48, 52, 226, 259
    patterns of, 52–53
    prevention, 91
    research, 103–104
    surveillance systems, 4, 60, 64, 66, 71, 72
Occupational Safety and Health Act, 21, 217–218, 219, 221, 223, 261
Occupational Safety and Health Administration (OSHA). *See also* National Institute for Occupational Safety and Health
    accomplishments, 222–223
    enforcement activities, 220–221, 222
    mission and focus, 21, 207, 218, 261
    outcome studies of regulation, 222–223
    reforms, 218–219, 223
    regulatory activities, 218, 219–220, 222
    research priority setting, 226
    resources and structure, 217–218, 219
    state programs, 182, 218
    surveillance activities, 218, 221–222
    technical assistance from, 219
    training activities, 222

Office of Justice Programs, 90, 128, 130, 207, 234–235. *See also* National Institute of Justice

Office of Juvenile Justice and Delinquency Prevention, 195, 207

Office of Safe and Drug-Free Schools, 195

Office of Technology Assessment, 220

Omnibus Crime Control Act of 1968, 235

Osteoarthritis, 99, 245

Outcomes
and costs, 157
managed care and, 165, 166
measures of effectiveness, 101, 149, 154–156
modeling, 154
nonfatal, measures of, 154–156
of occupational safety regulation, 222
prediction of, 152–154
surveillance systems, 76
trauma systems, 149, 150–156, 161, 165, 166, 261

Passive protection, 33, 121–122

Pathophysiology, 6, 99

Patient care, financing, 161–163

Patient-oriented measures of health status, 155

Patient risk factors, 156

Patterns of injury
by age, 49–52
by cause, 52
by gender, 49–52
occupational, 52–53
by race/ethnicity, 49–52

Pew Charitable Trust, 196

Physical environments, engineered safety features, 94

Playground safety, 85, 232, 241

Poison control centers, 21, 78, 84, 183, 193

Poisoning Prevention Packaging Act of 1970, 84, 212 n.6

Poisonings
age and, 48, 52
gender and, 52
mortality rates, 45, 46, 48, 84
nonfatal, 49
research, 84, 85, 245
surveillance systems, 76, 84

Police reports, 4, 65, 73, 78, 187, 209

Prevention of injury. *See also* Interventions; Research on prevention
accident prevention distinguished from, 24
Accidental Death and Disability recommendations, 18
barriers to, 104
core program elements, 181

cost-benefit analysis, 33
defined, 29, 30
federal role in, 35–36
firearm-related, 2, 7–8, 24, 86, 89, 126–128, 130, 132–134
integration into existing programs, 191
intentional injury, 25–26, 86–90
literature, 105–106
managed care and, 165
model programs, 85–86
pediatric programs, 142
public health role, 23
social action, 21, 26
state programs, 21
trauma systems role, 146–147
treatment linked to, 31–32, 146–147

Privacy and confidentiality issues, 76, 78, 187

Private-sector organizations, 179, 180, 260

Product safety. *See also* Consumer Product Safety Commission
corporate role, 180, 214
deaths, 212
design interventions, 26, 93
regulations and legislation, 34, 212 n.6
research, 214, 216–217
surveillance systems, 3, 67, 70, 213–214, 216

Professional organizations, 179, 180, 186, 265. *See also individual organizations*

Psychological trauma, 27

Public awareness, raising, 178, 180, 198–199, 201, 259

Public education. *See* Education interventions

Public health departments
funding of injury prevention, 7, 104, 183
perspective on injury prevention, 22, 23, 24, 33, 260
program placement, 181
state infrastructure strengthening, 181–191
on violence prevention, 26, 89

Public support
for motor vehicle safety, 120, 122, 133
for firearm safety, 133–134
nurturing, in injury field, 259, 265–266

Qualitative research, 101

Quality-adjusted life years (QALYs), 57

Quality of life
costs of injury, 53, 56, 57–58
measures of, 57, 154
and suicide, 86

Quality of Well-Being Scale, 57, 155

Race and ethnicity
and deaths from injuries, 50

and emergency department visits, 51–52
and hospitalizations, 50–51
patterns of injury by, 49–52
Rand Health Insurance Measures for Child
    Health Status, 155
Randomized controlled trials (RCTs), 6, 102,
    103
Recommendations
    of *Accidental Death and Disability*, 18–19
    coding, 3, 15, 64
    fatal intentional injury surveillance sys-
        tem, 4–5, 15, 73–74
    federal role, 6, 10, 11-12, 16, 104, 196,
        212, 217, 226–227, 230, 238, 245–249,
        250
    firearm-related injuries, 7, 8, 15, 131, 134
    of *Injury Control*, 104, 195
    of *Injury in America*, 12, 19–20, 104, 251
    occupational injuries, 11, 16, 226–227
    outcomes research, 9, 15, 161, 167
    research on prevention, 6–7, 15, 98, 99,
        101, 103, 104–105, 212, 217, 226–227,
        247-248
    state infrastructure building, 10, 16, 190,
        196, 250
    summary of, 15–16
    surveillance systems, 3, 4–5, 15, 64, 71–
        72, 73–74, 212
    technical assistance, 10
    training, 3, 10, 15, 16, 64, 104–105, 196,
        212, 230, 238
    trauma care systems, 8–9, 15, 161, 167,
        230
    violence prevention, 11, 12, 16, 238, 248
Recreational activities, injury prevention, 85–
    86, 106, 244, 245–246, 247–248, 264
Refrigerator Safety Act, 212 n.5
Regulation
    child-resistant packaging, 93
    cost-benefit balancing, 222
    firearm safety, 7, 126–128, 132, 134
    flammability standards, 87, 93
    motor vehicle safety, 118–119
    occupational health and safety, 218, 219–
        220, 222
    paternalism controversy, 33, 34–35
    water heater temperatures, 87
Rehabilitation, 9, 29, 30, 140, 150, 152, 155,
    157, 158, 161, 165, 167, 184, 228, 240,
    243
Remediation of injuries, 23
Remove Intoxicated Drivers (RID), 21, 120
Research on prevention. *See also* Evaluation
    of interventions; *individual disciplines*
    Accidental Death and Disability recom-
        mendations, 18

accomplishments, 5, 82, 83–95
animal experiments, 97, 98
on assaultive injuries, 24, 129
behavioral, 91–92
bias, 36, 102
cadaver use, 97, 98
capacity building, 2, 259, 262–264
centers, 2, 6, 19–20, 103, 148, 195, 240–
    241, 243, 244–245
challenges in, 6, 83, 88, 93, 95, 97
childhood injury, 142
collaborative approach, 238–239
communicating results, 105–106, 198,
    201, 265
cost-effectiveness, 104, 159
extramural, 6, 104, 148, 208, 211, 212,
    223, 226, 228, 230, 235, 236, 238, 240,
    243–244, 245, 263
federal funding, 8, 14, 18, 19, 103–105,
    106, 130, 148, 208, 210–212, 240, 243
firearm injuries, 7, 128–130, 134, 243,
    247
Injury in America recommendations, 19–
    20
investigator-initiated, 104, 142, 208, 211,
    224, 226, 228, 236, 240, 243, 245, 247,
    262–263
motor vehicle safety, 6, 21, 83, 84, 99–
    100, 119–120, 123, 208, 210–212, 243,
    247
multidisciplinary nature of, 5, 7, 95–103,
    119, 129–130, 134, 198, 224–225, 230
occupational safety and health, 223–226
opportunities, 95–106, 123
organization of researchers, 106
peer review of, 6, 104, 105, 211, 224, 228,
    236, 240, 244
priority setting, 224, 225–226, 242, 245–
    248, 262, 267–268
product safety, 214, 216–217
qualitative, 101
recommendations, 6, 7, 14, 98, 99, 101,
    103, 104–105, 212, 226, 230, 247–248
rehabilitation, 228
state and community sponsorship of, 180,
    185
training for, 6, 103–105, 106, 212, 230,
    238, 243, 262
trauma care, 8, 9, 19, 119, 120, 129, 148,
    149, 150–156, 159, 168, 224, 226, 227,
    230, 245, 247 n.17
validation, 98
violence prevention, 235, 236–237, 238,
    239
Residential injury prevention, 21, 244, 245–
    246, 247–248, 264

Resource libraries, 198
Revised Trauma Score (RTS), 153, 154
Risk
  analysis, 34, 85
  factors, patient, 156
  perception, 100–101, 122, 215
  regulation, 34
  significant, 220
Risk-taking behavior, 34
  age and, 100
  identification of, 101–102
  monitoring, 67
  perception of risk and, 6, 100–101, 122, 215
  response to safety improvements, 100–101, 122, 215
  research on, 120, 243
Robert Wood Johnson Foundation, 1, 20
Royal Society for the Prevention of Accidents (England), 21

Safe America Conference, 31
Safe Communities program, 193, 209
Safety-belt use laws, 34–35, 78, 91–92, 120, 122, 123, 209
Safety innovation, 23
Scaling multiple injuries, 151, 152–154
Self-inflicted injuries, 29. *See also* Suicides
Self-protection, 92, 122
Severity Index, 97
Sheppard-Towner Act of 1922, 231
Sickness Impact Profile, 155
SIDS Alliance, 215
Skylights, 60
Smoke detectors/alarms, 61, 84, 87, 91, 189, 242
Snell Memorial Foundation, 185
Social Security Act, Title V, 231
Society of Automotive Engineers databases, 105
Society of Trauma Nurses, 146
Socioeconomic environments, 94–95
Space heaters, unvented, 215
Special Crash Investigation (SCI) program, 61
Special Projects of Regional and National Significance, 231, 232–233
Speed limit, national maximum, 46 n.3, 82, 120, 121, 123
Sport-utility vehicles, 123
Sports injuries, 87, 185
State and Community-Based Injury Control Programs, 242 n.15
State and Community Formula Grant Program, 208
State and Community Highway Safety Grant Program, 120

State and Territorial Injury Prevention Directors' Association (STIPDA), 10, 77, 181, 188, 190, 196
State and community response
  advocacy, 180, 185, 199–201
  agencies and organizations, 180, 182–183
  barriers to, 9–10, 186, 194
  coalition building, 185, 190, 192, 193, 201
  collaboration, 191–193, 201
  educational, 179, 180, 185, 190, 192, 197 n.3, 199, 200, 201, 225
  evaluation of programs, 197–198, 209
  federal role, 10, 189, 191, 192, 194, 197, 200, 201, 241
  firearm regulation, 127–128, 130
  funding for programs, 10, 179, 180, 181, 182–183, 184, 186, 188–190, 196, 198, 201, 209, 232–234, 241, 242
  grassroots organizations, 180, 193, 200
  implementation of programs, 9, 178–180, 197
  injury prevention programs, 21, 118, 120, 130, 181, 187–188, 191, 192, 209, 241
  motor vehicle accident related programs, 120, 209
  nonprofit organizations, 180, 184–185, 199–200
  occupational safety and health programs, 218
  private-sector organizations, 179, 180, 185
  professional organizations, 179, 180, 186
  public awareness, raising, 178, 180, 198–199, 201
  public health infrastructure, 181–191, 242, 249–250, 264
  recommendations, 10, 190, 196
  research sponsorship, 180, 185, 198, 209
  strategic planning, 10, 187–188
  surveillance systems, 3, 61, 74–78, 85, 117, 125, 128, 147, 187, 189
  technical assistance, 10, 179, 187, 188, 190, 194, 197, 201, 209, 241
  training, 10, 179, 185, 191, 194–197, 201
  trauma systems management, 8, 143–145, 147, 149
Steps to Prevent Firearm Injury (STOP) Program, 196–197
Substance abuse, and violence, 89, 130. *See also* Alcohol use
Substance Abuse and Mental Health Services Administration, 69, 206
Sudden Infant Death Syndrome, 215
Suffocation, 45, 46, 48, 52, 53, 76, 85, 87, 214, 215

Suicides
   age and, 47, 86, 124
   carbon monoxide and, 87–88
   clusters, 87, 88
   firearm-related, 8, 45, 47, 48, 73, 86, 132
   gender and, 47
   magnitude of, 58
   mortality rates, 45, 86, 259
   prevention, 24, 26, 86–88, 106, 191, 246,
      247–248, 252
   race/ethnicity and, 50
   research, 88, 101, 106, 246, 247–248
   risk factors, 86, 94, 246
   surveillance systems, 4, 72, 73, 74, 125,
      246
   trends, 46, 58
Surveillance systems, 3. *See also specific*
      systems
   coding issues, 62–64, 147–148, 187
   defined, 60
   evaluation of, 71, 72
   fire and burn injuries, 75, 189
   firearm-related injuries, 7, 71, 73, 125–
      126, 134, 187, 189
   funding, 187, 241, 242, 245, 249, 259
   intentional injury data, 4, 72–74, 79
   intentionality issue, 25–26
   limitations, 3, 70, 74, 75, 76
   linkages between, 70, 77, 78, 79, 105–
      106, 117, 147–148, 239
   motor vehicle injuries, 4, 65, 68, 71, 72,
      78, 117–118
   national data sources, 3, 61, 64–74
   needs, 3–5, 61–62, 76, 78–79, 125–126
   occupational injuries, 53, 66, 72, 218,
      221–222, 223–224
   privacy and confidentiality issues, 76, 78,
      187
   product-related injuries, 3, 67, 70, 213–
      214, 216
   quality of data, 3, 76
   recommendations, 3, 4, 62, 71–72, 73
   research on, 226, 243, 259
   software, 77, 78
   state and local data sources, 3, 61, 74–78,
      85, 117, 125, 128, 147, 187, 189
   structure of database, 64
   technical assistance, 187
   trauma care, 147–148, 149, 187, 189
   uniform data sets, 3, 75, 77–78, 147, 148
   uses, 3, 4, 60–62, 70, 72, 74–75, 76, 83,
      85, 117–118, 125, 266
Survey of Occupational Injuries and Illnesses,
      66, 72, 221

Technical assistance, 10, 179, 187, 188, 190,
      194, 197, 201, 209, 219, 241, 249
Terminology, 28–30
The Injury Prevention Program (TIPP), 196
Timeline, 284-295
Time-series study designs, 103
Tolerance to injury, 96–97, 119
Toy Manufacturers of America, 185
Toy standards, 217
Training
   burn program, 228–229, 262
   coding, 3, 64, 71
   funding for, 6, 103–105, 106, 224–225,
      241, 243, 248–249, 262
   health care professionals, 196–197, 226,
      241
   injury prevention practitioners, 10, 179,
      185, 201, 243, 262
   interdisciplinary model, 195
   occupational safety, 222, 224–225
   peer, 92
   recommendations, 3, 10, 64, 104–105,
      196, 248–249, 262
   of researchers, 6, 103–105, 106, 211–212,
      238, 240, 248–249, 243, 262
   trauma-care providers, 145–147, 191,
      228–229, 243, 262
   violence prevention, 195, 235, 237, 238
Transportation Research Information Services,
      105
Trauma and Injury Severity Score, 151, 154
Trauma care systems. *See also* Acute care;
      Emergency department visits; Emer-
      gency medical services; Rehabilitation
   case mix, 152–154
   components, 8, 139, 140, 167–168
   computer applications in, 105
   cost-effectiveness, 9, 158–159, 168
   costs of, 9, 154, 156–159, 168
   criteria to identify, 150
   evaluation of effectiveness of, 9, 146, 147,
      148, 149, 150–152, 154–156
   exclusive, 139
   federal support for, 8, 147, 149, 159–161,
      168, 188, 261
   financing of, 9, 138, 143, 149, 159–163,
      167, 168
   growth in, 138, 145, 148–150
   inclusive, 139–140
   injury severity, 152–154
   legislation, 139–140, 143, 144, 145, 149,
      159–161
   limits on number of centers, 144–145, 149
   managed care and, 150, 162, 163, 164–
      167, 168
   management, 139, 143–145

outcomes of, 9, 149, 150–156, 161, 165, 166, 168, 261
overview of, 139–146
patient-care financing, 161–163
pediatric, 142
personnel, 145–146
prevention role, 146–147
recommendations, 8–9, 161, 167
research, 8, 9, 19, 119, 120, 129, 148, 149, 150–156, 159, 168, 244, 247 n.17
special populations, 142–143, 168, 245
state and regional agencies, 8, 143–145, 147, 149
state support for, 149, 159–161
surveillance systems, 147–148, 149
training, 145–147
unreimbursed care, 157, 162, 166
utilization measures, 165
volume of patients, 144–145
Trauma Care Systems Planning and Development Act, 139–140, 143, 144, 149, 160, 161
Trauma centers, 140, 141–142, 144, 147, 148, 149, 150, 151, 157, 163
Trauma Foundation, Injury and Violence Prevention Library, 198
Trauma registries, 75–77, 79, 85, 142, 144, 147, 149, 151, 155–156
Traumatic Brain Injury Program, 231
Treatment of injuries, 29. *See also* Trauma care systems
costs, 55, 154
prevention linked to, 31–32
research on, 99, 104
surveillance systems, 76
training, 104
Triage, 140, 151, 159, 166–167

Understanding Violence Against Women report, 236
Undetectable Firearms Act, 127
Uniform Crime Reporting (UCR) System, 72, 125
Uniform data sets, 147, 148
Uniform Data System for Medical Rehabilitation, 147
Uniform hospital discharge data, 3, 75, 77–78, 187, 209
Unintentional injuries, 28–29
deaths, 83
research accomplishments, 83–86, 87
University of North Carolina Injury Prevention Research Center, 195
U.S. Coast Guard, 207
U.S. Fire Administration, 185, 207
U.S. Public Health Service Act, 227, 233

U.S. Surgeon General, 88
Workshop on Violence and Public Health, 89

Vehicle Research Center, 184
Vermont Healthy Vermonters 2000 program, 192
Violence. *See also* Assaultive injuries; Homicides
against women, 236–237, 238–239
defined, 25 n.2
domestic, 75, 88, 128, 191, 232, 237, 239
evaluation of programs, 235
magnitude of, 58
prevention, 2, 24–25, 26–27, 85–86, 88–90, 94, 106, 184, 191, 195, 196–197, 232, 235, 238, 246, 247–248, 252
public health perspective, 89
research, 101, 106, 128, 130, 235, 246, 247–248
risk factors, 89, 94, 95, 128
surveillance systems, 66, 67, 72
workplace, 128
Violence Against Women Act of 1994, 236
Violence in Families report, 90, 237
Violent Crime Control and Law Enforcement Act of 1994, 89, 127, 234, 235, 246
Vital statistics system, 65, 67, 75, 77, 125, 209
Voluntary Protection Program, 221

Walsh-Healy Act of 1936, 218
War Revenue Act, 127
Whiplash, 97–98
Whitaker Foundation, 185
W.K. Kellogg Foundation, 1, 20, 21
Worker safety, 21, 180, 225, 226–227. *See also* Occupational injuries
Workers' compensation, 91, 158, 162, 163
World Bank, 57
World Conference on Injury Prevention and Control, 64
World Health Organization, 57, 62. *See also* International Classification of Diseases
Working Group on Injury Surveillance Methodology, 64

Years of potential life lost (YPLL), 1
by cause of death, 53, 54, 263
research investment relative to, 18, 19
Young Worker Community-Based Health Education Project, 225
Youth Risk Behavior Surveillance System, 67

Zero-tolerance laws, 36